EARLY DEFIBRILLATION

EARLY DEFIBRILLATION

Robert J. Huszar

Former Medical Director
Emergency Medical Services Program
New York State Department of Health

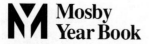 **Mosby**
Year Book

St. Louis Baltimore Boston Chicago London Philadelphia Sydney Toronto

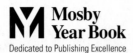

Editor: Claire Merrick
Editorial Assistant: Sandra Becker
Project Manager: John Rogers
Production Editor: Celeste Clingan
Cover Design: Julie Taugner
Cover Art: © Ron Boisvert

Printed in the United States of America

Mosby–Year Book, Inc.
11830 Westline Industrial Drive
St. Louis, MO 63146

Library of Congress Cataloging-in-Publication Data

Huszar, Robert J.
    Early defibrillation / Robert J. Huszar.
      p.   cm.
    Includes index.
    ISBN 0-8016-2927-6
    1. Electric countershock. 2. Cardiovascular emergencies.
  3. Emergency medical technicians. I. Title.
    [DNLM: 1. Allied Health Personnel. 2. Arrhythmia—therapy.
  3. Electric Countershock. 4. Heart Arrest—therapy. WG 330 H972e]
RC684.E4H87 1991
616.1′025—dc20
DNLM/DLC
for Library of Congress   90-13665
                                     CIP

CL/VH 9 8 7 6 5 4 3 2 1

Acknowledgements

During the three years that it has taken to produce the first edition of *Early Defibrillation,* many have helped to make it possible. First, I would like personally to thank **Richard A. Weimer,** Executive Editor, for having faith in its undertaking and **Adrianne Williams,** Assistant Editor, who helped to initiate the project. As the text took shape, **Claire Merrick,** Senior Editor, stepped in and helped to guide me in the development of its form and content. I especially would like to thank Claire for this. Also, **Sandra M. Becker,** Editorial Assistant, and **Nancy Peterson,** Assistant Editor, need recognition and thanks for their preparation of the manuscript for production.

Celeste Clingan, Senior Production Editor at Mosby–Year Book, Inc., must be acknowledged for her skill in producing and coordinating the text, art, and tables and **Julie Taugner,** for her cover design.

For their patience and tolerance, I would like to thank the photogenic EMS professionals who posed for the scans in Chapter 8. They include **Sandra J. Dougherty, EMT-P** (New York City Emergency Medical Services), **John J. O'Donnell** (District Manager, Laerdal Medical Corp.), **Alan A. St. Onge, EMT** (Security and Emergency Services, Fox Run Mall, Newington, NH), and **Peter Wahl, Firefighter, EMT** (Emergency Medical Services, Newington Fire Department, Newington, NH). The photography for this book was provided by **Phillip Noury,** Austin Studios, Fox Run Mall, Newington, NH.

I would also like to acknowledge with gratitude the following for their time, effort, and expertise in the field of early defibrillation in reviewing the manuscript in its various phases of development:

Mark P. Adams
Executive Director
Central Shenandoah EMS Council
Fisherville, Virginia

Douglas Austin, Jr.
EMT Program Coordinator
King County Division of Emergency Medical Services
Seattle/King County
Department of Public Health
Seattle, Washington

Robert Davis
President
EMS/Associates
Pawling, New York

Chris Eldridge
Hightstown, New Jersey

Robert Elling, EMT-P
Associate Director
Emergency Medical Services Program
New York State Department of Health
Albany, New York

Richard H. Hillman
Marketing Manager
Space Labs
First Medic Division
Redmond, Washington

Ward Hamilton
Director of Business Development
Paul Kiely
Region Manager
John J. O'Donnell
Distric Manager
Wayne Reval
Marketing Manager, Defibrillator
Laerdal Medical Corp.
Armonk, New York

Nancy Sue Hudson, R.N.
Arlington, Virginia

David Schlageter
U.S. Sales Office Manager
Steve Sperrazza, R.N.
Sales Representative
Emergency Care Division
Marquette Electronics Inc.
Milwaukee, Wisconsin

Andrew Stern, NREMT-P
Paramedic Supervisor
Town of Colonie EMS
Albany, New York

Kyle D. Witt
Prehospital Group Product Manager
Mark T. Ungs
Capital District Sales Manager
Physio-Control
Redmond, Washington

This book is dedicated to my wife,
Jean

Prologue

A survey of the results of the early defibrillation programs in New York State in 1989 showed that of the 351 persons with cardiac arrest managed by emergency medical technicians trained in early defibrillation (Emergency Medical Technicians-Defibrillation [EMTDS]) during a three-year period, the initial electrocardiogram showed ventricular asystole in 151 (43%), ventricular fibrillation in 146 (42%), electromechanical dissociation (EMD) in 43 (12%), idioventricular rhythm in 9 (3%), and ventricular tachycardia and bradycardia in 1 each (<1%). Twenty-three patients with ventricular fibrillation (16%), 3 with electromechanical dissociation (7%), and 1 with ventricular asystole (<1%) were reported to have been discharged from the hospital.

The out-of-hospital lives saved in persons experiencing ventricular fibrillation occurred primarily in those whose cardiac arrest was either witnessed by the EMTD or whose cardiopulmonary resuscitation was performed immediately by a medical professional before early defibrillation was administered. Other studies have shown similar results, that is, early defibrillation is most effective when applied in the early minutes of cardiac arrest from ventricular fibrillation.

This book is dedicated to providing a basis for training emergency medical technicians, first responders, and other first-responding emergency personnel in early defibrillation in the hope that patients suffering unexpected cardiac arrest may not die needlessly.

Robert J. Huszar, M.D.
Former Medical Director
Emergency Medical Services Program
New York State Department of Health

Introduction

Early Defribrillation is intended to be used as a text in the training of **first responders** and **emergency medical technicians** in the use of the automated external defibrillator (AED), including the semi-automatic external defibrillator (SAED) and the fully automatic external defibrillator, in **early defibrillation programs.**

Chapters 1, 2, and **3** provide general information regarding the basic anatomy of the chest and heart, including the physiology of the heart, acute myocardial infarction, and cardiac arrest.

Chapters 4 and **5** describe the electrocardiogram and the basic rhythms and dysrhythmias and in particular ventricular tachycardia and ventricular fibrillation in simple terms. These chapters are primarily intended to provide the necessary information to enable the first responders and emergency medical technicians involved in early defibrillation programs using the semi-automatic external defibrillator to analyze and interpret certain basic rhythms and dysrhythmias if so required by local protocol.

Chapters 6 and **7** present the fundamental principles and use of defibrillatory shock in the management of prehospital cardiac arrest and the description of the basic components of the automated external defibrillator. Chapter 7 also presents the features of different manufacturers' models of automated external defibrillators.

Chapter 8 contains detailed standard generic algorithms and protocols for using the automated external defibrillator in managing pre-arrival and post-arrival cardiac arrest, with and without bystander CPR, by a first responder or an emergency medical technician alone or aided by another rescuer trained in cardiopulmonary resuscitation.

The appendix provides detailed protocols in using specific semi-automatic and fully automatic external defibrillators.

In the absence of a standard curriculum for training programs for first responders and emergency medical technicians in early defibrillation, there was a tendency to include material in this manual that was felt to be somewhat more advanced than required by some early defibrillation training programs. To offset this, a check-off list of objectives is included at the beginning of each chapter to aid the instructor at the beginning of the course to identify for the students the **"need-to-know"** material and that which is **"nice-to-know."**

In addition, the electrocardiograms of those dysrhythmias that are considered treatable by defibrillatory shock and cardiopulmonary resuscitation, if necessary, and those, by cardiopulmonary resuscitation alone are identified by appropriate logos recently established by the American Heart Association in such emergencies in emergency cardiac care. Dysrhythmias requiring shock are identified by a "shock" logo*, and those requiring only CPR, a "CPR" logo†.

---

*

†

Contents

Chapter 1

Anatomy and Physiology of the Chest and Its Contents

OBJECTIVES

Upon completion of all or part of this chapter as required by your early defibrillation program, you should be able to complete the following objectives indicated by your instructor:

☐ Name and identify the three major parts of the skeletal frame of the chest.
☐ Name and identify the parts of the rib cage.
☐ Define and use the following directional terms: midline, medial, lateral, anterior, posterior, and parallel.
☐ Locate, on your own body, the three major landmarks of the chest.
☐ Name and locate, on an anatomical drawing, the following major structures found in the chest: the lungs, heart, aorta, pulmonary artery, and superior and inferior vena cavae.
☐ Label the four chambers, the four heart valves, and two septa of the heart.
☐ Describe the two major functions of the right heart and the left heart.
☐ Define ventricular systole and diastole.
☐ Identify the two basic kinds of cardiac cells and their functions.
☐ Name and identify the parts of the electrical conduction system of the heart.
☐ Define and locate the primary, escape, and ectopic pacemakers of the heart.
☐ Define inherent firing rate and give the inherent firing rates of the following:
   • SA node
   • AV junction
   • Ventricles
☐ Describe the two major reasons why an escape pacemaker may take over the electrical activity of the heart.
☐ List three major heart conditions responsible for escape and ectopic beats and rhythms.
☐ Name an escape rhythm.
☐ List two ectopic dysrhythmias.

Anatomy of the Chest

The **chest** (or **thorax**) is located between the neck and diaphragm. Its skeletal frame consists of the **sternum,** the **rib cage,** and the **thoracic spine.** The **sternum** is the elongated, arrowhead-shaped bone in the center of the anterior part of the chest. It is divided into the upper part, the **manubrium;** the mid portion overlying the heart, the **body;** and the partially moveable triangular tip at the lower end of the sternum, the **xiphoid process.** Attached to the manubrium are the two **clavicles** (or **collar bones**), one on each side, forming part of the **shoulder girdle** (Figures 1-1 and 1-2).

The **rib cage** consists of twelve pairs of **ribs** and their **costal cartilages.** The point where the costal cartilage unites with the anterior (front) tip of the rib is called the **costochondral junction.** All the ribs are attached in the back to the thoracic spine. The upper seven ribs are attached in front by their costal cartilages directly to the sternum. The next three ribs are attached by their cartilages to the ribs above, and the last two ribs, being too short, are unattached. The spaces between the ribs are called **intercostal spaces.** They are numbered from the top down with the **first intercostal space** underneath the clavicle, between the first and second rib.

On each side of the chest is an imaginary line, used as a landmark, that bisects the clavicle on that side and runs parallel to the **midline of the ster-**

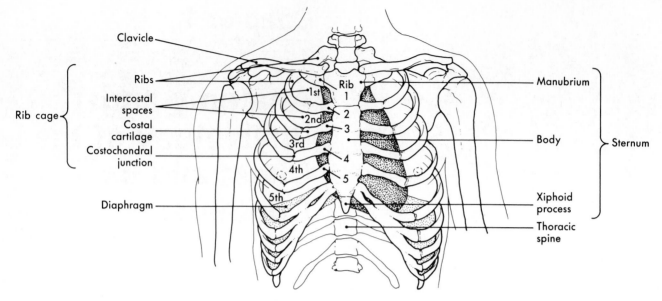

Figure 1-1. The chest.

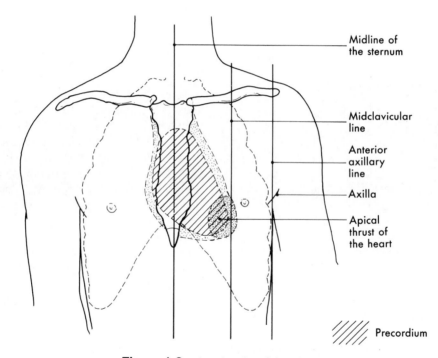

Figure 1-2. Landmarks of the chest.

num (see box). It is called the **midclavicular line.** Lateral to the midclavicular line is another imaginary line that begins at the anterior border of the **axilla (armpit)** and runs parallel to the midclavicular line. It is called the **anterior axillary line.**

In the chest itself are the **lungs,** the **heart,** and the **four major blood vessels of the body** which carry the blood to and from the heart—the two major veins (the **superior vena cava** and the **inferior vena cava**) and the two major arteries (the **aorta** and **pulmonary artery**) (Figure 1-3). The heart lies behind the sternum with the **base (or top) of the heart** at the level of the upper third of the sternum and the **apex of the heart** normally at

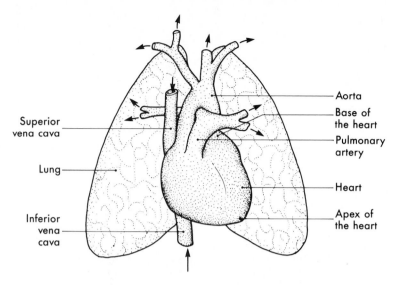

Figure 1-3. The heart and lungs.

Labels: Superior vena cava, Lung, Inferior vena cava, Aorta, Base of the heart, Pulmonary artery, Heart, Apex of the heart

Directional Terms	
Midline	An imaginary line that runs up and down the middle of the body.
Medial	Toward the midline.
Lateral	Away from the midline.
Anterior	Front.
Posterior	Back.
Parallel	Running alongside in the same direction at a constant distance.

the level of the fourth and fifth intercostal space just medial to the midclavicular line. The right ventricle, for the most part, lies directly behind the sternum; and the left ventricle, to the left of the sternum. The region of the lower anterior part of the thorax overlying the heart is called the **precordium,** an important landmark. Just within the midclavicular line and medial to the left nipple, at the level of the fourth and fifth intercostal space, can be felt the **apical thrust of the heart** produced by the forceful contractions of the ventricles.

Anatomy and Physiology of the Heart
Anatomy

The **heart,** a muscle whose sole purpose is to circulate blood through the **circulatory system** (the blood vessels of the body), consists of four hollow chambers. The two upper chambers are the thin-walled **right** and **left atria;** the two lower chambers are the thick-walled and muscular **right** and **left ventricles.** The muscular walls, or **myocardium,** of the **left ventricle** are about three times thicker than those of the **right ventricle.** The heart is frequently referred to as having a **base,** formed by the two atria, and an **apex,** the lower parts of the two ventricles.

The heart is surrounded by a thick fibrous cover, the **pericardium.** Between the pericardium and the heart is a fluid-filled space called the **pericardial cavity** (Figure 1-4).

The **interatrial septum** (a thin membranous wall) normally separates the two atria, and a thicker, more muscular wall, the **interventricular septum,** separates the two ventricles. The two septa, in effect, divide the heart into two pumping systems, the **right heart** and the **left heart,** each consisting of an atrium and a ventricle.

The **right heart** pumps blood into the **pulmonary circulation** (the blood vessels within the lungs and those carrying blood to and from the lungs). The **left heart** pumps blood into the **systemic circulation** (the blood vessels in the rest of the body and those carrying blood to and from the body including the heart itself—the **coronary circulation**) (Figure 1-5).

The **right atrium** receives **unoxygenated blood** from the body via two of the body's largest veins (the **superior vena cava** and **inferior vena cava**) and from the heart itself by way of the **coronary sinus.** The blood is delivered from the right atrium to the **right ventricle** through the **tricuspid valve.** The right ventricle then pumps the unoxygenated

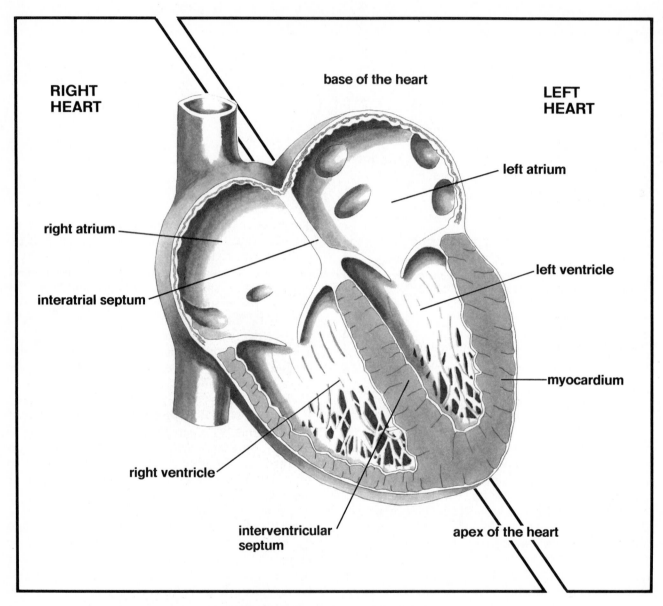

Figure 1-4.   Anatomy of the heart.

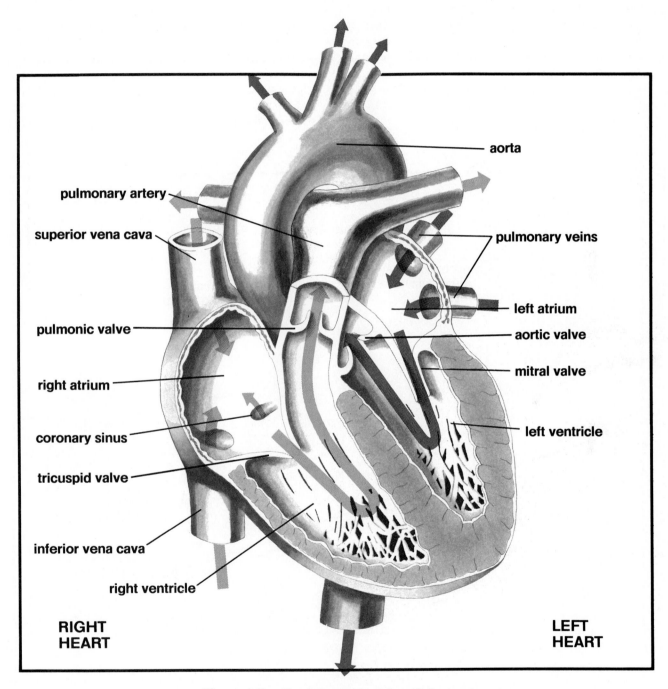

aorta

pulmonary artery

superior vena cava

pulmonary veins

left atrium

pulmonic valve

aortic valve

mitral valve

right atrium

coronary sinus

left ventricle

tricuspid valve

inferior vena cava

right ventricle

RIGHT HEART

LEFT HEART

Figure 1-5. Circulation of blood through the heart.

blood through the **pulmonic valve** into the lungs via the **pulmonary artery.** In the lungs, the blood picks up oxygen and releases excess carbon dioxide.

The **left atrium** receives the newly **oxygenated blood** from the lungs via the **pulmonary veins** and delivers it to the **left ventricle** through the **mitral valve.** The left ventricle then pumps the oxygenated blood out through the **aortic valve** into the **aorta,** the largest artery in the body. From the aorta, the blood is distributed throughout the body where the blood releases oxygen and collects carbon dioxide.

Physiology

The heart performs its pumping action over and over in a rhythmic sequence. First, the two atria relax, allowing the blood to pour in from the body and lungs. As the atria fill with blood, the atrial pressure rises and forces the tricuspid and mitral valves to open, allowing the blood to empty rapidly into the two relaxed ventricles. Then the atria contract, filling the ventricles to capacity. The period of relaxation, dilation, and filling of the ventricles with blood is called **ventricular diastole.**

Following the contraction of the atria, the pressures in the atria and ventricles equalize, and the

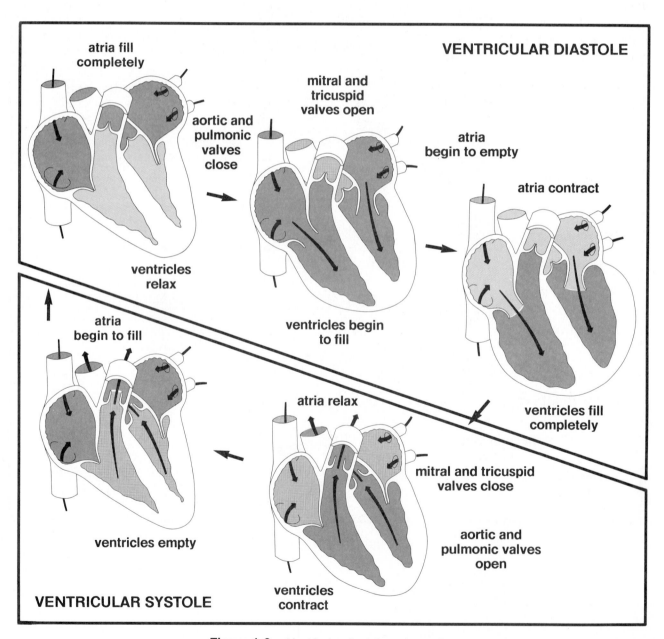

Figure 1-6. Ventricular diastole and systole.

tricuspid and mitral valves begin to close. Then the ventricles contract vigorously, causing the ventricular pressure to rise sharply. The tricuspid and mitral valves close completely, and the aortic and pulmonic valves snap open, allowing the blood to be ejected forcefully into the pulmonary and systemic circulation at about the same time. Meanwhile the atria are again relaxing and filling with blood. As soon as the ventricles empty of blood and begin to relax, the ventricular pressure falls, the aortic and pulmonic valves shut tightly, and the rhythmic cardiac sequence begins anew. The period during which the ventricles contract and empty of blood is called **ventricular systole.** Normally, the cycle of a ventricular systole followed by a ventricular diastole occurs **60 to 100 times a minute at rest** (Figure 1-6).

Cardiac Cells

The heart is composed of two basic kinds of cardiac cells—the **myocardial cells** and the **specialized cells of the electrical conduction system of the heart** (Figure 1-7).

The **myocardial cells** have the ability to contract when they are electrically stimulated. Such cells are said to have the **property of contractility.** These cells form the thin muscular layer of the atrial wall and the much thicker muscular layer of the ventricular wall (the **myocardium**).

The **specialized cells of the electrical conduction system,** which do not have the ability to contract, have two main functions:

- **Generation of tiny electrical impulses spontaneously.** The cells of the electrical conduction system that have this **property of automaticity** are called **pacemaker cells.**
- **Conduction of the electrical impulses** to the myocardial cells throughout the heart at an extremely rapid rate, causing the myocardial cells to contract. The rate of conduction of the electrical impulse through the electrical conduction system is at least six times faster than that through the myocardial cells themselves. The ability of cardiac cells to conduct electrical impulses is called the **property of conductivity.**

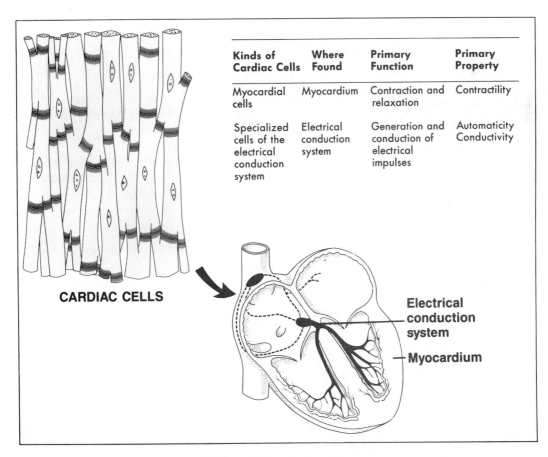

Kinds of Cardiac Cells	Where Found	Primary Function	Primary Property
Myocardial cells	Myocardium	Contraction and relaxation	Contractility
Specialized cells of the electrical conduction system	Electrical conduction system	Generation and conduction of electrical impulses	Automaticity Conductivity

CARDIAC CELLS

Electrical conduction system

Myocardium

Figure 1-7. Cardiac cells.

Electrical Conduction System of the Heart

At the head of the **electrical conduction system,** located in the right atrium near the inlet of the superior vena cava, is a group of pacemaker cells making up the **sinoatrial (SA) node.** The SA node is called the **primary (or dominant) pacemaker of the heart** because the **electrical impulses,** which cause the heart to contract, normally originate here. Below the SA node, in the area where the atria are attached to the ventricles, lies another group of specialized cells, the **atrioventricular (AV) node** (Figure 1-8).

Between the SA node and AV node is a network of electrical conductive fibers, the **internodal atrial conduction tracts,** through which the electrical impulses generated in the SA node are transmitted to the AV node. Immediately below the AV node, another group of specialized cells, the **bundle of His,** conducts the electrical impulse into the **right and left bundle branches** through which the impulses are then conducted into the ventricles. The atrioventricular (AV) node and bundle of His

form the **atrioventricular (AV) junction.** At the ends of the bundle branches is a fine network of fibers, the **Purkinje* network,** which conduct the electrical impulses directly to the muscle fibers of the ventricles.

Primary, Escape, and Ectopic Pacemakers of the Heart

As discussed previously, the electrical impulses normally arise in the **SA node, the primary (dominant) pacemaker of the heart,** producing a normal heart beat, the so-called **normal sinus rhythm.** This is because, under normal conditions, the SA node has the ability to generate electrical impulses at a higher rate than any other part of the heart. Under certain abnormal conditions, however, any part of the electrical conduction system can become a pacemaker and generate electrical

---

*Purkinje is pronounced **Purr-kin-gee.**

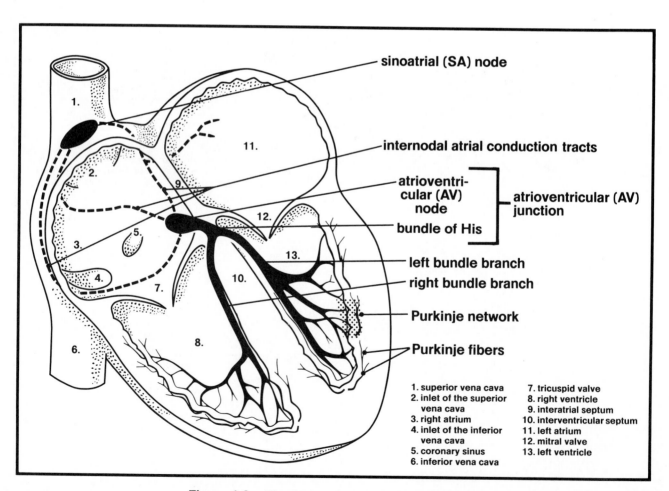

1. superior vena cava
2. inlet of the superior vena cava
3. right atrium
4. inlet of the inferior vena cava
5. coronary sinus
6. inferior vena cava
7. tricuspid valve
8. right ventricle
9. interatrial septum
10. interventricular septum
11. left atrium
12. mitral valve
13. left ventricle

Figure 1-8.   Electrical conduction system of the heart.

impulses. Such pacemakers are called either **escape or ectopic pacemakers,** depending on the factors responsible for their activation.

Escape pacemaker. Should the **SA node, the primary pacemaker,** cease to function or the electrical impulses fail to be transmitted to the AV junction or the ventricles, a pacemaker in the electrical conduction system below the SA node (i.e., in the AV junction or ventricles) normally takes over control of the heart. Such a pacemaker is called an **escape pacemaker.** The heart beat produced by an escape pacemaker is called an **escape rhythm** (Figure 1-9).

The rate at which an escape pacemaker generates electrical impulses depends on the site of the pacemaker. The farther away the escape pacemaker is from the SA node, the slower is the rate of its generation of electrical impulses. The rate at which an escape pacemaker and, for that matter,

the SA node usually generate electrical impulses is called the **inherent firing rate.** The SA node has an inherent firing rate of 60 to 100 times per minute; the AV junction, 40 to 60 times per minute; and the ventricles, 20 to 40 times per minute.

Under certain heart conditions, parts of the electrical conduction system may be damaged, causing a disruption of conduction of the electrical impulses to the ventricles. These heart conditions include the following:
- **Significant coronary heart disease**—obstructive disease of the heart's own blood supply.
- **Myocardial ischemia**—decreased blood flow to the myocardium.
- **Acute myocardial infarction**—death of portion of the heart muscle caused by the sudden partial or complete occlusion of the artery to the affected heart muscle.

If an escape pacemaker in the ventricles takes

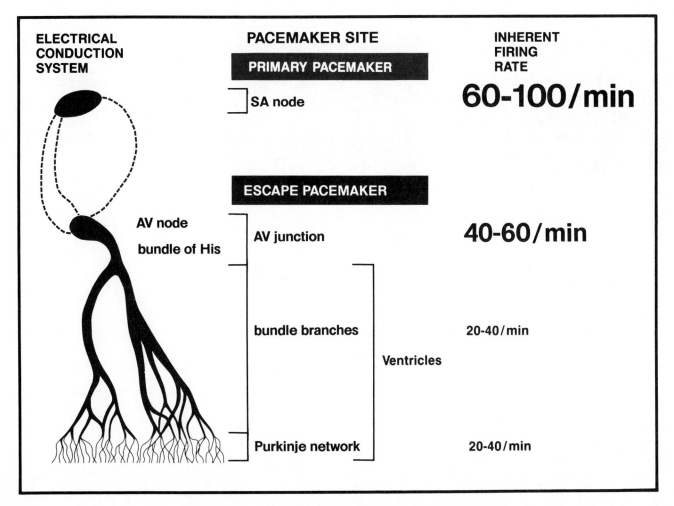

Figure 1-9.   Primary and escape pacemakers of the heart.

Coronary heart disease

Myocardial ischemia

Acute myocardial infarction

Figure 1-10. Causes of escape and ectopic beats and rhythms.

over, a very slow heart beat called **ventricular escape rhythm** results. If an escape pacemaker fails to take over, the heart stops beating completely **(ventricular asystole*),** resulting in **cardiac arrest** (Figure 1-10).

Ectopic pacemaker. Under the same conditions that can produce an escape rhythm (i.e., significant coronary heart disease, myocardial ischemia, and acute myocardial infarction) and sometimes without apparent cause, the cells of any part of the electrical conduction system (and even the myocardial cells in some instances) may become abnormally excitable and begin generating electrical impulses automatically. Such a group of cells is called an **ectopic* pacemaker.** Ectopic pacemakers can arise in the atria, AV junction, or ventricles.

The heart beat produced by an ectopic pacemaker is called an **ectopic beat** or **rhythm. Ectopic beats** may occur one at a time; in groups of two, three, or more; or they may occur continuously as an **ectopic rhythm.** An **ectopic rhythm** may be slow, normal, or very rapid, occurring at a regular or irregular rate. Ectopic beats and rhythms usually disrupt normal or escape rhythms; an ectopic rhythm may even override them completely, taking control of the heart.

If an ectopic pacemaker in the ventricles with an extremely rapid heart rate takes over **(ventricular tachycardia),** the blood flow may decrease or stop completely, resulting in cardiac arrest. The reason for this is that a rapid ventricular ectopic rhythm is usually very inefficient. If the ventricular ectopic rhythm becomes extremely irregular and chaotic **(ventricular fibrillation),** cardiac arrest always occurs.

Escape and ectopic beats and rhythms are generally grouped together under the term **dysrhythmia,** a term meaning **abnormal rhythm.** The specific dysrhythmias noted previously, i.e., **ventricular tachycardia, ventricular fibrillation,** and **ventricular asystole** are described in **Chapters 4** and **5.**

***Asystole** means absence of a heartbeat.

***Ectopic** means being **"out-of-place,"** that is, occurring in an abnormal location.

Chapter 2

Acute Myocardial Infarction

OBJECTIVES

Upon completion of all or part of this chapter as required by your early defibrillation program, you should be able to complete the following objectives indicated by your instructor:

☐ Define the term coronary heart disease.
☐ Name three complications of coronary heart disease.
☐ Define sudden cardiac death.
☐ Define life-threatening dysrhythmia.
☐ Define angina pectoris.
☐ List the three major causes of occlusion of a coronary artery resulting in an acute myocardial infarction.
☐ Name the four major causes of death in acute myocardial infarction.
☐ Describe the typical candidate for an acute myocardial infarction.
☐ Describe the chest pain present in acute myocardial infarction, including the incidence, location, intensity, radiation, and duration.
☐ List two common early symptoms of acute myocardial infarction in each of the following categories:
  • General symptoms
  • Cardiac symptoms
  • Respiratory symptoms
  • Gastrointestinal symptoms
☐ Describe the patient's general appearance and skin in acute myocardial infarction.
☐ Describe the patient's vital signs (pulse, respirations, and blood pressure) in acute myocardial infarction.
☐ Describe the normal course of an AMI.
☐ List four complications of AMI.
☐ List two complications for each of the following categories of complications:
  • Benign complications.
  • Serious, treatable complications.
  • Lethal complications.
☐ Define a dysrhythmia.
☐ List four life-threatening dysrhythmias responsible for the majority of deaths during the prehospital phase of AMI.
☐ List five causes of dysrhythmias.
☐ Define bradycardia and tachycardia.

☐ List four life-threatening dysrhythmias of particular concern for EMTs and first responders involved in early defibrillation programs.
☐ Name the single most important cause of congestive heart failure, cardiogenic shock, and ventricular aneurysm.
☐ Describe the mechanism of left heart failure.
☐ Define pulmonary congestion and pulmonary edema, indicating the difference between them.
☐ Describe the primary and classic symptom of left heart failure.
☐ Define the following signs of left heart failure and list two additional signs of left heart failure:
  • Cyanosis
  • Tachycardia
  • Tachypnea
  • Rales
  • Hemoptysis
☐ Name the most common cause of right heart failure.
☐ Describe the mechanism of right heart failure.
☐ Define the terms edema and effusion and list where each can be found in the body.
☐ List five signs of right heart failure.
☐ Describe the mechanism of cardiogenic shock.
☐ List eight signs of cardiogenic shock.
☐ Describe the mechanism of the development of ventricular aneurysm.
☐ List the three common sites of cardiac rupture.
☐ Define cardiac tamponade.
☐ List six consequences of rupture of the anterior wall of the left ventricle.

Cardiovascular disease is the number one killer in the United States today with about 540,000 persons dying of **coronary heart disease (CHD)** each year. **Coronary heart disease** is the result of a slow, progressive narrowing, hardening, and eventual obstruction (**occlusion**) of the coronary arteries supplying blood to the muscle of the heart (myocardium). This aging and destructive disease process of coronary arteries caused by repeated blood clots, tissue scarring, and cholesterol deposits

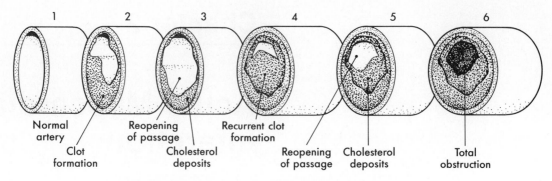

Figure 2-1. Coronary heart disease and atherosclerosis.

within the arteries is called **atherosclerosis** (Figure 2-1).

The **three major complications** of coronary heart disease are **sudden cardiac death, angina pectoris,** and **acute myocardial infarction** (Figure 2-2).

Sudden Cardiac Death

Sudden cardiac death is **cardiac arrest from a life-threatening (or lethal) dysrhythmia* in a person without earlier signs or symptoms of coronary heart disease, in one who was not expected to die.** The cause of the life-threatening dysrhythmia is said to be a sudden obstruction of a

---

*A **life-threatening (or lethal) dysrhythmia** is a disturbance in the heart rate (extremely slow or fast) or rhythm (extremely irregular), which, if not treated immediately, can cause death.

narrowed segment of an atherosclerotic coronary artery by a blood clot **(thrombus).**

Angina Pectoris

Angina pectoris is a clinical syndrome characterized by recurring chest pain which occurs when the demand for blood in an area of the myocardium during physical exertion or emotional stress is greater than that available through a partially obstructed atherosclerotic coronary artery supplying the area. The anginal pain produced by the lack of blood in the myocardium **(ischemia)** is usually of short duration, typically 3 to 5 minutes. Like the chest pain of acute myocardial infarction, in the following discussion, anginal pain usually appears behind the middle or upper part of the sternum **(substernally)** and radiates to the same areas of the upper body as does the pain of AMI. Angina, un-

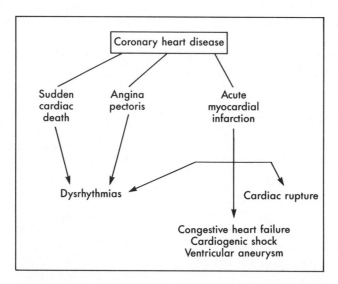

Figure 2-2. Complications of coronary heart disease.

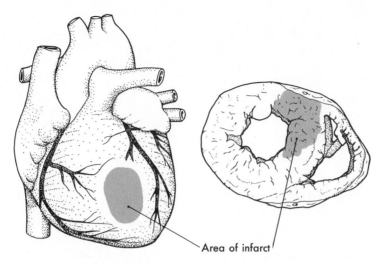

Figure 2-3. Acute myocardial infarction.

like the pain of AMI, however, disappears within a few minutes after rest or alleviation of emotional stress or shortly after administration of **nitroglycerin** tablet under the tongue. A complication of angina pectoris is **cardiac arrest,** the result of a life-threatening dysrhythmia brought on by the ischemia.

Acute Myocardial Infarction

Acute myocardial infarction (AMI) is the sudden partial or complete obstruction **(occlusion)** of one or more atherosclerotic coronary arteries, causing a marked decrease of blood flow to the myocardium **(ischemia)** followed by death **(necrosis)** of the affected myocardium (Figure 2-3). The **three major causes** of a coronary artery occlusion resulting in an acute myocardial infarction are:
- **Formation of a blood clot (thrombosis, thrombus)** in the coronary artery
- **Hemorrhage under an existing partial obstruction (plaque)**
- **Rupture and displacement of a plaque** into the main passage **(lumen)** of the coronary artery

About two thirds of the patients with an **acute myocardial infarction** die before they reach the hospital. The majority of those dying outside the hospital do so within the first 2 hours after the onset of symptoms when the incidence of **life-threatening dysrhythmias** is the highest. Consequently, life-threatening dysrhythmias are the major cause of death during the prehospital phase of AMI (Figure 2-4).

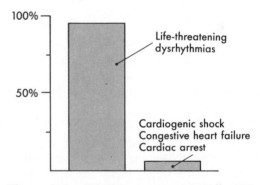

Figure 2-4. Principle causes of death in AMI.

The chances of survival for the hospitalized patient with an AMI have improved greatly over the past 30 to 40 years. This is primarily the result of the use of hospital coronary care units, which continuously monitor the patient's electrocardiogram (ECG), and improved patient care procedures, particularly in the prevention and treatment of life-threatening dysrhythmias. **Cardiogenic shock, severe congestive heart failure,** and **cardiac rupture** have replaced life-threatening dysrhythmias as the major cause of hospital deaths in AMI following the introduction of coronary care units. These complications will be described in the following discussion.

Clinical Picture of AMI

The person suffering an AMI is often pictured as a white, middle-aged, aggressive male who is heavy set, overweight, inactive, and has a stressful job. This person also smokes excessively and has hypertension or diabetes (or both), a family history of coronary artery disease, and elevated blood cholesterol or lipids (or both). **Although this picture represents the typical AMI patient, older and younger persons both male and female, especially those who smoke, can also suffer an AMI regardless of family history or past illness.**

Symptoms of AMI

Although an AMI is often preceded by repeated episodes of **angina pectoris,** an AMI can occur suddenly and without previous symptoms. Sudden exertion such as climbing stairs, running, mowing a lawn, or shoveling snow by a person not used to such physical activity; a heavy meal; or severe emotion can trigger an AMI. On the other hand, an AMI can occur at rest and even during sleep.

Chest pain is the most common symptom of an acute myocardial infarction. In 80 to 90 percent of all AMI patients, a painful sensation is felt behind the middle or upper part of the sternum (**substernally),** varying in intensity from a mild discomfort, easily ignored, to a severe and terrifying constricting or crushing pain, lasting about an hour or longer. In about less than a third of the patients, the pain radiates to the left shoulder, elbow, forearm, wrist, and little finger, and sometimes to the right shoulder. Occasionally, the pain radiates to the neck, jaw, and upper teeth; the upper back; or the midline of the upper abdomen (**epigastrium).** A few patients, who are most likely experiencing their first attack, have no pain. They are having a **"silent" myocardial infarction** (Figure 2-5).

Other common symptoms present during an acute myocardial infarction (whether or not pain is experienced) are:

- **General symptoms:** the patient is **extremely fatigued** and **weak; restless, anxious,** and **apprehensive with a sense of impending doom;** or **confused, disoriented, lightheaded,** or **drowsy.**
- **Cardiac symptoms:** the patient usually has **chest pain,** as described previously, and, in addition, may experience **palpitations or "skipping of the heart."**
- **Respiratory symptoms:** the patient may have **difficulty in breathing (dyspnea) with a sensation of suffocation** and a **cough** which may be **productive of blood-tinged sputum (hemoptysis).**
- **Gastrointestinal symptoms:** the patient may complain of a **loss of appetite (anorexia) with nausea and vomiting** and an **urge to defecate** (Figure 2-6).

Pain	Angina	AMI
Incidence	100%	80-90%
Description	Mild discomfort to severe, terrifying constriction or crushing pain	Same
Location	Substernal	Same
Radiation	Left shoulder, elbow, forearm, wrist, and little finger. Occasionally to right shoulder, neck, jaw, back, or epigastrium	Same
Duration	Few minutes, relieved by rest and nitroglycerin	1 hour or longer

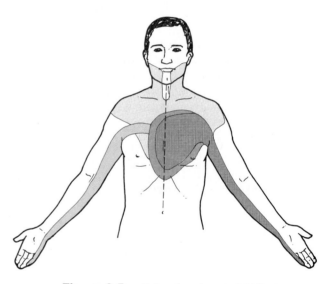

Figure 2-5.   Pain of angina and AMI.

Signs of AMI

The patient's physical signs vary in acute myocardial infarction, depending on the site and extent of the damage to the heart muscle and on the reaction of the patient's body to the AMI (Figure 2-7). The following are some of the signs that may be seen in acute myocardial infarction:

- **General appearance:** the patient may appear **alert and oriented but restless; anxious and apprehensive; confused and disoriented;** or **unconscious with or without convulsions.**
- **Vital signs:** the **pulse** may be **normal** (60 to 100 beats/minute), **rapid** (over 100 beats/

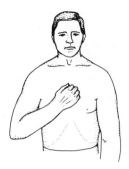

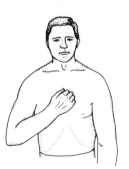

General

Fatigue and weakness

Restlessness, anxiety, and apprehensiveness with a
   sense of impending doom

Confusion, disorientation, light headedness, or
   drowsiness

Cardiac   **Gastrointestinal**

Chest pain   Anorexia
Palpitations   Nausea and vomiting
                                   Urge to defecate
Respiratory

Dyspnea
Cough
Hemoptysis

Figure 2-6. Common early symptoms in AMI.

minute—**tachycardia**), or **slow** (less than 60
beats/minute—**bradycardia**).

The **respiratory rate** may be **normal** (12
to 16 breaths/minute), **rapid** (greater than 16
breaths/minute—**tachypnea**), or **slow** (less
than 12 breaths/minute).

The **systolic blood pressure** may be **normal** (90 to 140 mm Hg), **elevated** (above 140
mm Hg), or **low** (less than 90 mm Hg) if hypotension or shock is present.

• **Skin:** the patient's skin usually appears **pale,**
often with a **bluish, grayish, or purplish**

tinge to it **(cyanosis). The skin is usually **cold**
and clammy** to the touch.

Even when many of the classic signs and symptoms of acute myocardial infarction are present, diagnosis of an AMI cannot be confirmed without
significant **changes in the patient's ECG** and an
increase in certain chemical compounds normally
present in the patient's blood, called **serum enzymes,** resulting from an abnormal release of these
enzymes from dead heart tissue. Both of these
changes occur later in the course of the AMI.

General Appearance

Alert and oriented, but restless
Anxious and apprehensive
Confused and disoriented
Unconscious with or without convulsions

Pulse

Normal (60 to 100 beats/min), rapid, or slow

Respiratory Rate

Normal (12 to 16 breaths/min), rapid, or slow

Systolic Blood Pressure

Normal (90 to 140 mm Hg), elevated, or low

Skin

Pale
Cyanotic
Cold and clammy

Figure 2-7. Common early signs in AMI.

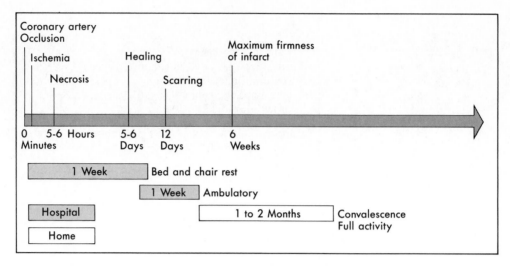

Figure 2-8. Normal course of an AMI.

Normal Course of an AMI

The myocardial tissue beyond the obstruction of the coronary artery supplying it becomes deficient in blood, a condition called **ischemia,** within minutes after the **coronary artery occlusion.** Five to six hours later, the ischemic tissue begins to show cellular changes of death called **necrosis.** These changes are at their height on the fifth or sixth day following an AMI, at which time **healing** of the area of dead tissue, the so-called **infarct,** begins. On about the twelfth day, as connective tissue begins to be deposited, **scarring** begins. Maximum firmness of the scar tissue is achieved by the sixth week (Figure 2-8).

During the first week, the injured myocardium is susceptible to complications such as cardiac rupture if it is subjected to tachycardia or elevated blood pressure. For these reasons, bed and chair rest and prevention of excitement and anxiety, as well as constipation, are necessary during this period. Before being discharged from the hospital, the patient is permitted to become ambulatory for about a week. An AMI patient who does not have serious complications generally remains in the hospital for several weeks. Following discharge, the patient continues convalescence for 1 to 2 months before resuming full activity.

Complications of AMI

Some kind of complication almost always occurs with an AMI. The complications of AMI may be electrical or mechanical in nature. They include:

Electrical complications:
• **Dysrhythmias**
Mechanical complications:
• **Congestive heart failure, cardiogenic shock, ventricular aneurysm**
• **Rupture of the heart**

Many of these complications are insignificant and have a favorable outcome (**benign complications**). Other complications are more serious but treatable (**serious, treatable complications**). A small number of complications, no matter how treated, almost always cause death (**lethal complications**) (Figure 2-9). The following complications of AMI will be discussed below:

Benign complications:
• **Non life-threatening dysrhythmias**
• **Mild congestive heart failure**
Serious, treatable complications:
• **Certain life-threatening dysrhythmias, such**

Electrical Complications

Dysrhythmias
    Nonlife-threatening dysrhythmias
    Life-threatening dysrhythmias
        Pulseless ventricular tachycardia
        Ventricular fibrillation
        Ventricular asystole
        Electromechanical dissociation (EMD)

Mechanical Complications

Congestive heart failure
Cardiogenic shock
Ventricular aneurysm
Rupture of the heart

Figure 2-9. Major complications in AMI.

as **ventricular tachycardia and ventricular fibrillation of short duration**
- **Severe congestive heart failure**

Lethal complications:
- **Certain life-threatening dysrhythmias such as prolonged pulseless ventricular tachycardia, ventricular fibrillation, ventricular asystole, and electromechanical dissociation (EMD)**
- **Cardiogenic shock**
- **Rupture of the heart**

Dysrhythmias

Dysrhythmias, the most common complication of AMI, are **disturbances in heart rate or rhythm.** They have been detected in over 90 percent of patients with AMI whose ECGs have been continuously monitored during hospitalization. Some dysrhythmias appear only once, briefly, whereas others recur often or persist for a long time. The majority of the dysrhythmias are not life-threatening and do not result in cardiac arrest. Only about 10 percent are life-threatening and cause cardiac arrest if not treated.

The prevention of life-threatening dysrhythmias using **antidysrhythmic drugs** and the termination of these dysrhythmias, should they occur, primarily by **defibrillation, the delivery of a direct-current (DC) shock,*** have reduced the mortality rate in hospitalized patients by about 50 percent. In the majority of AMI patients who die before reaching the hospital, the cause of death is also a life-threatening dysrhythmia—**pulseless ventricular tachycardia, ventricular fibrillation, ventricular asystole,** and **electromechanical dissociation (EMD).**

It is estimated that two-thirds of the patients who die from AMI do so within the first 2 hours of their AMI and before reaching the hospital. Most of these deaths are from life-threatening dysrhythmias that result in cardiac arrest. One of the prime reasons for this high prehospital mortality rate from dysrhythmias is that life-threatening dysrhythmias occur more frequently during the first few hours following the onset of AMI than later in the course. The other reason is that patients experiencing an AMI often deny the existence of their illness and wait too long before requesting **basic life support services that offer early defibrillation** or **advanced life support services** if such emergency medical services indeed exist in their community.

Dysrhythmias in AMI are the result of disturbances in the normal functioning of the heart's pacemakers or electrical conduction system. These can increase or decrease the heart rate or stop it completely or cause the heart to beat erratically. The following are some of the causes of dysrhythmias:
- Ischemia of or direct damage to portions of the heart and its electrical conduction system from partial or complete coronary artery occlusion
- Distention of the chambers of the heart because of congestive heart failure
- Release of toxic substances from damaged heart muscle
- Electrical instability at the junction of normal and damaged heart muscle
- Irritation or inflammation of the heart and its electrical conduction system

The dysrhythmias that may be life-threatening and must be considered for treatment in the prehospital and hospital phase of AMI are:
- Dysrhythmias with a heart rate 35 to 60 beats per minute or less (**bradycardias**)
- Dysrhythmias with a heart rate above 100 to 140 beats per minute (**tachycardias**)
- Dysrhythmias originating in the ventricles (**ventricular dysrhythmias**)

The life-threatening dysrhythmias that are of particular concern for EMTs and first responders (**EMT/FR-Ds**) involved in early defibrillation programs are:
- Ventricular asystole and electromechanical dissociation (EMD), which require CPR alone
- Ventricular fibrillation, which requires defibrillation and, if defibrillation is not effective, CPR also
- Pulseless ventricular tachycardia, which requires either defibrillation and CPR as in ventricular fibrillation or CPR alone

The recognition and management of these life-threatening dysrhythmias are discussed in **Chapters 4** and **5** (Figure 2-10).

Dysrhythmia	Treatment
Ventricular asystole	CPR
Electromechanical dissociation (EMD)	CPR
Pulseless ventricular tachycardia	Defibrillation and CPR or CPR alone
Ventricular fibrillation	Defibrillation and CPR

Figure 2-10. Management of life-threatening dysrhythmias in early defibrillation.

*Referred to as **"defibrillatory shock"** or simply as **"shock"** in this book.

Congestive Heart Failure, Cardiogenic Shock, and Ventricular Aneurysm

Some degree of weakness and disability of the myocardium occurs in the majority of patients with AMI since there is always some damage to the myocardium, usually the left ventricle. Once a segment of the left ventricular wall, for example, is damaged by an AMI, it soon becomes lifeless and unable to contract, becoming "dead weight" and interfering with the effective contraction of the rest of the ventricle. Thus, the ability of the left ventricle to pump blood is reduced (the so-called **pump failure**), causing **left heart failure.** If the disability is slight, it may result in little or no symptoms; if it is more severe, it usually results in **congestive heart failure.** If pump failure is very severe, **cardiogenic shock** and even **death** may result.

If the damaged segment in the left ventricle is large and badly weakened, it will balloon outward during ventricular contractions (**ventricular systole),** eventually producing a bulge in the ventricular wall similar to that produced in a weakened area of an inner tube. Such a defect is known as a **ventricular aneurysm.**

Congestive Heart Failure

Some degree of congestive heart failure occurs in the majority of patients with AMI because of left heart failure. It may be mild and produce no symptoms, or it may be severe, causing severe pulmonary congestion and edema and right heart failure.

Left Heart Failure

When congestive heart failure is present in AMI, its cause is most likely failure of the left ventricle brought on by damage to its myocardium. As the right ventricle continues to contract normally, it delivers more blood to the failing left ventricle via the pulmonary circulation than the left ventricle can handle. Since the blood cannot be completely emptied from the left ventricle each time it contracts, the left ventricle begins to distend and the blood to back up, first into the left atrium, then into the pulmonary veins and capillaries, and finally into the pulmonary arteries. At the point when the pulmonary blood vessels become engorged and rigid with excess blood, **pulmonary congestion** is present. This process is known as **backward failure of the left heart.**

As the pressure and blood volume continue to increase within the lungs, the liquid part of the

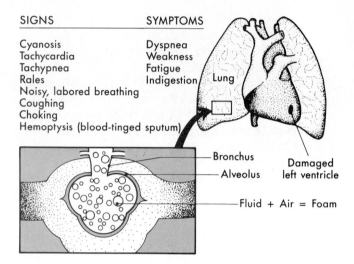

SIGNS	SYMPTOMS
Cyanosis	Dyspnea
Tachycardia	Weakness
Tachypnea	Fatigue
Rales	Indigestion
Noisy, labored breathing	
Coughing	
Choking	
Hemoptysis (blood-tinged sputum)	

Figure 2-11.   Left heart failure.

blood, called **serum,** is forced out of the blood within the capillaries into the tiny air sacs in the lung (**alveoli**) which they surround. Here it mixes with air, producing foam. When this occurs, **pulmonary edema** is present.

Signs and Symptoms of Left Heart Failure

In left heart failure, the congestion and edema within the lung prevent adequate oxygenation of arterial blood and elimination of carbon dioxide. The primary and classic **symptom** of left heart failure is **difficulty in breathing with a frightening feeling of suffocation accompanying the shortness of breath (dyspnea).** Other symptoms such as **weakness, fatigue,** and **indigestion** may also be present (Figure 2-11).

The **signs** seen in severe left heart failure include:

- Bluish discoloration of the skin, fingernail beds, and mucous membranes (**cyanosis**)
- Rapid heart rate (**tachycardia**)
- Rapid, shallow breathing (**tachypnea),** often noisy and labored
- Fine "popping" sounds in the lungs caused by fluid and foam in the small air passages of the lungs (**rales**)
- Coarse, dry rattling sounds in the throat
- Coughing
- Choking
- Blood-tinged sputum (**hemoptysis**)

Right heart failure often follows severe left heart failure. When this occurs, the signs and symptoms of left heart failure are lessened, since the right heart can no longer pump as much blood into the lungs as it did previously. The decrease in the output of the right heart often brings about a decrease in pulmonary congestion and edema.

Right Heart Failure

Right heart failure is most commonly caused by left heart failure. It can also occur without left heart failure in certain heart or lung diseases, a common one being chronic lung disease (**chronic obstructive pulmonary disease [COPD]**).

As the pressure in the pulmonary vascular system increases because of left heart failure, resistance to blood flow through the pulmonary vasculature also increases. The right heart can initially increase its work capacity to overcome the increased pulmonary pressure. Eventually, however, the right ventricle cannot keep up with the work load and fails to function properly. When this occurs, the blood first backs up into the **veins of the body,** followed by a rise in the venous pressure. The veins, including the superficial veins such as the **jugular veins** in the neck, become distended and the **body organs (liver, spleen,** and **kidney)** become engorged. Finally, the blood serum escapes from the blood in the capillaries into the surrounding tissue producing **edema** and an accumulation of fluid (called **effusion**) in the abdominal cavity, in the thoracic cavity (**pleural effusion**), and in the sac surrounding the heart (**pericardial effusion**). When edema involves the extremities, particularly the legs, it is called **peripheral edema.**

Signs and Symptoms of Right Heart Failure

The **signs** of right heart failure are:
- Rapid heart rate (**tachycardia**)
- Distended and pulsating neck veins
- Edema of the lower extremities (**peripheral edema**) or entire body
- Engorged liver and spleen
- Fluid in the abdominal cavity

When left heart failure and right heart failure occur together, the signs and symptoms of both are present (Figure 2-12).

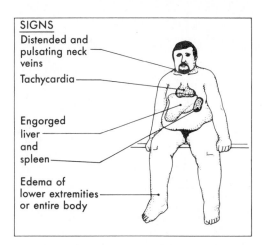

Figure 2-12. Right heart failure.

100 mm Hg or to a level 30 mm Hg below the patient's previous systolic blood pressure may indicate shock.
- A **rapid, weak and thready pulse** (usually over 110 beats/minute) (**tachycardia**)
- **Rapid, shallow respirations** (30 to 40 breaths/minute) (**tachypnea**)
- **Cold, clammy skin**
- **Collapsed veins**
- **Delayed capillary refill over 2 seconds**
- **Abnormal mental status** ranging from extreme anxiety and apprehensiveness to confusion, disorientation, and drowsiness (but still verbally responsive) to unconsciousness
- **Glassy, staring eyes**

When congestive heart failure accompanies shock, the signs and symptoms of both complications are present.

If the course of cardiogenic shock is not reversed within several hours of its onset, 80 to 100 percent of patients in shock will die. A life-threatening dysrhythmia is usually the final complication (Figure 2-13).

Cardiogenic Shock

Cardiogenic shock occurs in about 15 percent of all hospitalized AMI patients, caused primarily by extensive damage to the left ventricle. This results in ineffective contractions of the left ventricle and a marked decrease in the **stroke volume** (blood volume emptied from the heart with each beat), **cardiac output,** and **blood pressure.**

Signs typical of cardiogenic shock include:
- A **low systolic blood pressure of 90 mm Hg or less.** In patients with previous hypertension, a drop in the systolic pressure to about

Ventricular Aneurysm

A small number of patients with an AMI will develop a **ventricular aneurysm** in the late stages of recovery. An aneurysm is a thin-walled bulge in the ventricular wall in the area of weakened, dead (**necrotic**) tissue. It is usually located in the wall of the left ventricle. Because an aneurysm cannot contract, it bulges outward during ventricular systole, filling up with blood. This results in a decrease in **stroke volume** and **cardiac output.** When the aneurysm takes up more than one-fourth of the left ventricular wall, congestive heart failure

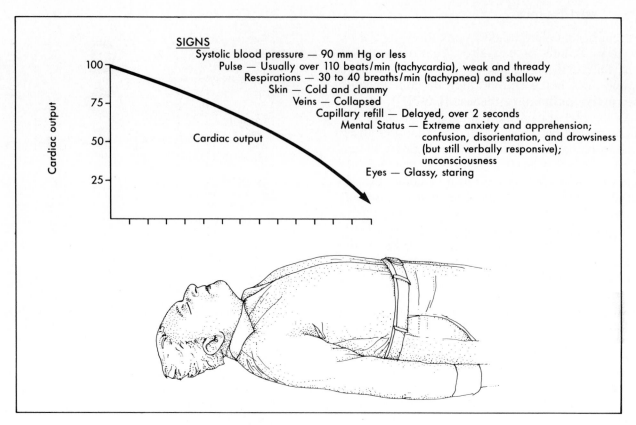

SIGNS
Systolic blood pressure — 90 mm Hg or less
Pulse — Usually over 110 beats/min (tachycardia), weak and thready
Respirations — 30 to 40 breaths/min (tachypnea) and shallow
Skin — Cold and clammy
Veins — Collapsed
Capillary refill — Delayed, over 2 seconds
Mental Status — Extreme anxiety and apprehension; confusion, disorientation, and drowsiness (but still verbally responsive); unconsciousness
Eyes — Glassy, staring

Figure 2-13. Cardiogenic shock.

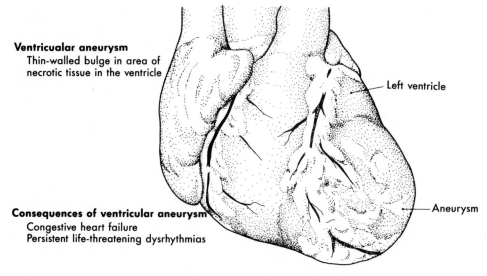

Ventricualar aneurysm
Thin-walled bulge in area of necrotic tissue in the ventricle

Left ventricle

Consequences of ventricular aneurysm
Congestive heart failure
Persistent life-threatening dysrhythmias

Aneurysm

Figure 2-14. Ventricular aneurysm.

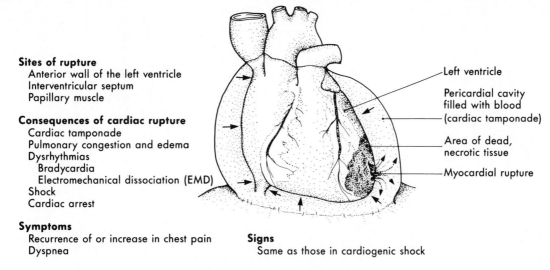

Sites of rupture
Anterior wall of the left ventricle
Interventricular septum
Papillary muscle

Consequences of cardiac rupture
Cardiac tamponade
Pulmonary congestion and edema
Dysrhythmias
Bradycardia
Electromechanical dissociation (EMD)
Shock
Cardiac arrest

Symptoms
Recurrence of or increase in chest pain
Dyspnea

Left ventricle
Pericardial cavity
filled with blood
(cardiac tamponade)
Area of dead,
necrotic tissue
Myocardial rupture

Signs
Same as those in cardiogenic shock

Figure 2-15. Cardiac rupture.

usually develops. Persistent life-threatening ventricular dysrhythmias often accompany an aneurysm (Figure 2-14).

Cardiac Rupture

Rupture of the heart is a rare lethal complication in AMI. About two-thirds of the ruptures occur within the first two weeks of the AMI. The usual site of the rupture is within the myocardial infarction in an area of dead, necrotic tissue (**myocardial rupture**) (Figure 2-15).

The anterior wall of the left ventricle is the most frequent site of rupture. When it occurs, it is inevitably fatal, causing sudden death. Immediately upon rupture of the ventricular wall, blood escapes into the **pericardial cavity,** completely filling and distending it, preventing normal filling and emptying of the heart, a condition called **cardiac tamponade.** The patient may experience the **recurrence of chest pain** or an **increase in its severity.**

Severe shortness of breath (dyspnea) and **slowing of the heart rate (bradycardia)** may also occur. Inevitably, the patient goes into **shock,** followed rapidly by **cardiac arrest.** A common complication is **electromechanical dissociation (EMD),** a condition in which an ECG is present but a pulse is absent. Cardiopulmonary resuscitation is usually not effective in this instance. Unless the diagnosis is made immediately and mechanical circulatory assistance and emergency surgical repair are provided, death is inevitable.

Other parts of the heart, such as the wall between the ventricles (the **interventricular septum**) and the strands of muscle that anchor the heart valves in place (**papillary muscles**) may also rupture, but the incidence is low and sudden death within minutes is less likely. When this occurs, the patient usually develops **acute severe pulmonary congestion and edema,** and in some cases, **shock** and may eventually **die** if the rupture is not surgically repaired.

Chapter 3

Cardiac Arrest

OBJECTIVES

Upon completion of all or part of this chapter as required by your early defibrillation program, you should be able to complete the following objectives indicated by your instructor:

☐ Define cardiac arrest.
☐ List nine situations or conditions in which cardiac arrest can occur.
☐ List the four life-threatening dysrhythmias responsible for cardiac arrest in the order of their decreasing incidence.
☐ Describe briefly:
  • Ventricular fibrillation
  • Ventricular asystole
  • Electromechanical dissociation (EMD)
  • Pulseless ventricular tachycardia
☐ Explain the role of respiratory arrest in cardiac arrest.
☐ Differentiate between clinical death and biological death.
☐ Describe the sequence of biological events that take place between the occurrences of clinical death and biological death.
☐ Define apnea and hypoxia.
☐ Describe the signs of cardiac arrest as they relate to the following:
  • State of consciousness and neurological status
  • General appearance
  • Skin and mucous membranes
  • Respirations and breath sounds
  • Vital signs and heart sounds
  • Eyes
☐ List the three most important signs in recognizing cardiac arrest.
☐ State the indications for using an automated external defibrillator and CPR upon arrival on the scene of a cardiac arrest.
☐ Identify two circumstances under which both CPR and the automated external defibrillator may not be effective.
☐ Define obviously dead.
☐ Define livor mortis and rigor mortis.
☐ Describe two traumatic conditions which may possibly prevent CPR from being performed but still allow the use of the automated external defibrillator.

Definition of Cardiac Arrest

Cardiac arrest is the sudden, unexpected loss of an effective pumping action of the heart caused by a life-threatening dysrhythmia. It results in an abrupt cessation of circulation of blood to the vital organs, causing death. Cardiac arrest can occur in the following situations and conditions:

• Unexpectedly without previous signs or symptoms of coronary heart disease, the so-called **sudden cardiac death**
• In a patient with obvious **coronary heart disease** such as **angina pectoris** or **acute myocardial infarction with or without any of its complications—congestive heart failure, cardiogenic shock, ventricular aneurysm, or cardiac rupture**
• **Respiratory insufficiency or arrest**
• **Hypothermia**
• **Drowning**
• **Multiple trauma, especially if hypovolemia is present**
• **Electrocution**
• **Drug overdose**
• **Poisoning**

Life-threatening Dysrhythmias and Cardiac Arrest

The **life-threatening dysrhythmias** recorded at the time of prehospital resuscitation of cardiac arrest are, in the order of decreasing incidence, **ventricular fibrillation, ventricular asystole, electromechanical dissociation (EMD),** and **pulseless ventricular tachycardia** (Figure 3-1).

The most commonly seen life-threatening dysrhythmia in the prehospital setting of cardiac arrest is **ventricular fibrillation,** the chaotic, uncoordinated beating of the ventricles which produces no cardiac output and, consequently, no pulse or

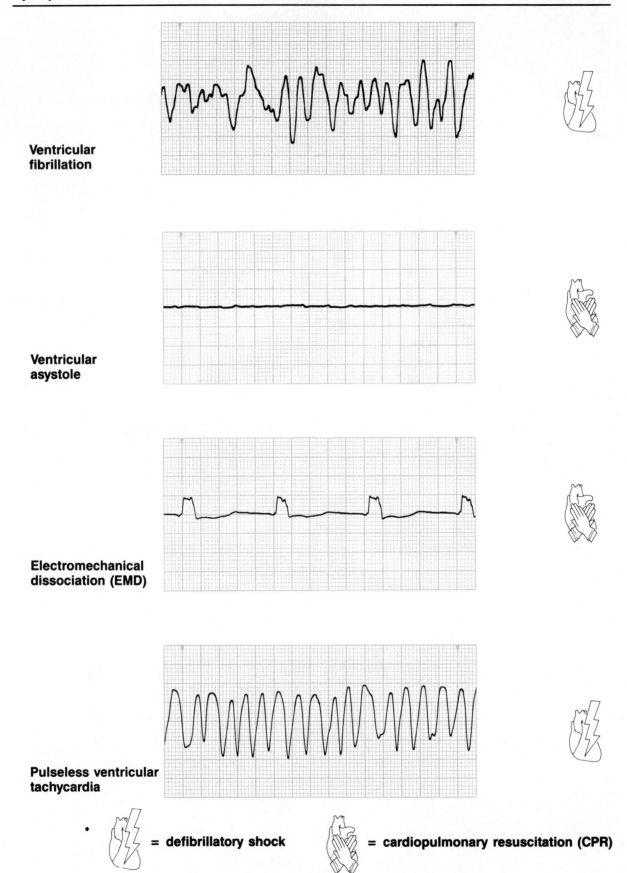

Ventricular fibrillation

Ventricular asystole

Electromechanical dissociation (EMD)

Pulseless ventricular tachycardia

* = **defibrillatory shock** = **cardiopulmonary resuscitation (CPR)**

Figure 3-1. The four most common dysrhythmias resulting in cardiac arrest.

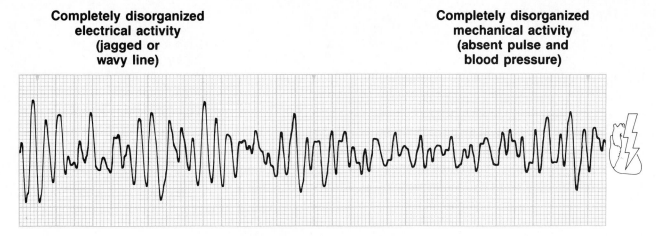

Completely disorganized electrical activity (jagged or wavy line)

Completely disorganized mechanical activity (absent pulse and blood pressure)

Figure 3-2. Ventricular fibrillation.

blood pressure. In ventricular fibrillation, **electrical and mechanical activity are present but they are completely disorganized and ineffectual.** The electrocardiogram in ventricular fibrillation is recorded as a jagged or wavy line (Figure 3-2).

Ventricular fibrillation usually occurs in the setting of severe coronary heart disease, often following an acute myocardial infarction or a previous myocardial infarction, especially if a complication, such as congestive heart failure, or rarely, ventricular aneurysm or cardiac rupture is present. The cause may be acute myocardial ischemia from partial or total coronary artery occlusion, or it may be electrical instability of the ventricles from whatever cause. A small number of patients who develop ventricular fibrillation do so without any apparent cause or premonitory signs or symptoms, the so-called **"sudden cardiac death."** Since studies have shown that ventricular tachycardia often degenerates into ventricular fibrillation after a vari-

able length of time, many of the patients with ventricular fibrillation may have had ventricular tachycardia initially. Other causes of ventricular fibrillation, not primarily related to coronary heart disease, although it may be present, are:

- **Decreased blood volume (hypovolemia)** caused by trauma
- **Electrocution** from contact with 110 to 220 volt AC current lasting 2 to 3 seconds or longer
- **Respiratory insufficiency** from any cause, resulting in decreased amount of oxygen (hypoxia) in the tissues of the body
- **Drowning**
- **Hypothermia**
- **Excess of certain cardiac drugs**
- **Imbalance of certain chemicals in the blood,** such as calcium or potassium, the so-called **blood electrolytes**

The second most commonly seen dysrhythmia in

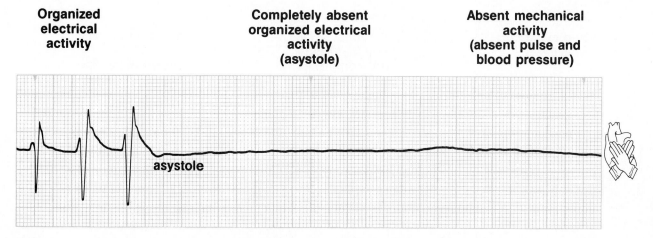

Organized electrical activity

Completely absent organized electrical activity (asystole)

Absent mechanical activity (absent pulse and blood pressure)

asystole

Figure 3-3. Ventricular asystole.

**Organized electrical
activity**

**Absent mechanical
activity
(absent pulse and
blood pressure)**

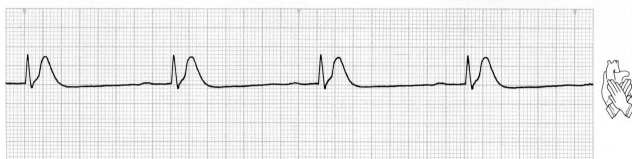

Figure 3-4. Electromechanical dissociation (EMD).

the prehospital setting is **ventricular asystole.** It occurs when **organized electrical activity of the ventricles ceases,** and the ventricles stop beating (i.e., the **mechanical activity** of the heart stops). Ventricular asystole can occur in an acute myocardial infarction or in drowning, or it may be the final result of other life-threatening dysrhythmias. The ECG in ventricular asystole is a flat, sometimes gently waving line (Figure 3-3).

The third most common dysrhythmia is **electromechanical dissociation (EMD),** a condition in which an **organized electrical activity** of some kind is present, but for some reason the ventricles cannot contract and pump the blood effectively so as to produce a pulse and blood pressure (i.e., the **mechanical activity** of the heart is absent) (Figure 3-4).

Electromechanical dissociation can occur in AMI, but the mechanism is not completely understood in this setting. Electromechanical dissociation also results from hypovolemia, tension pneu-

mothorax, cardiac tamponade, and blood electrolyte imbalance (e.g., decrease in blood calcium, increase in blood potassium).

The least common dysrhythmia in prehospital cardiac arrest is **pulseless ventricular tachycardia,** in which a specific **organized electrical activity,** consisting of a series of rapidly occurring, abnormal wide and distorted **QRS complexes,** is present, but where, as in electromechanical dissociation, mechanical activity is absent. Ventricular tachycardia, like ventricular fibrillation, also occurs in the setting of severe coronary heart disease, often following an acute myocardial infarction or a previous myocardial infarction and when an excess of certain drugs has been taken. The causes of ventricular tachycardia are generally the same as those of ventricular fibrillation (Figure 3-5). (**QRS complexes** are described in **Chapter 4.**)

Respiratory arrest lasting several minutes can also result in cardiac arrest if left untreated. The

**Organized electrical
activity**

**Abnormal wide
and distorted
QRS complexes**

**Absent mechanical
activity
(absent pulse and
blood pressure)**

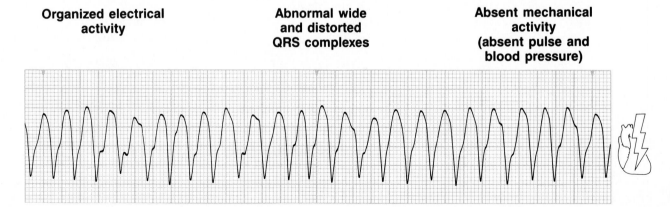

Figure 3-5. Pulseless ventricular tachycardia.

reason for this is that lack of oxygen causes the heart to develop ventricular tachycardia or fibrillation and finally within minutes, if untreated, ventricular asystole. Causes of respiratory arrest include drowning, suffocation, airway obstruction, certain drugs or anesthetic agents that depress the respiratory center, and asthma.

Consequences of Cardiac Arrest

Immediately at the onset of cardiac arrest, as the blood pressure and pulse cease, circulation to the **vital organs** (e.g., brain, heart, lungs) stops. At the moment this occurs, **clinical death** is present. The patient experiences a moment of faintness followed within seconds by loss of consciousness. Momentary gasping breathing **(agonal gasping)** occurs within seconds, followed by complete absence of breathing **(apnea)** in about 15 to 30 seconds. As the brain becomes devoid of oxygen **(hypoxic)**, **convulsions** may occur briefly. The pupils begin to dilate 30 to 40 seconds after the circulation stops and are usually completely dilated within 1½ to 2 minutes. In certain instances, pupils may dilate only partially or not at all because of eye disease or drugs (Figure 3-6).

Within 4 to 5 minutes after clinical death, if cardiopulmonary resuscitation is not provided, some of the brain cells begin to die, followed by irreversible brain damage within 5 to 10 minutes or

sooner. At the moment irreversible brain damage has occurred, **biological death** is present.

When respiratory arrest occurs first, the heart continues to beat for about 3 to 6 minutes as long as there is a supply of oxygen in the body, particularly in the lungs. As severe hypoxia develops and carbon dioxide and other acids accumulate because of the lack of oxygen, producing **acidosis,** life-threatening ventricular dysrhythmias appear, rapidly terminating in cardiac arrest. The onset of cardiac arrest is therefore delayed for several minutes following primary respiratory arrest.

Signs of Cardiac Arrest

The following signs appear in cardiac arrest regardless of its cause. The patient becomes unconscious within seconds, assumes a deathlike appearance, and may convulse. The skin becomes pale, cold, sweaty, and clammy, and the mucous membranes, pale or cyanotic. Respirations slow, become gasping, and then stop. Breath sounds, when present, may be noisy or bubbling. The pulse, blood pressure, and heart sounds disappear immediately. **It is a waste of time to try to obtain the blood pressure or listen for heart sounds when cardiac arrest occurs.** The surface of the eyes dries up, assuming a ground-glass appearance, and the pupils soon become dilated (Figure 3-7).

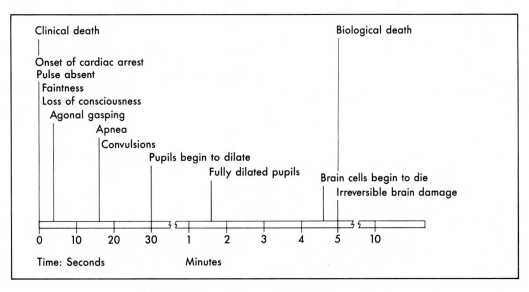

Figure 3-6. Sequence of events in cardiac arrest.

Mental status:	Unconsciousness
	Deathlike appearance
	Brief convulsions possible
Pulse:	Absent
Respirations:	Slow, becoming absent
	Gasping, noisy, or bubbling while
	present
Skin:	Pale cyanotic, sweaty, cold and clammy
Eyelids:	Drooping
Eyes:	Dull with a vacant stare, glazed with a
	ground-glass appearance
Pupils:	Dilated

Figure 3-7.   Signs of respiratory and cardiac arrest.

Recognition of Respiratory and Cardiac Arrest

The signs of respiratory and cardiac arrest are as follows:

- The patient is unconscious and has a deathlike appearance. Brief convulsions may occur at the onset of cardiac arrest.
- The pulse is absent immediately. This, of all signs, is the most important one in determining whether or not cardiac arrest is present.
- The respirations slow and become absent within 15 to 30 seconds. When present, they may be gasping, noisy, or bubbling.
- The skin becomes pale, cyanotic, sweaty, and cold and clammy.
- The eyelids begin to droop.

- The eyes assume a dull vacant stare and become glazed over with a ground-glass or hazy appearance as their surface dries up.
- The pupils begin dilating within 30 to 40 seconds, becoming fully dilated by 1½ to 2 minutes. One or both pupils may already be dilated from drugs, prescribed medications, surgery, or other causes. Conversely, the pupils may not dilate because of disease or drugs.

The three most important signs in the recognition of cardiac arrest, in the order in which they are determined, are **unresponsiveness, absent respirations,** and **absent pulse.**

Indications for Application of the Automated External Defibrillator and CPR

The use of the **automated external defibrillator** (AED) for the analysis of the ECG rhythm and, when necessary, the administration of a **defibrillatory shock** to terminate pulseless ventricular tachycardia and ventricular fibrillation (**defibrillation**) is indicated immediately in all patients with cardiac arrest except those who are **obviously dead.** Obviously dead patients are defined as those with **decapitation** and those with **widespread livor mortis, rigor mortis,** or **evidence of tissue decomposition.**

Livor mortis (also known as **post-mortem lividity** and **dependent lividity**) is the dull red discoloration of the skin that appears approximately 20 to 30 minutes after death in the parts of the body closest to the surface on which the body is lying, the so-called dependent part of the body. This is the result of accumulation of blood in the blood

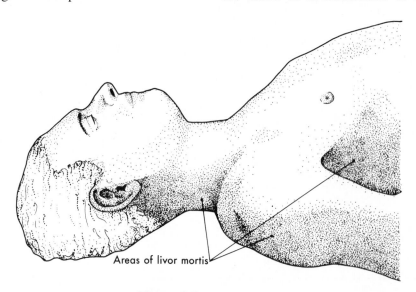

Areas of livor mortis

Figure 3-8.   Livor mortis.

CPR and Automated External Defibrillator (AED) Ineffective

Obviously dead patient
   Decapitation
   Widespread livor mortis
   Rigor mortis
   Tissue decomposition
Documented cardiac arrest of over 10 minutes without CPR

CPR Ineffective, but AED may be effective

Traumatic conditions
   Severe crushing injuries to the face and neck
   Severe fractures to the sternum and ribs

Figure 3-9. Circumstances under which CPR or the AED or both may not be effective.

vessels, especially the veins and venules, in these parts of the body because of gravity (Figure 3-8).

Rigor mortis is the stiffening of the muscles of the body caused by chemical changes following death. It begins to appear within 30 minutes to 6 hours or more after death, most commonly within 2 to 4 hours, following an initial period of limpness (flaccidity), and lasts 16 to 24 hours. Stiffness of the body resulting from exposure to cold and the muscular spasm and rigidity sometimes associated with electrocution may mimic rigor mortis.

CPR is indicated immediately upon arrival at the scene of a cardiac arrest while the defibrillator electrodes are being applied and the AED is being set up. CPR is stopped as soon as the defibrillator electrodes have been applied and the AED is turned on. Under no condition should the application of the defibrillator electrodes and initial analysis of the patient's ECG by the automated external defibrillator be delayed. An exception to this rule is when a single rescuer, the EMT/FR-D, arrives at the scene where no bystander CPR is being performed. Application of the electrodes and set up of the AED takes preference over CPR! A detailed description of the AED is presented in **Chapter 7.** The application of the AED and performance of CPR under various circumstances are detailed in **Chapter 8.**

CPR is restarted immediately after the AED determines that a shock is not indicated or after three or up to six consecutive shocks have been delivered, depending on the local early defibrillation system's protocol, and a shockable rhythm is still present.

It may not be possible to perform CPR if the following traumatic conditions are present: **severe crushing injuries to the face and neck** or **severe fractures to the sternum or ribs** (i.e., injuries which prohibit the proper performance of resuscitative procedures). The AED, however, can still be used in these circumstances.

In addition, use of both the AED and CPR may **not** be indicated **if true cardiac arrest has been documented to have been present for more than 10 minutes without CPR being applied.** Under these conditions, the patient cannot be resuscitated successfully, nor his or her central nervous system be restored to its **prearrest condition. If this interval cannot be determined with reasonable accuracy, especially if hypothermia is present or drowning has occurred, the patient should be given the benefit of the doubt, and CPR started and/or the AED applied immediately** (Figure 3-9).

IMPORTANT!
THE DECISION OF WHETHER OR NOT CPR SHOULD BE PERFORMED IN THE ABOVE CIRCUMSTANCES, HOWEVER, SHOULD BE THAT OF THE LOCAL MEDICAL CONTROL!

Chapter 4

The Electrocardiogram (ECG) and Basic Rhythms and Dysrhythmias

OBJECTIVES

Upon completion of all or part of this chapter as required by your early defibrillation program, you should be able to complete the following objectives indicated by your instructor:

☐ Define an ECG.
☐ Describe how the mechanical activity of the heart is best assessed.
☐ Define the following components of the ECG:
  • P wave
  • QRS complex
  • T wave
☐ Define organized ECG rhythm.
☐ Describe the relationship between the P wave, QRS complex, and T wave and the mechanical activity of the atria and ventricles.
☐ Define the term ECG artifact, describe how they may interfere with the automated external defibrillator's analysis of the patient's ECG, and list five common artifacts.
☐ Describe a pacemaker spike.
☐ List the four major categories of ECG rhythms and dysrhythmias.
☐ Define the following:
  • A perfusing rhythm
  • A nonperfusing rhythm
☐ List four nonperfusing rhythms.
☐ List five perfusing rhythms.
☐ Define the following:
  • A shockable rhythm
  • A nonshockable rhythm
☐ List three nonshockable rhythms.
☐ List two shockable rhythms.

☐ Describe the following rhythms and dysrhythmias and their treatment in an early defibrillation program:
  • Organized ECG rhythm
  • Normal sinus rhythm
  • Ventricular tachycardia with a pulse
  • Ventricular tachycardia without a pulse
  • Ventricular fibrillation
  • Ventricular asystole
  • Electromechanical dissociation (EMD)

This chapter is primarily intended for those early defibrillation programs where semi-automatic external defibrillators (SAEDs) are used and where the EMT/FR-Ds may be required to have some knowledge of the electrocardiogram and several **basic rhythms and dysrhythmias** (e.g., **normal sinus rhythm, ventricular tachycardia, ventricular fibrillation, ventricular asystole,** and **electromechanical dissociation [EMD]**) in the management of prehospital cardiac arrest.

The Electrocardiogram (ECG)

The **electrocardiogram (ECG)** is a graphic representation of the **electrical activity of the heart** which causes the atria and ventricles to contract (the **mechanical activity of the heart**). The ECG can be used only to evaluate the electrical activity of the heart and not the mechanical activity. To evaluate the mechanical activity of the heart, the pulse and blood pressure must be assessed.

Components of the Electrocardiogram

As soon as an electrical impulse is generated in the SA node, it spreads across the atria producing the **P wave** in the ECG. This is immediately followed by the contraction of the atria. The electrical impulse continues through the AV node, bundle of His, and the bundle branches to the ventricles. The impulse then rapidly spreads across the ventricles producing the **Q, R,** and **S waves** (collectively called the **QRS complex**), which follow the P wave, causing the ventricles to contract. Following the QRS complex, while the ventricles are finishing contracting and beginning to relax, the **T wave** is produced (Figure 4-1 and 4-2).

An ECG in which QRS complexes can be recognized, each followed by a T wave in most instances, is called an **organized ECG rhythm.** P waves need not be present for an ECG to be called an organized ECG rhythm. When QRS complexes

are absent, the ECG is either **ventricular fibrillation** or **ventricular asystole.** Ventricular fibrillation is present when the ECG looks like a **jagged or wavy line.** When the ECG is a **flat line,** ventricular asystole is present. These dysrhythmias will be described later in this chapter (Figure 4-9).

Summary

- The **P wave** represents the **electrical activity of the atria** just before they contract.
- The **QRS complex** represents the **electrical activity of the ventricles** just before they contract.
- The **T wave** represents the **electrical activity of the ventricles** while they are finishing contracting and beginning to relax.
- The **contractions of the atria and ventricles** are the **mechanical activity of the heart.**

It is extremely important to understand the sequence of electrical and mechanical (**electromechanical**) events relative to the electrocardiogram

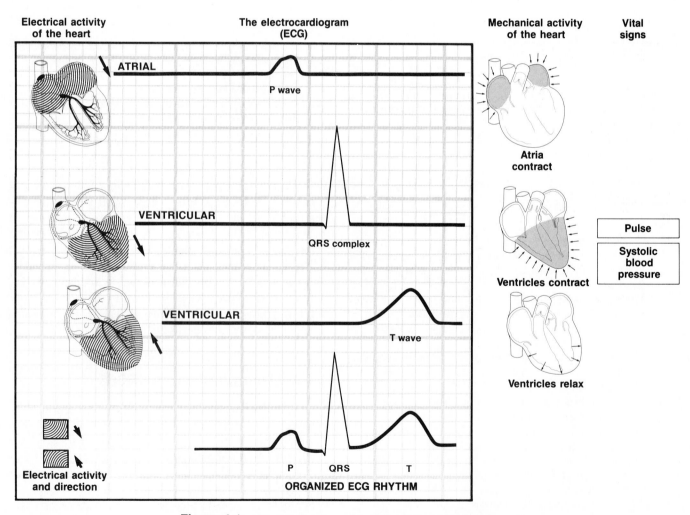

Figure 4-1.   Electrical and mechanical activity of the heart.

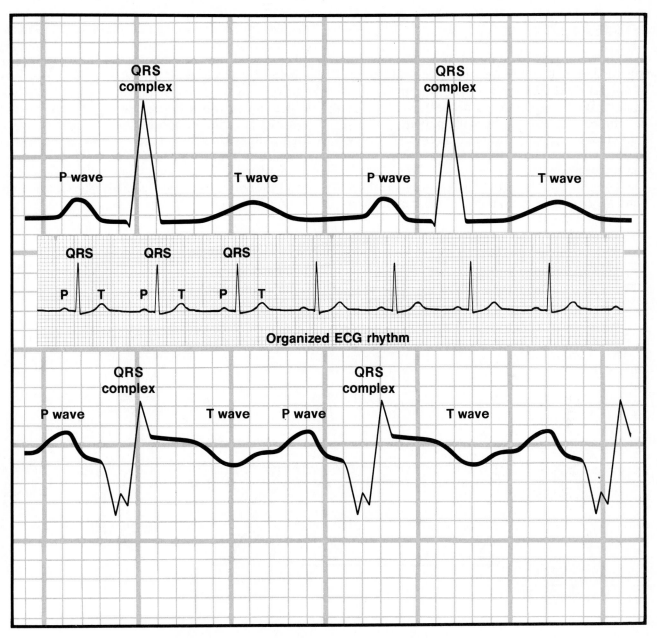

Figure 4-2. Components of the electrocardiogram (ECG).

and the cardiovascular system. **Normally, the ventricles contract immediately following the onset of the QRS complex, producing a pulse.** Should a pulse not follow each QRS complex, a life-threatening condition called **electromechanical dissociation (EMD)** is present (Figure 4-3).

Artifacts

Abnormal waves and spikes in an ECG that result from sources other than the electrical activity of the heart and interfere with or distort the components of the ECG are called **artifacts.** The causes of artifacts are **muscle tremor, patient or ECG cable movement, alternating current (AC) interference, loose electrodes,** and **external chest compression.**

When an ECG is being analyzed by the **ECG analysis circuit** of the automated external defibril-

lator and ventricular fibrillation or ventricular tachycardia is not present, artifacts may cause the ECG analysis circuit to mistake the artifacts for ventricular fibrillation or ventricular tachycardia, resulting in an incorrect interpretation calling for **"SHOCK."** Conversely, when ventricular fibrillation is present, artifacts such as those produced by external chest compression or patient or ECG cable movement, for example, may cause the ECG analysis circuit to mistake the artifacts for a rhythm other than ventricular fibrillation, resulting in a possible **"NO SHOCK"** instruction. This can also occur in a patient with a permanently implanted artificial pacemaker whose pacemaker continues to generate **pacemaker spikes** after the onset of ventricular fibrillation.

Muscle tremor can occur in tense or nervous patients or those shivering from cold and give the ECG a finely or coarsely jagged appearance (Figure 4-4).

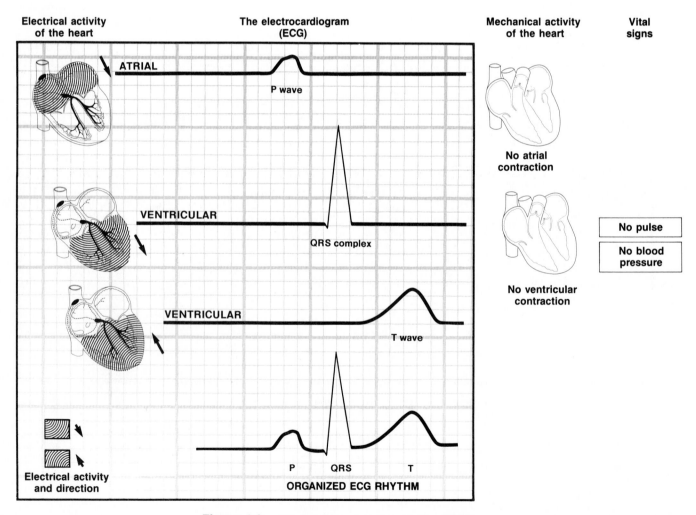

Figure 4-3.   Electromechanical dissociation (EMD).

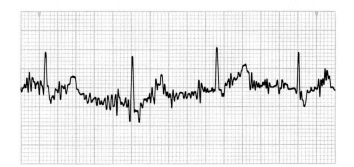

Figure 4-4. Muscle tremor.

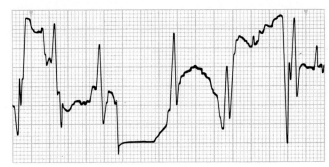

Figure 4-5. Patient or ECG cable movement or electrode problems.

Patient or ECG cable movement can produce a coarsely jagged appearance of the ECG with sharp spikes and waves. **Loose electrodes or electrodes that are in poor electrical contact with the skin** because of insufficient or dried electrode paste or jelly can also cause multiple, sharp spikes and waves in the ECG (Figure 4-5).

AC interference can occur when a poorly grounded, AC-operated ECG machine is used or when an ECG is obtained near high tension wires, transformers, electric heaters, or neon lights. This results in a thick baseline composed of 60-cycle waves (Figure 4-6).

External chest compressions during cardiopulmonary resuscitation in most instances cause regularly spaced, wide, upright waves, synchronous with the downward compressions of the chest (Figure 4-7).

Pacemaker spikes, although technically not artifacts, are included here for completeness. They are the small electrical impulses generated by an artificial pacemaker at a rate usually between 60 and 75 beats per minute (Figure 4-8).

Basic ECG Rhythms and Dysrhythmias

The ECG rhythms and dysrhythmias that the EMT/FR-D should be able to identify are grouped into the following four major categories:
- **Organized ECG rhythms**
- **Ventricular tachycardia**
- **Ventricular fibrillation**
- **Ventricular asystole** (Figure 4-9)

Perfusing and Nonperfusing Rhythms

The basic ECG rhythms and dysrhythmias are further categorized as to whether or not they produce a palpable peripheral pulse. Rhythms and dysrhythmias that **DO** produce a palpable peripheral pulse and a blood pressure are identified as **perfusing rhythms;** those that **DO NOT,** are identified as **nonperfusing rhythms** (Figure 4-10).

Certain dysrhythmias typically never produce a pulse, i.e., **ventricular fibrillation** and **ventricular asystole.** All the other rhythms and dysrhyth-

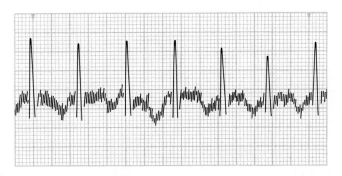

Figure 4-6. AC interference.

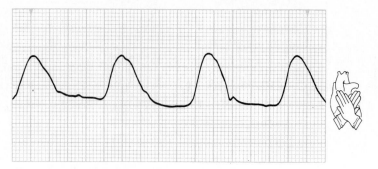

Figure 4-7.   External chest compression.

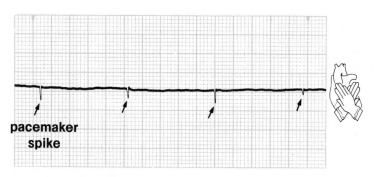

pacemaker
spike

Figure 4-8.   Pacemaker spikes.

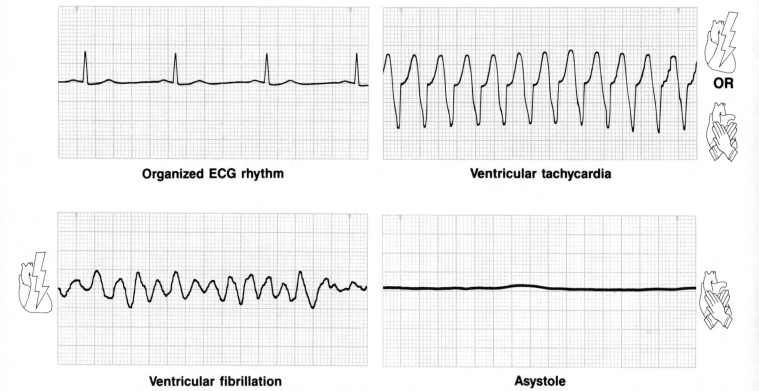

Organized ECG rhythm

Ventricular tachycardia

OR

Ventricular fibrillation

Asystole

Figure 4-9.   Four major categories of ECG rhythms and dysrhythmias.

mias, which usually produce a pulse, may not do so under certain conditions, such as an **extremely rapid heart rate, hypovolemia,** and **cardiac tamponade.*** When a rhythm or dysrhythmia which should produce a pulse is pulseless, the condition is called **electromechanical dissociation (EMD).** When ventricular tachycardia occurs without a pulse, although it is technically an electromechanical dissociation, it is specifically identified as **pulseless ventricular tachycardia.**

***Cardiac tamponade** is a serious cardiac condition in which a collection of blood is present within the pericardial sac, constricting the ventricles and causing the amount of blood pumped out by the heart to decrease.

Shockable and Nonshockable Rhythms

Finally, the basic rhythms and dysrhythmias are categorized into those that **ARE** treatable by a **defibrillatory shock** in the context of an early defibrillation program—the **shockable rhythms,** and those that **ARE NOT** treatable by shock—the **nonshockable rhythms.**

- **Organized ECG rhythms, electromechanical dissociation (EMD),** and **ventricular asystole** are **nonshockable rhythms** (Figure 4-11).
- **Ventricular fibrillation** is a **shockable rhythm** (Figure 4-12).
- **Ventricular tachycardia may or may not be a shockable rhythm** depending on the analy-

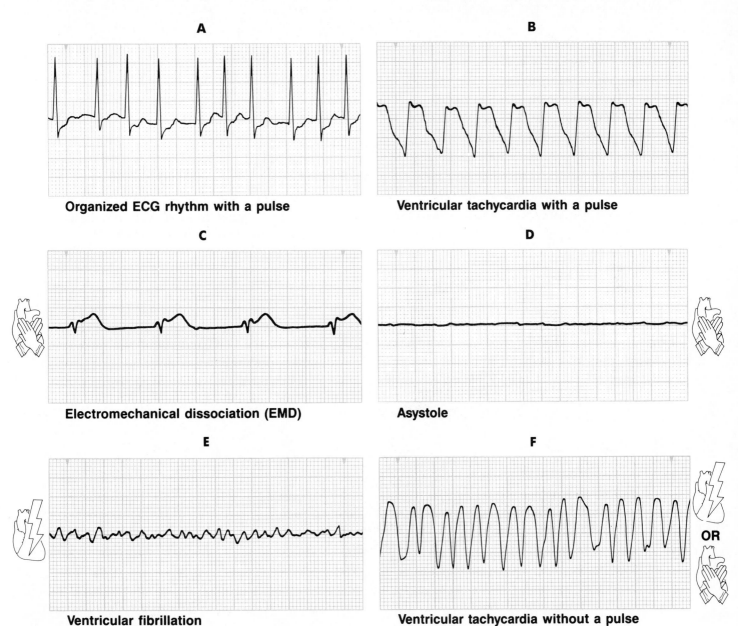

A
Organized ECG rhythm with a pulse

B
Ventricular tachycardia with a pulse

C
Electromechanical dissociation (EMD)

D
Asystole

E
Ventricular fibrillation

F
Ventricular tachycardia without a pulse

OR

Figure 4-10.   **A** and **B,** Perfusing rhythms. **C, D, E,** and **F,** nonperfusing rhythms.

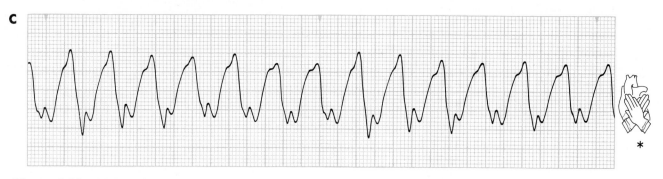

A

P   T

QRS

**Organized ECG rhythm with
or without a pulse**

B

P

Ventricular asystole

C

Figure 4-11. Nonshockable rhythms. **C,** Nonshockable ventricular tachycardia with or without a pulse and shockable ventricular tachycardia with a pulse. Asterisk denotes CPR indicated when pulse is absent.

sis of the dysrhythmia by the automated external defibrillator and on whether or not a pulse is present as determined by the rescuer. In its analysis of ventricular tachycardia, the ECG analysis circuit of the automated external defibrillator uses the rate of the ventricular tachycardia in its determination of whether or not the dysrhythmias is shockable. If the rate is above a certain value, the ventricular tachycardia is **shockable;** if below this value, it is **nonshockable.** This rate value varies amongst the various automated external defibrillator

models, ranging from 120 to 200 beats per minute. Because of this, a ventricular tachycardia with a rate of 160 beats per minute, for example, may be determined to be shockable by one automated external defibrillator and nonshockable by another. **The bottom line is that a ventricular tachycardia with a pulse as determined by the rescuer is *NOT SHOCKABLE* regardless of the interpretation of the automated external defibrillator** (Figure 4-12).

The following outline identifies the rhythms and

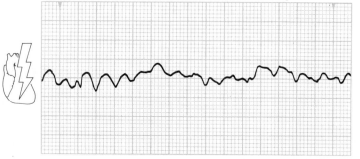

Ventricular fibrillation

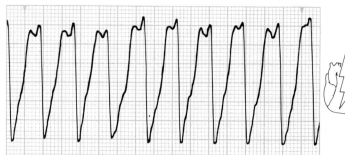

Shockable ventricular tachycardia without a pulse

Figure 4-12. Shockable rhythms.

Table 4-1 The relationship of perfusion and the need to deliver a shock in the basic rhythms and dysrhythmias described in this manual.

Rhythm/dysrhythmia	Perfusing	Nonperfusing	Nonshockable	Shockable
Perfusing/nonshockable				
Organized ECG rhythms with a pulse (including normal sinus rhythm)	+		+	
Nonshockable or shockable* ventricular tachycardia, with a pulse	+		+	
Nonperfusing/nonshockable				
Electromechanical dissociation (EMD)		+	+	
Nonshockable* pulseless ventricular tachycardia		+	+	
Ventricular asystole		+	+	
Nonperfusing/shockable				
Shockable* pulseless ventricular tachycardia		+		+
Ventricular fibrillation		+		+

*Shockability as determined by the automated external defibrillator.

dysrhythmias described in this chapter that are nonshockable and those that are shockable:

Nonshockable rhythms
  A. **Organized ECG rhythms with a pulse**
      • **Normal sinus rhythm**
  B. **Electromechanical dissociation (EMD)**
  C. **Nonshockable* ventricular tachycardia with or without a pulse**
  D. **Shockable* ventricular tachycardia with a pulse**
  E. **Ventricular asystole**
Shockable rhythms
  A. **Shockable* pulseless ventricular tachycardia without a pulse**
  B. **Ventricular fibrillation**

Table 4-1 shows the relationship between perfusion and the need to deliver a shock in the basic

*Shockability as determined by the automated external defibrillator.

rhythms and dysrhythmias described in this manual.

Dysrhythmia Interpretation

The description of the following rhythms and dysrhythmias includes the **heart rate, rhythm, pacemaker site, P waves, QRS complexes,** and **pulse. Specific treatment** of each rhythm and dysrhythmia is also indicated. Although basic life support treatment modalities, such as positioning the patient, opening and maintaining an open airway, administering high concentration oxygen, and so forth, are not specified in the treatment section, it is assumed that they are provided whenever appropriate. **Table 4-2** summarizes the heart rate and pacemaker sites of four rhythms and dysrhythmias described in this chapter.

Table 4-2 The heart rate and pacemaker sites of four rhythms and dysrhythmias described in this chapter.

	Rhythms and dysrhythmias	
Rhythm or dysrhythmia	Heart rate beats/min	Pacemaker site
Normal sinus rhythm	60 to 100	SA node
Ventricular tachycardia	>100	Ventricles
Ventricular fibrillation	0	Ventricles
Ventricular asystole	0	None

Organized ECG Rhythm

The term **organized ECG rhythm** is used to indicate the presence of QRS complexes and, in most instances, T waves on the ECG, with or without P waves, indicating **organized electrical activity of the heart** (Figure 4-13). An organized ECG rhythm includes all the rhythms and dysrhythmias **except** ventricular tachycardia, ventricular fibrillation, and ventricular asystole. All **organized ECG rhythms** are **nonshockable** regardless of whether or not a pulse is present.

Heart rate. The heart rate according to the ECG is 60 to 100 beats per minute, but it may be as low as 20 or as high as 160 or more beats per minute.

Rhythm. The rhythm may be regular or irregular.

Pacemaker site. The pacemaker site may be above the ventricles or in the ventricles.

P waves. P waves may be present or absent.

QRS complexes. QRS complexes are present. They may be narrow or wide, distorted, and bizarre.

Pulse. A pulse is usually present, but it may be absent. If a pulse is absent, **electromechanical dissociation (EMD)** is present.

Specific treatment. No specific treatment is indicated for an **organized ECG rhythm with a pulse. Cardiopulmonary resuscitation** and **immediate transport** are indicated if **electromechanical dissociation (EMD)** is present.

SHOCK IS NOT INDICATED!

Notes

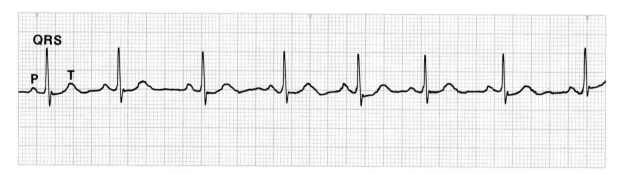

Figure 4-13. Components of an organized ECG rhythm.

Organized ECG Rhythm

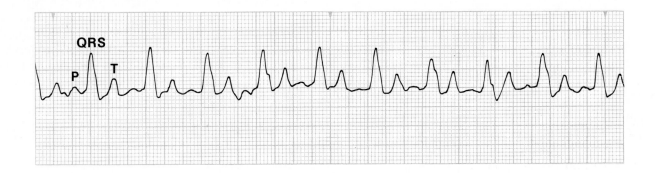

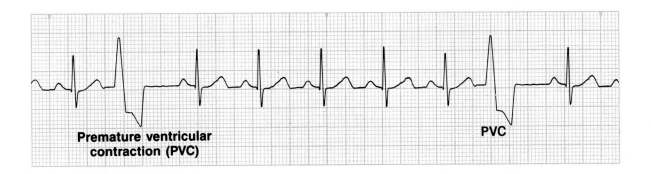

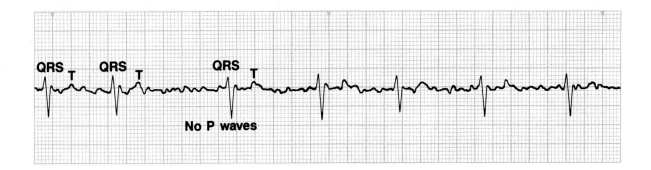

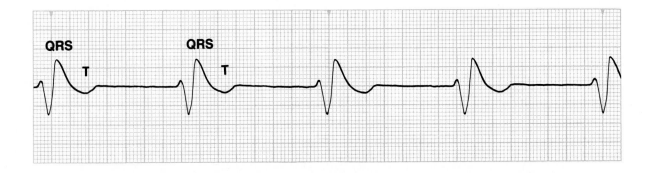

Normal Sinus Rhythm (NSR)

Heart rate. The heart rate according to the ECG is 60 to 100 beats per minute (Figure 4-14).

Rhythm. The rhythm is essentially regular.

Pacemaker site. The pacemaker site is the **SA node.**

P waves. The identical P waves are positive (upright) and precede each QRS complex.

QRS complexes. The QRS complexes are normally narrow but may be wide. A QRS complex follows each P wave.

Pulse. A pulse is normally present after every QRS complex. If a pulse is absent, **electromechanical dissociation (EMD)** is present.

Specific treatment. No specific treatment is indicated for a **normal sinus rhythm with a pulse. Cardiopulmonary resuscitation** and **immediate transport** are indicated if **electromechanical dissociation (EMD)** is present.

SHOCK IS NOT INDICATED!

Notes

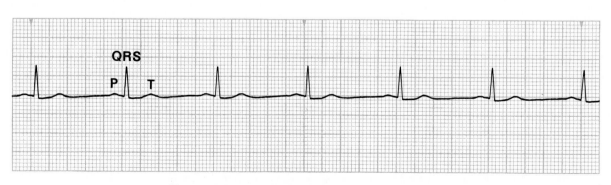

Figure 4-14.   Components of normal sinus rhythm.

Normal Sinus Rhythm (NSR)

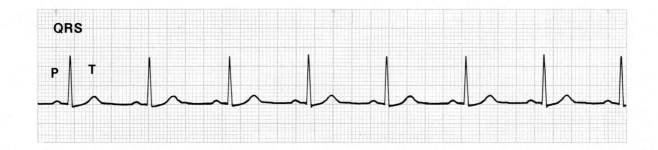

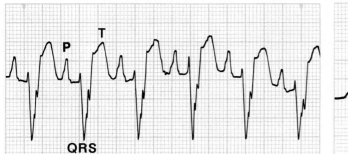

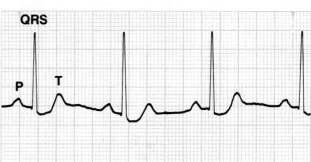

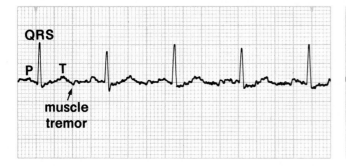

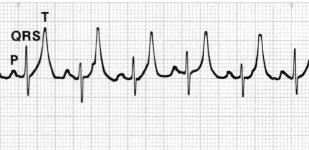

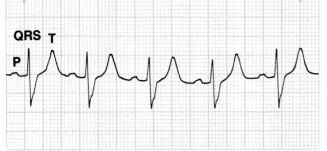

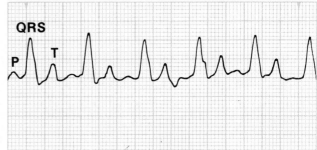

Ventricular Tachycardia (VT, V-TACH)

Heart rate. The heart rate according to the ECG is over 100 beats per minute, usually between 110 and 250 beats per minute. Ventricular tachycardia may occur in short bursts of three or more beats separated by the underlying ECG rhythm **(paroxysmal or nonsustained ventricular tachycardia)** or continuously for a period of time **(sustained ventricular tachycardia)** (Figure 4-15).

Rhythm. The rhythm is essentially regular.

Pacemaker site. The pacemaker site of ventricular tachycardia is an ectopic pacemaker in the ventricles.

P waves. P waves may be present or absent.

QRS complexes. The QRS complexes are always wide and usually distorted and bizarre.

Pulse. A pulse may be present or absent. When a pulse is absent, **electromechanical dissociation (EMD)** is present. In this instance, the electromechanical dissociation is specifically identified as **pulseless ventricular tachycardia** since this is the only form of electromechanical dissociation that is **shockable,** i.e., treated by defibrillatory shock.

Specific treatment. No specific treatment is indicated for **ventricular tachycardia with a pulse, whether it is shockable or nonshockable** as determined by the automated external defibrillator. A **pulseless ventricular tachycardia,** however, must be treated immediately; the treatment varies, depending on whether the ventricular tachycardia is **shockable** or **nonshockable** as determined by the automated external defibrillator.

Cardiopulmonary resuscitation and **immediate transport** are indicated if a **nonshockable pulseless ventricular tachycardia** is present. A **shockable pulseless ventricular tachycardia,** however, must be treated immediately by **defibrillatory shock** and, if shock is unsuccessful, by **cardiopulmonary resuscitation,** followed by **immediate transport.**

SHOCK IS INDICATED IMMEDIATELY FOR SHOCKABLE PULSELESS VENTRICULAR TACHYCARDIA!

Notes

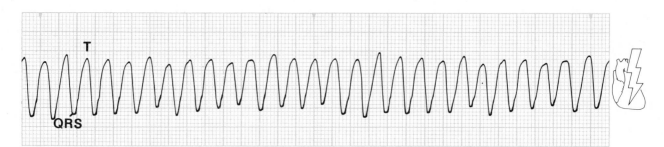

Figure 4-15.   Components of ventricular tachycardia (VT, V-TACH).

Ventricular Tachycardia (VT, V-TACH)

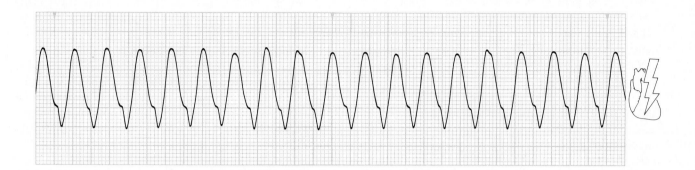

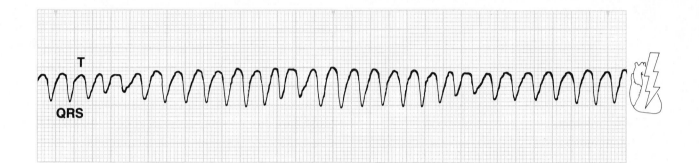

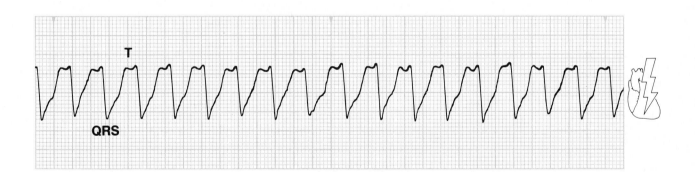

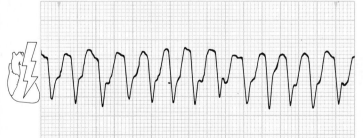

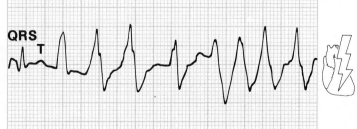

Ventricular Fibrillation (VF, V-FIB)

Heart rate. The heart rate according to the ECG is zero. The ventricles contract from about 300 to 500 times a minute in an unsynchronized, uncoordinated, and haphazard manner without producing a pulse. A fibrillating heart has been described as looking like a **"bag of worms"** or a **"quivering bowl of jelly"** (Figure 4-16).

Rhythm. The rhythm is grossly irregular.

Pacemaker site. The pacemaker sites of ventricular fibrillation are multiple ectopic pacemakers in the ventricles.

QRS complexes. QRS complexes are absent. Instead, numerous, markedly dissimilar, bizarre, jagged, or rounded or pointed **fibrillation waves** are present. They may be large (**"coarse"**) or small (**"fine"**), resembling an almost flat, wavy line which may be mistaken for ventricular asystole.

Pulse. A pulse is **always absent.**

Specific treatment. Ventricular fibrillation must be treated immediately by **defibrillatory shock** and, if shock is unsuccessful, by **cardiopulmonary resuscitation,** followed by **immediate transport.**

SHOCK IS INDICATED IMMEDIATELY!

Notes

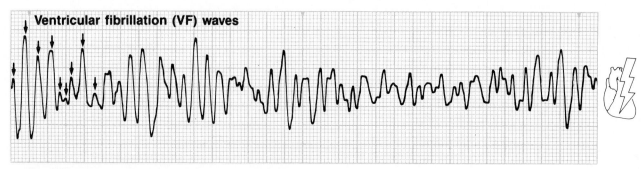

**No P waves, QRS complexes, or T waves
(Coarse VF)**

Figure 4-16.   Components of ventricular fibrillation (VF, V-FIB).

Ventricular Fibrillation (VF, V-FIB)

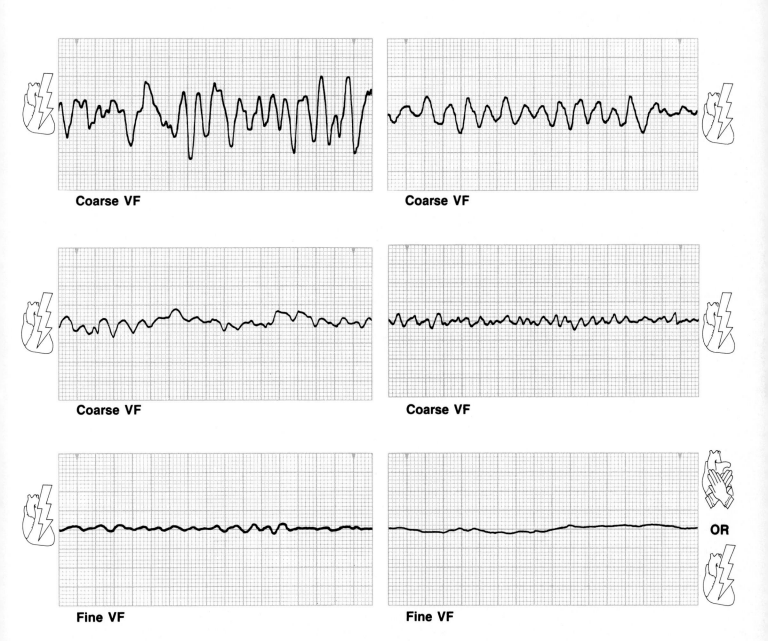

Coarse VF

Coarse VF

Coarse VF

Coarse VF

Fine VF

Fine VF

Ventricular Asystole (Cardiac Standstill)

Heart rate. The heart rate according to the ECG is zero (Figure 4-17).

Rhythm. Rhythm is absent.

Pacemaker site. The electrical conduction system of the heart is not functioning, and a pacemaker site in the ventricles is absent.

P waves. P waves may be present or absent.

QRS complexes. QRS complexes are absent. Instead, a flat, sometimes wavy, line is present.

Pulse. A pulse is **always absent.**

Specific treatment. Cardiopulmonary resuscitation and **immediate transport** are indicated if **ventricular asystole** is present.

SHOCK IS NOT INDICATED!

Notes

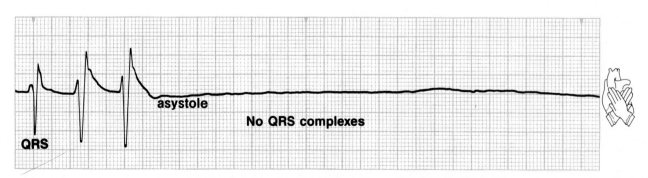

Figure 4-17.   Components of ventricular asystole.

Ventricular Asystole
(Cardiac Standstill)

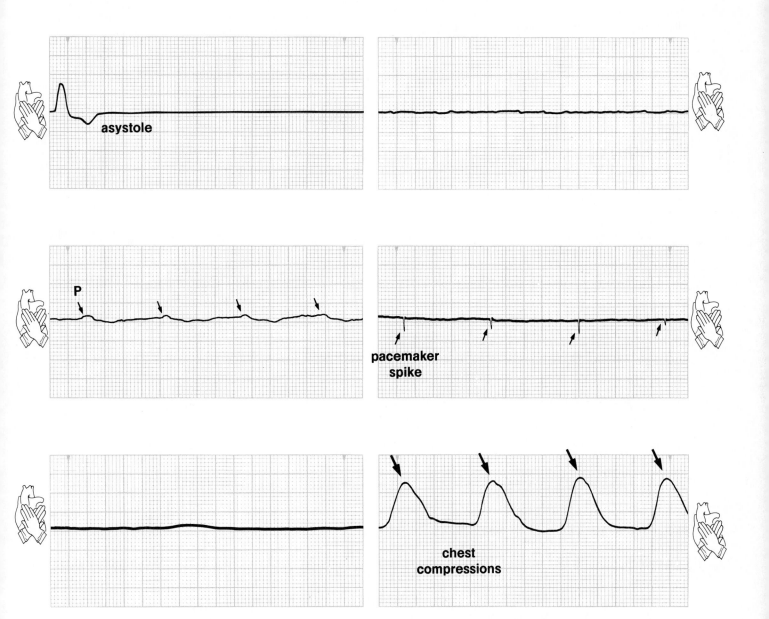

asystole

P

pacemaker
spike

chest
compressions

Electromechanical Dissociation (EMD)

Heart rate. The heart rate according to the ECG is usually 60 to 100 beats per minute, but it may be as low as 20 or as high as 160 or more beats per minute (Figure 4-18).

Rhythm. The rhythm may be regular or irregular.

Pacemaker site. The pacemaker site may be above the ventricles or in the ventricles.

P waves. P waves may be present or absent.

QRS complexes. QRS complexes are present. They may be narrow or wide, distorted, and bizarre.

Pulse. Although an ECG rhythm is present on the ECG, the pulse is **absent.**

Specific treatment. Cardiopulmonary resuscitation and **immediate transport** are indicated if **electromechanical dissociation (EMD)** is present.

SHOCK IS NOT INDICATED!

Notes

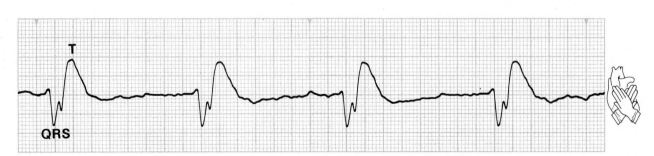

Figure 4-18.   Components of electromechanical dissociation (EMD).

Electromechanical Dissociation (EMD)

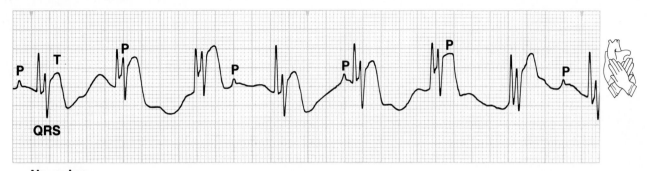

No pulse

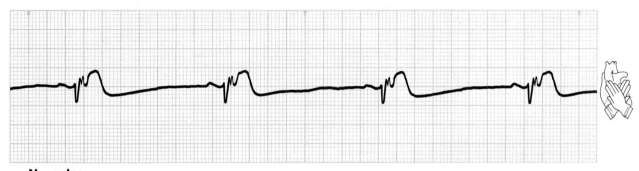

No pulse

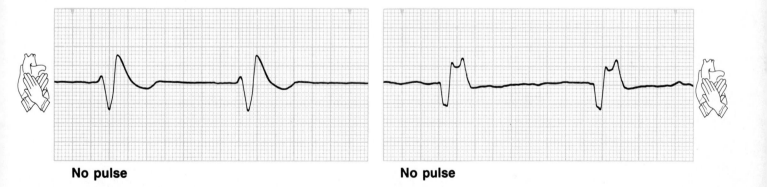

No pulse   **No pulse**

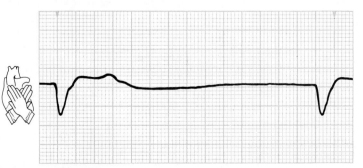   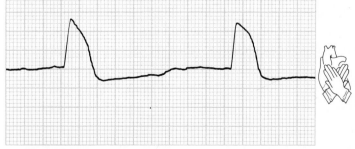

No pulse   **No pulse**

Chapter 5

Ventricular Fibrillation and Ventricular Tachycardia

OBJECTIVES

Upon completion of all or part of this chapter as required by your early defibrillation program, you should be able to complete the following objectives indicated by your instructor:

☐ Describe the heart in ventricular fibrillation.
☐ State the appropriate treatment of ventricular fibrillation and how it works.
☐ Describe the different types of ventricular tachycardia.
☐ State the treatment of:
  • Shockable pulseless ventricular tachycardia.
  • Nonshockable ventricular tachycardia with or without a pulse.
☐ List the nonshockable rhythms with a pulse and indicate their treatment.
☐ List the nonshockable rhythms without a pulse and indicate their treatment.
☐ List the shockable rhythms without a pulse and indicate their treatment.

Ventricular Fibrillation

Ventricular fibrillation is a life-threatening dysrhythmia in which the numerous individual muscle fibers of the ventricles contract independently in a spasmodic, uncoordinated manner rather than in a smoothly synchronized contractile fashion (Figure 5-1). This gives the nonbeating heart a bloated, quivering appearance, often graphically described as a **"bag of worms"** or a **"quivering bowl of jelly."** The ineffectual twitchings that result are incapable of circulating blood to sustain life or of producing a heartbeat, pulse, and blood pressure. Such a dysrhythmia is called **a nonperfusing rhythm.**

Although it does sustain life, **cardiopulmonary resuscitation (CPR)** by itself cannot convert ventricular fibrillation into a **perfusing rhythm,** an organized ECG rhythm with a pulse. A **defibrillatory shock (defibrillation)** is the only means by which ventricular fibrillation can be terminated (Figure 5-2).

Ventricular Tachycardia

Ventricular tachycardia is a life-threatening dysrhythmia in which the ventricles are contracting extremely rapidly, between 100 and 250 beats per minute. It results when an ectopic pacemaker in the ventricles overrides the underlying ECG rhythm. Ventricular tachycardia may occur in short bursts of three or more beats separated by the underlying ECG rhythm (**paroxysmal or nonsustained ventricular tachycardia**) or continuously for a period of time (**sustained ventricular tachycardia**) (Figure 5-3).

When the ventricular rate rises above 180 beats per minute, the cardiac output begins to fall because of the decrease in the filling time of the ventricles between contractions (**ventricular diastole).** This can be compared to trying to empty a container of water with a bulb syringe. The faster one tries to squeeze and empty the bulb, the less efficient it becomes.

With the decrease in the cardiac output, the pulse becomes weak and the blood pressure falls.

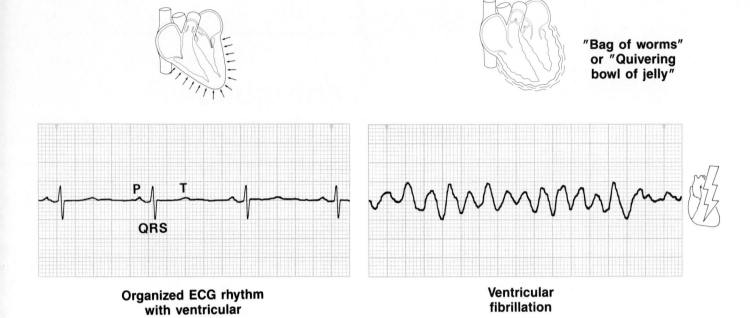

"Bag of worms"
or "Quivering
bowl of jelly"

Organized ECG rhythm
with ventricular
contraction

Ventricular
fibrillation

Figure 5-1.   Ventricular fibrillation.

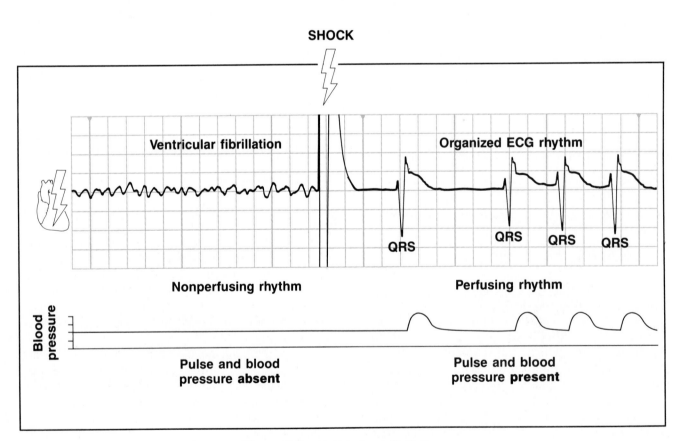

Figure 5-2.   Ventricular defibrillation.

**Paroxysmal
(nonsustained)
V-TACH**

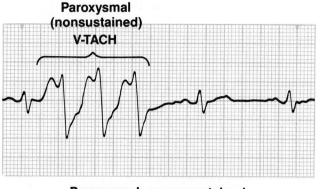

**Paroxysmal or nonsustained
ventricular tachycardia**

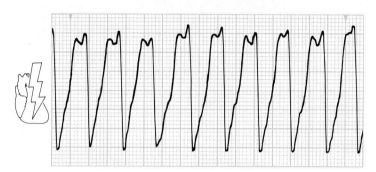

Sustained ventricular tachycardia

Figure 5-3. Types of ventricular tachycardia.

At the point the pulse and blood pressure disappear, **pulseless ventricular tachycardia** is present (Figure 5-4). Such a dysrhythmia is called a **nonperfusing rhythm.** Once ventricular tachycardia becomes pulseless, it rapidly degenerates into ventricular fibrillation if not converted into a perfusing rhythm by **defibrillation.**

Summary of the Management of Ventricular Fibrillation and Ventricular Tachycardia

Ventricular fibrillation and shockable pulseless ventricular tachycardia. Immediately upon determination by the automated external defibrillator in a patient who is in cardiac arrest that **ventricular fibrillation** or a **shockable ventricular tachycardia** is present (i.e., a **shockable pulseless rhythm**), a defibrillatory shock is delivered in an attempt to terminate the life-threatening dysrhythmia **(defibrillation).** If early defibrillation is provided by a single rescuer, the **EMT/FR-D,**

defibrillation takes precedence over cardiopulmonary resuscitation. If two rescuers, **one trained in CPR** and the other the **EMT/FR-D,** are providing early defibrillation, the **CPR-trained rescuer** performs cardiopulmonary resuscitation while the **EMT/FR-D** readies the automated external defibrillator and attaches the defibrillator electrodes prior to defibrillation. In any event, defibrillation and, if applicable, cardiopulmonary resuscitation must be provided as soon as possible after arrival of the rescuer(s) at the scene of a cardiac arrest.

The longer cardiac arrest is permitted to continue without defibrillation and, if applicable, CPR, the more difficult it is to defibrillate the heart because of the adverse effects of anoxia and acidosis on the automaticity, conductivity, and contractility of the heart.

In case of defibrillation-resistent ventricular fibrillation or pulseless ventricular tachycardia, certain drugs, such as **epinephrine, lidocaine,** and **bretylium tosylate,** may have to be administered by paramedics or emergency department personnel before defibrillation will be successful.

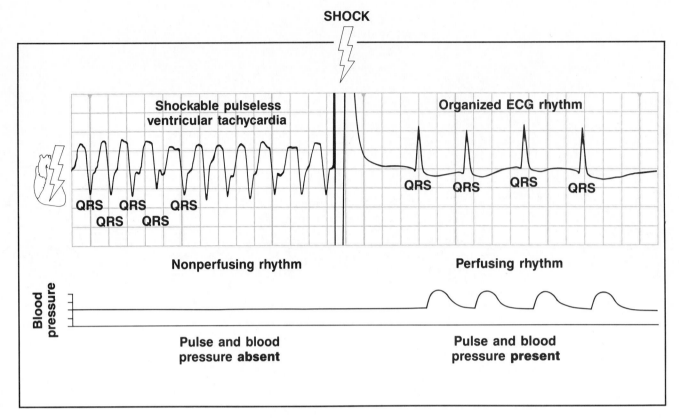

Figure 5-4. Defibrillation of shockable pulseless ventricular tachycardia.

The techniques of defibrillation using the automated external defibrillator are described in detail in **Chapter 8** and **Appendix A.**

Nonshockable pulseless ventricular tachycardia. If a patient is in cardiac arrest and a **nonshockable ventricular tachycardia** is present as determined by the automated external defibrillator, indicating a **nonshockable pulseless rhythm** CPR must be started immediately. The ECG is then analyzed periodically, while CPR is being performed, to detect the possible transformation of the **nonshockable ventricular tachycardia** into a **shockable rhythm,** i.e., **shockable ventricular tachycardia** or **ventricular fibrillation.** Should this occur, a **defibrillatory shock** is indicated immediately. A **nonshockable pulseless rhythm** also includes

electromechanical dissociation (EMD) and **ventricular asystole.**

Nonshockable or shockable ventricular tachycardia with a pulse. If a **nonshockable** or a **shockable ventricular tachycardia,** as determined by the automated external defibrillator, and a **pulse** is present (i.e., a **nonshockable rhythm with a pulse**), providing close observation, obtaining vital signs, and monitoring the ECG are required because of the threat of impending loss of the pulse or degeneration of the ventricular tachycardia into ventricular fibrillation. Should either one occur, a **defibrillatory shock** is indicated immediately. A **nonshockable rhythm with a pulse** also includes **all organized ECG rhythms,** including **normal sinus rhythm,** with a pulse (Figure 5-5).

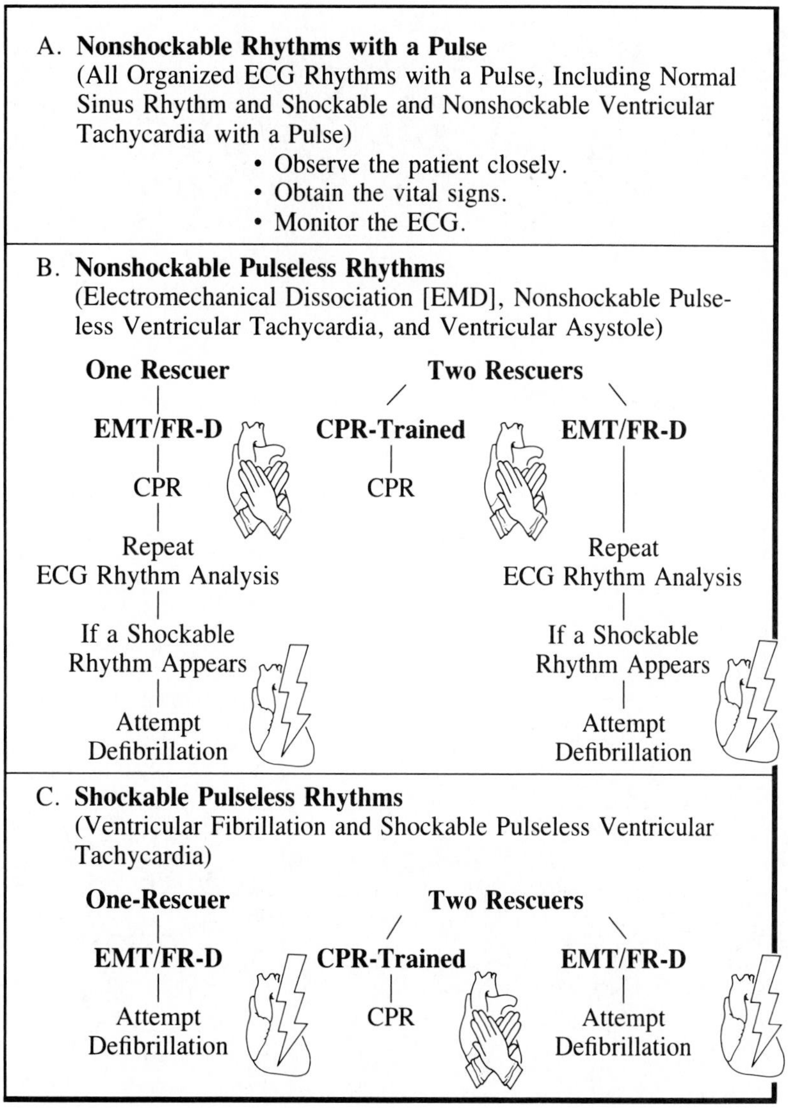

A. **Nonshockable Rhythms with a Pulse**
(All Organized ECG Rhythms with a Pulse, Including Normal Sinus Rhythm and Shockable and Nonshockable Ventricular Tachycardia with a Pulse)
- Observe the patient closely.
- Obtain the vital signs.
- Monitor the ECG.

B. **Nonshockable Pulseless Rhythms**
(Electromechanical Dissociation [EMD], Nonshockable Pulseless Ventricular Tachycardia, and Ventricular Asystole)

One Rescuer

EMT/FR-D

CPR

Repeat
ECG Rhythm Analysis

If a Shockable
Rhythm Appears

Attempt
Defibrillation

Two Rescuers

CPR-Trained   EMT/FR-D

CPR

Repeat
ECG Rhythm Analysis

If a Shockable
Rhythm Appears

Attempt
Defibrillation

C. **Shockable Pulseless Rhythms**
(Ventricular Fibrillation and Shockable Pulseless Ventricular Tachycardia)

One-Rescuer

EMT/FR-D

Attempt
Defibrillation

Two Rescuers

CPR-Trained   EMT/FR-D

CPR

Attempt
Defibrillation

Figure 5-5. Management of shockable and nonshockable rhythms.

Chapter 6

Defibrillatory Shock

OBJECTIVES

Upon completion of all or part of this chapter as required by your early defibrillation program, you should be able to complete the following objectives indicated by your instructor:

☐ Describe how a defibrillatory shock converts ventricular fibrillation into a perfusing rhythm.
☐ List and describe the seven basic components of a portable defibrillator.
☐ Define joules (watt seconds) and joules of delivered energy.
☐ List seven major causes of ineffective defibrillation.
☐ Describe the following hazards and side effects to the patient:
  • Arcing and its prevention
  • Chest burns
  • Myocardial damage
☐ Describe the following hazards to the rescuer or bystander and their prevention:
  • Accidental shocking
  • Accidental exposure to nitroglycerin ointment
☐ Describe the precautions in using the automated external defibrillator in the following conditions and circumstances:
  • Permanent implanted artificial pacemaker
  • Automatic implantable cardiovascular defibrillator (AICD)
  • Presence of other chest electrodes
  • Vibration/motion
  • Hypothermia
  • Traumatic or hypovolemic cardiac arrest
  • Restricted environments such as helicopters

Development of Defibrillatory Shock

Experimentation in the late 1920s showed that a high-energy **alternating-current (AC) shock** delivered across a patient's chest to the heart was effective in terminating ventricular fibrillation **(defibrillation).** It was found that the AC shock caused all of the muscle fibers of the ventricles to contract simultaneously, putting a stop to their fibrillating. After a brief period of inactivity, the SA node or some other pacemaker of the heart took over, resulting in an organized ECG rhythm. If the myocardium was still able to function, the ventricles responded to the organized electrical impulses and began to contract rhythmically, producing a pulse. Thus, it was shown that **defibrillation** could convert ventricular fibrillation into a **perfusing rhythm.** Later, in the 1960s, **direct-current (DC) shock** replaced alternating current for defibrillation, since it was found to be more effective and less traumatic to the patient.

Subsequently, direct-current (DC) defibrillatory shock was found useful in terminating certain dysrhythmias other than ventricular fibrillation in the hospital and prehospital setting, including ventricular tachycardia, with and without a pulse. In the prehospital setting, as far as the early defibrillation programs are concerned, only certain dysrhythmias without a pulse are considered for defibrillation, i.e., **ventricular fibrillation** and **pulseless ventricular tachycardia.**

Prehospital Ventricular Defibrillation

In the late 1960s, portable manual defibrillators and ECG monitoring equipment made it possible for highly trained advanced emergency medical technicians (AEMTs) to terminate ventricular fibrillation in the prehospital setting. Because of this, the number of prehospital deaths from ventricular fibrillation has been substantially reduced. Later, in the 1970s, automated external defibrillators were developed with the capability of electronically determining whether or not a shock should be delivered. This permitted rescuers, such as Emergency Medical Technicians (EMTs) and First Responders (FRs) without advanced life support training, but with specialized training in operating automated external defibrillators, to manage cardiac arrest in the field as effectively as with manual defibrillators.

Portable Defibrillator

The portable manual or automated external defibrillator is a device consisting of the following basic components:
- A heavy-duty rechargeable battery.
- A capacitor for storage of electrical energy.
- A capacitor charging circuit which charges the capacitors to a preset energy level just before the capacitor is discharged to delivery the stored energy. It usually takes 8 to 10 seconds to charge the capacitor with a fully-charged battery, depending on the energy level to which the capacitor is to be charged.
- A variable discharge control calibrated in units of electrical energy called joules (or watt-seconds) (manual defibrillator) or a preset discharge control (automated external defibrillator).

- Two defibrillator paddles with large metal electrode plates, handles, and manually controlled discharge buttons (manual defibrillator) or two defibrillator electrodes (automated external defibrillator). Usually, one defibrillator paddle or electrode is identified as positive, the other as negative.
- Two defibrillator paddle or electrode cables.
- An oscilloscope or similar device, such as a liquid crystal display (LCD), for ECG monitoring (Figure 6-1).

When the **charge circuit** is turned on, the battery charges the capacitor to the energy level selected by the joules or watt-seconds control. **Joules** are the units of measurement used to designate the amount of electrical energy stored in the capacitor. The stored energy is generally greater than the energy delivered to the patient's chest across the defibrillator paddles or electrodes because of a loss of energy through the paddles or electrodes, connecting cables, and connectors and across the chest wall due to electrical resistance. After the capacitor is discharged, delivering the direct-current (DC) shock, the defibrillator's capacitor requires recharging before the next discharge (Figure 6-2).

The energy delivered in defibrillatory shock is indicated as **joules of delivered energy.** The energy delivered is approximately 80% of the energy actually stored in the defibrillator's capacitor.

Manual defibrillator

Automated external defibrillator (AED)

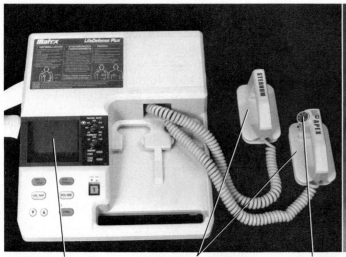
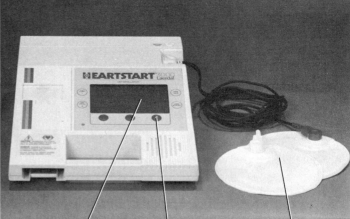

Oscilloscope or liquid crystal diode (LCD) Defibrillator paddles with metal electrode plates, handles, manually controlled discharge buttons, and cables Variable discharge control

Liquid crystal diode (LCD) Preset discharge control Disposable defibrillator electrodes with cables

Figure 6-1. Portable manual and automated external defibrillators. Common components are rechargeable battery, capacitor, and capacitor charging circuit.

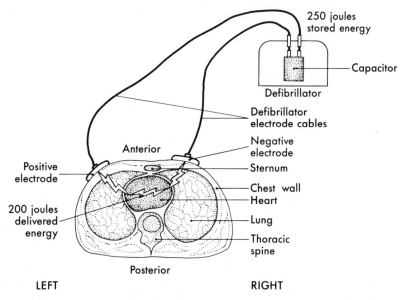

Figure 6-2. The path of the defibrillatory shock from the defibrillator to the heart.

Causes of Ineffective Defibrillation

Defibrillation is not always effective in terminating ventricular fibrillation or pulseless ventricular tachycardia. Some of the major causes of ineffective defibrillation are:

Poor patient condition
- Enlarged heart
- Hypovolemia (low blood volume), usually from trauma
- Massive myocardial infarction
- Myocardial rupture and cardiac tamponade
- Severe pulmonary or respiratory disease
- Trauma

Prolonged cardiac arrest
Delay in initiating CPR and defibrillation
Inadequate CPR
- Hypoxia
- Acidosis
- Hypercarbia (excessive blood carbon dioxide)

Inadequate electrical current delivered to the heart
- Barrel-shape of the patient's chest
- Defective equipment (defibrillator, cables, or defibrillator electrodes)
- Electrically conductive material between the defibrillator electrodes, i.e., nitroglycerin ointment, salt water; or excessive sweat
- Improper placement of the defibrillator electrodes

- Placement of defibrillator electrodes too close to a permanent implanted artificial pacemaker
- Inadequate contact between the patient's chest and the defibrillator electrodes.

Operator inexperience or error
Drug toxicity

Hazards and Side Effects to the Patient

Arcing

Arcing is the leaping of the current from one defibrillator electrode to another when the automated external defibrillator is discharged, shortcircuiting the current of the shock away from the heart. This can occur in the following situations:
- If electrically conductive material such as nitroglycerin ointment, salt water, or excessive sweat are present on the chest wall between the two defibrillator electrodes
- If the metal conductive plates of the defibrillator electrodes are too close together (i.e., less than 5 inches apart)
- If the edges of the defibrillator electrodes are not securely attached to the chest wall

A drop in the DC current delivered across the chest to the heart because of arcing may make effective defibrillation unlikely. Arcing may also cause skin burns.

To prevent arcing, the following precautions should be taken:

- Wipe all conductive material such as nitroglycerin ointment, salt water, and excessive sweat off the chest and remove any nitroglycerin patches before applying the defibrillator electrodes. If the chest is excessively wet, apply an anti-perspirant such as Arrid Extra Dry and then wipe it off after it has dried, before attaching the electrodes.
- Ensure that the edges of the metal conductive plates of the two defibrillator electrodes are at least 5 inches apart and at least the same distance from a permanent implanted artificial pacemaker.
- Attach the edges of the defibrillator electrode pads securely to the chest wall, shaving any coarse hair on the chest wall under the electrode pads if necessary.

Chest Burns

Chest burns can result from any of the following:

- Multiple shocks, especially if there has been poor contact between the defibrillator electrodes and the skin
- Chest deformities, excessive hair, or other matter between the skin and the electrodes or poor technique in applying the defibrillator electrodes, causing poor contact between the skin and the electrodes
- Discharge of the shocks through a defibrillator electrode applied over a medical device such as a nitroglycerin patch which may result in the electrical current being primarily conducted through the device, concentrating the current delivered to a small area and resulting in chest burns
- Arcing

Myocardial Damage

Although a defibrillatory shock can revive a dying heart, it can also cause myocardial damage. The extent of the damage depends on the cumulative amount of energy delivered to the myocardium from repeated shocks. Such myocardial damage may result in pump failure and dysrhythmias, i.e., premature ventricular contractions, various tachycardias, and even ventricular fibrillation. Pump failure can result in left heart failure with pulmonary congestion and edema, hypotension, or shock.

Hazards to the Rescuer or Bystander

Accidental Shocking of Rescuers or Bystanders

Rescuers and bystanders may receive an electric shock while the patient is being defibrillated if they are touching any part of the patient's body or any metal object, such as a metal stretcher or bed frame, in contact with the patient. This may also occur if the patient is lying directly on the same conductive surface on which the rescuers and bystanders are kneeling or standing. This may be a puddle, a stretch of ocean water or damp sand, or a wet wooden structure, such as a damp porch, a dock, or the deck of a ship or boat.

To prevent accidental shocking of the rescuers and bystanders during defibrillation **always ensure** the following precautions:

- That there is no contact between the rescuers and bystanders and any part of the patient's body or any metal object, such as a metal stretcher or bed frame, in contact with the patient.
- That there is no conductive substance between the patient and the rescuers and bystanders, i.e., ocean water, damp sand, or wet wooden boards. To remedy this, put the patient on a wooden backboard with wooden runners to insulate the patient from the environment. If necessary, a second wooden backboard may have to be used for full protection of the rescuers and bystanders. It would be best, however, to avoid a wet environment, if possible, during the defibrillation of the patient.

Accidental Exposure to Nitroglycerin Ointment

Often, patients with angina pectoris are administered nitroglycerin for the treatment and prevention of angina pectoris. Nitroglycerin can be administered orally or as an ointment applied to the chest or extremities over an area from about 1 × 3 inches to over 4 × 5 inches. Sufficient absorption of nitroglycerin occurs through the skin (1) to cause vasodilation of the blood vessels of the body, especially the veins and consequent decrease in the venous return of blood to the heart and lowering of the blood pressure, thereby reducing the workload of the heart, and (2) to dilate the coronary blood vessels. Clinical studies have shown that it takes about 30 minutes before any detectable plasma levels of nitroglycerin appear after the application of nitroglycerin ointment to the skin. Because of this, there is little chance that a rescuer accidentally coming in contact with nitroglycerin ointment will develop any significant reactions from nitroglycerin, such as headache, hypotension, increased heart rate, and faintness, if the nitroglycerin ointment is removed from the rescuer's skin as soon as possible by wiping or washing.

Precautions and Special Advice

Permanent Implanted Artificial Pacemaker

The defibrillator electrodes should not be attached to the patient over or too close to a implanted artificial pacemaker. If placement is too close to certain pacemakers, the energy delivered by the automated external defibrillator may concentrate or localize at one or more sites in the myocardium where the pacemaker electrodes are positioned, resulting in myocardial burns or local electrical injury. The presence of an implanted pacemaker is suspected if there is a history of pacemaker implantation or if a bulge of about 2 inches in diameter is present beneath the skin, overlaid by a scar, in the right (or less frequently the left) upper anterior chest wall just below the clavicle.

To prevent any interaction with an implanted pacemaker, ensure that the negative defibrillator electrode is positioned so that the edge of its metal conductive plate is at least 5 inches from the implanted pacemaker. An acceptable alternate placement is in the right anterior axillary line just below the axilla (Figure 6-3).

NOTE: The small electrical impulses (**pacemaker spikes**) generated by the artificial pacemaker, which usually continue to be generated in the presence of ventricular fibrillation, may be misinterpreted by the automated external defibrillator as organized electrical activity of the heart. This would inhibit the automated external defibrillator from delivering a shock while informing the rescuer that a shock is not indicated, even when one should be delivered.

Automatic Implantable Cardiovascular Defibrillator (AICD)

Rarely, the patient managed by the EMT/FR-D will have an implanted **automatic implantable cardiovascular defibrillator (AICD).** The presence of an AICD is suspected if there is a history of an AICD implantation or if a bulge of about 3 × 4.5 inches is present beneath the skin, overlaid by a scar, left of the midline near the umbilicus. A Medic Alert tag worn by the patient may indicate the presence of this device.

The AICD is protected from external shocks. The AICD may discharge and deliver an internal shock while the EMT/FR-D is preparing to deliver

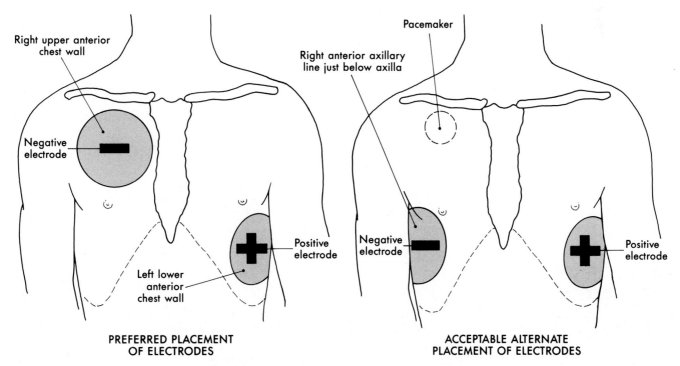

Figure 6-3. Placement of defibrillator electrodes.

an external shock. The maximum level of energy delivered to the patient's ventricles by the AICD is 30 joules. This may be felt on the skin surface by the rescuer as a 2-joules tingling sensation. Such a shock, however, will not harm the rescuer.

Presence of Other Chest Electrodes

The defibrillator electrodes should not be placed in contact with other electrodes attached to the patient because of the possibility of damaging the equipment to which the electrodes are attached or inadvertently conducting the shock to anyone touching this equipment.

Vibration/Motion

Shaking or movement of the defibrillator electrode cables or the patient may produce artifacts on the ECG which may be interpreted by the ECG analysis circuit of the automated external defibrillator as follows:

- With an organized ECG present, such artifacts may be interpreted by the ECG analysis circuit as ventricular fibrillation or ventricular tachycardia, prompting the automated external defibrillator to prepare for defibrillation. This is considered to be a **false-negative** interpretation.
- With ventricular fibrillation present, the artifacts caused by vibration or motion may be interpreted by the automated external defibrillator as an organized ECG rhythm, causing the defibrillator to abandon preparation for defibrillation and instruct the rescuer that "No Shock" is indicated. Such a determination is **false-positive.**

For these reasons the ECG should not be analyzed by the ECG analysis circuit in moving vehicles or environments with high vibration, e.g., factories, moving elevators. Certain automated external defibrillator models, however, have motion detector circuits which, when artifacts on the ECG caused by motion or vibration are detected, stop the analysis of the patient's ECG and warn the rescuer "Check Electrodes" or "Do not Touch Patient"—"Motion Detected." In general, the patient's ECG can be monitored, but not analyzed,

while the ambulance is in motion. If the ECG needs to be analyzed, it should be done after the ambulance has been pulled over to the curb and temporarily stopped.

Another reason for not analyzing the ECG while the ambulance is in motion is that, should the automated external defibrillator detect a shockable rhythm and instruct the rescuer to deliver a shock, the ambulance may encounter a rough, bumpy road, throwing the rescuers onto the patient at the moment the shock is being delivered and exposing them to a potentially life-threatening electric shock.

Hypothermia

Ventricular fibrillation and cardiac arrest is a recognized complication in hypothermic patients. Defibrillation may be futile, however, if the patient's core temperature is less than 87° F (31° C).

Traumatic or Hypovolemic Cardiac Arrest

Since the treatment in traumatic and hypovolemic cardiac arrest is blood volume replacement and surgery, the management of choice is basic life support, initial resuscitation at the scene, and immediate transport to the appropriate trauma center. However, if the driver involved in a motor vehicle accident is in cardiac arrest and is suspected of having had an acute myocardial infarction while driving, the use of the automated external defibrillator is indicated.

Patient Weight

The American Heart Association recommends that the automated external defibrillator only be used to deliver shock to patients in cardiac arrest who weigh more than 90 lb. This is based on the following: (1) that the maximum recommended level of energy of a defibrillatory shock should not exceed 4 J/kg of body weight in children and (2) that the lowest energy level which can be delivered by AED is 200 J.

Restricted Environments

Defibrillation is prohibited in helicopters by the Federal Aviation Agency (FAA).

Chapter 7

The Automated External Defibrillator

OBJECTIVES

Upon completion of all or part of this chapter as required by your early defibrillation program, you should be able to complete the following objectives indicated by your instructor:

☐ Define automated external defibrillator.

☐ Describe the difference between a semi-automatic external defibrillator and a fully automatic defibrillator.

☐ Name four life-threatening dysrhythmias and indicate which ones are treatable by defibrillatory shock.

☐ List eight common components of automated external defibrillators and briefly describe each.

☐ List nine optional features available in certain models of automated external defibrillators and briefly describe each.

☐ List six basic procedures common to all automated external defibrillators and one optional basic procedure, and briefly describe each.

☐ List the features of the automated external defibrillator used in your early defibrillation program.

☐ Outline the basic procedures in treating a persistent shockable rhythm using the automated external defibrillator designated for your early defibrillation program.

☐ Outline the generic protocols for the treatment of the following:

  • A persistent shockable rhythm (ventricular fibrillation or a pulseless ventricular tachycardia)

  • A nonshockable rhythm (ventricular asystole or electromechanical dissociation [EMD])

  • A shockable rhythm (ventricular fibrillation or a pulseless ventricular tachycardia) converting into a perfusing rhythm

The Automated External Defibrillator

The **automated external defibrillator** (AED) is an electrical device capable of delivering **direct-current (DC) shock** to a patient in cardiac arrest for the purpose of terminating ventricular fibrillation and pulseless ventricular tachycardia. The defibrillator may be completely **automatic,** delivering a shock without intervention by the rescuer once the defibrillator has been turned on and the patient's electrocardiogram (ECG) analyzed. If the defibrillator is semi-automatic, the delivery of the shock must be initiated manually by the rescuer on the advice of the defibrillator after it has analyzed the patient's ECG.

Components of an Automated External Defibrillator

Several **semi-automatic external defibrillator (SAED)** and **fully automatic external defibrillator** models are available from several manufacturers (Figure 7-1). The components common to all models include:

  • A **microprocessor** integrated circuit, programmed to analyze the patient's ECG, usually in the setting of a cardiac arrest. This **ECG analysis circuit** first determines if QRS complexes are present and, if they are, their width and rate of occurrence. In some models the ECG analysis circuit also determines if P waves are present. If QRS complexes are absent, the ECG analysis circuit determines if ventricular fibrillation waves are present. By this analysis the AED can, with a high degree of accuracy, determine if a **shockable ventricular tachycardia (i.e., ventricular tachycardia with a rate of 120 to 200 beats per minute or greater)** or **ventricular fibril-**

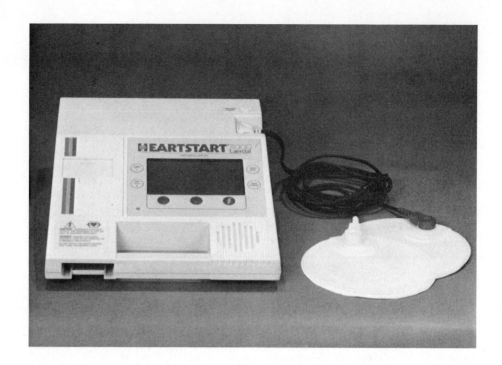

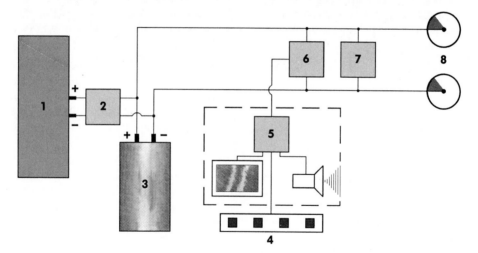

1. Battery

2. Capacitor charging circuit

3. Capacitor

4. Control panel

5. Audible and visual command circuit

6. Microprocessor ECG rhythm analyzing circuit

7. Impedance measuring circuit

8. Defibrillaor electrodes or pads

Figure 7-1.   Common components of AEDs.

lation is present. The rate used by the ECG analysis circuit in determining whether or not a ventricular tachycardia is shockable varies depending on the model of AED.* (See **Chapter 4** for a discussion of shockable and nonshockable ventricular tachycardia.) All other ECG rhythms and dysrhythmias, including **organized ECG rhythms** (e.g., **normal sinus rhythm**), **electromechanical dissociation (EMD), ventricular tachycardia with a rate of less than 120 to 200 beats per minute (nonshockable ventricular tachycardia),** and **ventricular asystole,** are considered to be **nonshockable** by the ECG analysis circuit (Table 7-1).

- An **audible and visual command circuit** to guide the rescuer in making a decision to deliver or not to deliver a shock in the setting of an absent pulse. This feature is found only in semi-automatic external defibrillators (SAEDs). Upon sensing the presence of ventricular fibrillation or a shockable ventricular tachycardia, the SAED instructs the rescuer to deliver a shock. When any other ECG rhythm or dysrhythmia is present, e.g., an organized ECG rhythm, ventricular asystole, or ventricular tachycardia with a rate of less than 120 to 200 beats per minute, the SAED instructs the rescuer not to deliver a shock. It is very important to understand that the decision to shock or not to shock made by the SAED is based on the analysis of the patient's ECG signal without regard to the presence or absence of the patient's pulse. **THE PATIENT'S PULSE MUST ALWAYS BE EVALUATED BEFORE THE INITIAL DECISION IS MADE BY THE RESCUER TO SHOCK OR NOT TO SHOCK AND PERIODICALLY THEREAFTER ACCORDING TO LOCAL PROTOCOL!**
- A **control panel,** usually a **liquid crystal display (LCD),** with low-power requirements, often backlit to enable viewing in low ambient light. The panel displays visual instructions to the rescuer, such as, **"NO SHOCK," "SHOCK," "ALERT," "STAND BACK,"** and so forth, depending on the model (Figure 7-2).
- A pair of disposable **defibrillator electrodes (or pads),** with easily removable backing.

Table 7-1 ECG rhythms and dysrhythmias considered to be shockable or nonshockable by the automated external defibrillator

Shockable	Nonshockable
Shockable ventricular tachycardia Ventricular fibrillation	All organized ECG rhythms (including normal sinus rhythm) Electromechanical dissociation (EMD) Nonshockable ventricular tachycardia Ventricular asystole

These may be pre-gelled or coated with an electrically conductive adhesive. The defibrillator electrodes, once applied to the patient's chest and the AED turned on, are used to sense the patient's ECG for analysis, to measure the impedance (or resistance) across the patient's chest, and to deliver the shocks. When properly attached (the negative defibrillator electrode attached to the upper right anterior chest, the positive electrode to the left lower anterior chest) an ECG lead commonly used for monitoring, **Lead II,** is displayed (Figure 7-3).

- An **impedance measuring circuit** to measure the **impedance** (or **resistance**) across the patient's chest wall between the two defibrillator electrodes after the electrodes have been applied. Before the AED will deliver a shock, a certain amount of impedance must be sensed between the defibrillator electrodes, indicating proper attachment of the electrodes to the chest wall. The impedance considered acceptable ranges from 30 to 200 ohms, depending on the AED model. Normally, the impedance across the chest wall is about 40 to 60 ohms, average 50 ohms.

If the impedance is below or above the specified range of 30 to 200 ohms, the rescuer is alerted to this fact, usually by an audible message, **"Check electrodes,"** indicating that the defibrillator electrodes are not properly applied. This may occur (1) if there is a bridge (or short circuit) between the electrodes, causing a very low impedance to be measured or none at all; (2) if the defibrillator electrodes are making poor electrical contact with the chest wall, causing a high impedance to be measured; or (3) if the electrodes are not making contact with the skin at all, a condition in which the impedance is said to be "infinite."

---

*The criteria used by at least one AED's ECG analysis circuit in determining the presence of a shockable ventricular tachycardia include (1) the presence of abnormally wide QRS complexes (0.16 second or greater) occurring at a rate of 120 to 140 per minute or greater and (2) the absence of P waves.

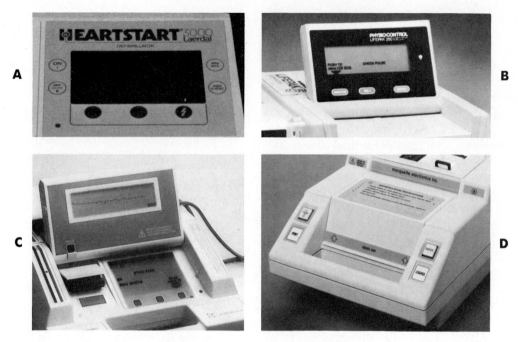

Figure 7-2.   Typical control panels.

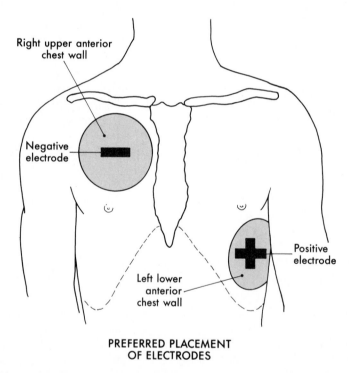

Right upper anterior chest wall

Negative electrode

Left lower anterior chest wall

Positive electrode

PREFERRED PLACEMENT OF ELECTRODES

Figure 7-3.   Defibrillator electrodes (pads) and their placement on the patient's chest.

- A heavy-duty, rechargeable long-life **battery.** Typically, a new, fully charged battery is capable of delivering about 50 shocks at maximum power, monitoring the ECG for 3.5 hours, or a combination of both: for example, 20 200-joule shocks and 10 360-joule shocks plus 2 hours of ECG monitoring. The capacity of a battery to provide full capability is significantly reduced in a cold environment.
- A **capacitor** for storage of electrical energy. It is charged to a preset energy level by the battery when the **charger circuit** is turned on **au-**

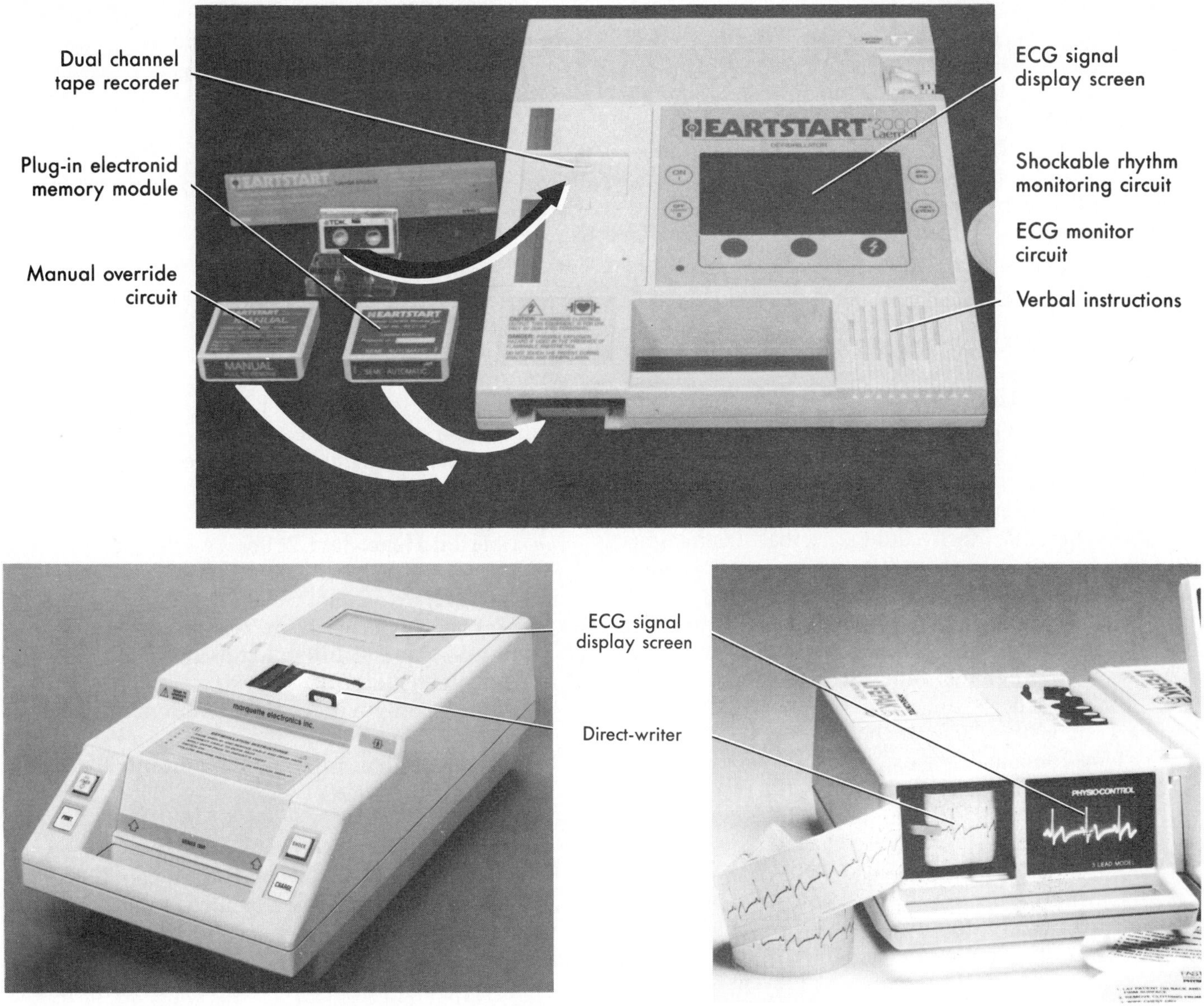

Dual channel
tape recorder

Plug-in electronid
memory module

Manual override
circuit

ECG signal
display screen

Shockable rhythm
monitoring circuit

ECG monitor
circuit

Verbal instructions

ECG signal
display screen

Direct-writer

Figure 7-4. Optional components of AEDs.

tomatically or **manually** by activation of a **"CHARGE" switch** and discharged automatically or upon manual activation of the **"SHOCK" switch,** depending on the AED model. The electrical energy stored in the capacitor is measured in units of electrical measure called **joules.** The energy levels to which the capacitor is charged is usually preset to deliver **200 joules** across the defibrillator electrodes for the **first shock, 200 or 300 joules** for the **second shock,** and **360 joules** for the **third shock.** Usually, if the charged capacitor is not discharged within 15 to 60 seconds or if the shockable rhythm analysis circuit does not sense a shockable rhythm while the capacitor is charging, causing **"NO SHOCK"** to be ad-

vised, the capacitor is automatically discharged (**"dumped"**) internally. **Because the shock is always "dumped" if it is not delivered within a certain period of time, the capacitor must be recharged each time the AED detects a shockable rhythm and advises "SHOCK."**

• A **capacitor charging circuit** which usually takes about 8 seconds to charge the capacitor to 200 or 300 joules and about 10 seconds to charge to 360 joules with a fully charged battery. The time to charge the capacitor to 360 joules increases to about 16 seconds after about 15 maximum energy discharges.

Optional features, available in certain models (Figure 7-4), include:

- An **ECG signal display screen,** usually a **liquid crystal display (LCD),** with low-power requirements, often backlit to enable viewing the ECG display in low ambient light. A **display freeze feature** which locks on a segment of the ECG being displayed to permit a more careful visual analysis of the ECG is an option in some models. In one model, the ECG signal display screen also displays the visual instructions.
- An **energy level switch** which permits the operator to switch the current energy level between 200 and 360 joules while the AED is charging.
- A **shockable rhythm monitoring circuit** which monitors the patient's ECG continuously for a shockable rhythm while the AED is turned on. If a shockable rhythm occurs (i.e., ventricular fibrillation or a shockable ventricular tachycardia), verbal instructions are issued in about 7 to 20 seconds, warning the rescuer to **"Check patient!"**
- **Verbal instructions** in addition to the visually displayed instructions on the control panel.
- A **dual channel tape recorder** which records the rescuer's voice and the patient's ECG continuously whenever the AED is turned on or on command.
- A **direct-writer** that permits the recording of the patient's ECG, a log of all the events, and the time they occurred on ECG paper, while the AED is in operation.
- A reusable **plug-in electronic memory module** which stores such data as the patient's ECG rhythm before and after each ECG analysis and shock, the time each event occurred, the messages and instructions generated by the AED, the date, and the serial number of the AED. The stored data is used to create a complete report of the EMT/FR-D intervention, including the patient's ECGs, results of the ECG analyses, recommended actions, actions taken, and the time each event occurred.
- An **ECG monitoring circuit** which permits the monitoring of the ECG, using regular disposable ECG electrodes. The ECG electrodes may be attached to the defibrillator electrode leads or to separate ECG monitoring leads, depending on the AED model. The defibrillator circuit is disabled when the AED is used primarily for ECG monitoring. If a shockable rhythm is detected while the patient's ECG is being monitored, the rescuer is alerted to the situation and instructed to apply the defibrillator electrodes.
- A **manual override circuit** to permit manual instead of automated defibrillation by more highly trained prehospital emergency care personnel.

Basic Procedures Common to Automated External Defibrillators

The basic procedures common to the **automated external defibrillators,** including the **semi-automatic external defibrillators (SAEDs)** and **fully automatic external defibrillators,** available at the time of publication of this manual and the generic alogrithms and protocols for using them in early defibrillation are presented in this section (Table 7-2). The SAEDs included in this review are:
- **First Medic 510**
- **First Medic 610**
- **Laerdal Heartstart 2000**
- **Laerdal Heartstart 1000/Rapid Zap 1000s**
- **Laerdal Heartstart 3000**
- **Marquette Series 1200 Responder**
- **Physio-Control Lifepak 200 automatic advisory defibrillator**
- **Physio-Control Lifepak 250 automatic advisory defibrillator**
- **Physio-Control Lifepak 300 automatic advisory defibrillator**

The fully automatic external defibrillators (Table 7-3) included in the review are:
- **Laerdal Heartstart 1000/Rapid Zap 1000**

The **basic procedures** common to the automated external defibrillators (Figure 7-5) **once cardiac arrest is verified** are:
- **Preparing and attaching the defibrillator electrodes**
- **Turning on the AED**
- **Analyzing the ECG rhythm**
- **Charging the defibrillator**
- **Delivering the shock**
- **Recording patient information and the patient's electrocardiogram (ECG) (optional)**

Preparing and attaching the defibrillator electrodes. The defibrillator electrodes used by all the AED models are similar—a conductive plate covered on one side by a conductive gel or adhesive, the other side attached to a nonconductive base. The area of the base surrounding the conductive plate is covered by an adhesive which makes the attachment of the defibrillator electrodes to the chest simple and reliable. The entire surface of the electrode is protected by a removable disposable backing.

Table 7-2 Features of semi-automatic external defibrillators (SAEDs)

Feature	Semi-automatic external defibrillator (SAED)							
	First Medic 610	First Medic 510	Heartstart 2000	Heartstart 3000 Lifepak 300*	Heartstart 1000s Rapid Zap 1000s	Lifepak 250*	Lifepak 200*	Responder 1200
ON/OFF switching	ON/OFF power switch	ON/OFF power switch	Swing-up cover	ON/OFF power switch	ON/OFF power switch	Swing-up cover	Swing-up cover	ON/OFF power switch
ECG signal display	Standard	None	Optional	Standard	None	Standard	None	Standard
Message display panel	Standard	Standard	Standard	Standard	Standard	Standard	Standard	Standard
Audio/visual messages	Beeps, visual messages, voice messages	Beeps, visual messages, voice messages	Beeps, visual messages, voice messages	Beeps, visual messages, voice messages	Beeps, visual messages, voice messages	Beeps, visual messages	Beeps, visual messages	Beeps, visual messages
ECG rhythm analysis	Manually, by pressing the "ANALYZE" button	Manually, by pressing the "ANALYZE" button	Manually, by pressing the "ANALYZE" button	Manually, by pressing the "ANALYZE" button	Continuous while "ON"	Manually, by pressing the "ANALYZE" switch	Manually, by pressing the "ANALYZE" switch	Continuous while "ON"
Continuous shockable rhythm monitoring	Standard	Standard	Standard	Standard	Standard	None	None	None
Charging of defibrillator	Automatic, following ECG rhythm analysis	Automatic, following ECG rhythm analysis	Automatic, following ECG rhythm analysis	Automatic, following ECG rhythm analysis	Automatic, following ECG rhythm analysis	Automatic, following ECG rhythm analysis	Automatic, following ECG rhythm analysis	Manually, by pressing the "CHARGE" key
Delivery of shock	Manually, by pressing the "SHOCK" button	Manually, by pressing the "SHOCK" button	Manually, by pressing the "SHOCK" button	Manually, by pressing the "SHOCK" button	Manually, by pressing the "SHOCK" button	Manually, by pressing the "SHOCK" switch	Manually, by pressing the "SHOCK" switch	Manually, by pressing the "SHOCK" switch
Recording options	Solid state memory, dual channel tape recorder	Solid state memory, dual channel tape recorder	Solid state memory, dual channel tape recorder	Solid state memory, dual channel tape recorder	Annotated dual channel tape recorder	Dual channel tape recorder	Dual channel tape recorder	Solid state memory, direct-writer, dual channel tape recorder

*Automatic advisory defibrillator.

Table 7-3   Features of a fully automatic external defibrillator

Feature	Fully automatic external defibrillator Heartstart 1000/Rapid Zap 1000
ON/OFF Switching	ON/OFF power switch
ECG Signal Display	None
Message Display Panel	Standard
Audio/Visual Messages	Beeps, visual messages, voice messages
ECG Rhythm Analysis	**Continuous** while "ON"
Continuous Shockable Rhythm Monitoring	None
Charging of Defibrillator	**Automatic,** following ECG rhythm analysis
Delivery of DC Shock	**Automatic,** following charging of the defibrillator
Recording Options	Annotated dual channel tape recorder

Turning on the AED. The AEDs are turned on either by activating an **ON/OFF switch** or by **swinging up the lid** with the screen to its fullest extent. Reactivating the ON/OFF switch or returning the lid down to its original position turns the AEDs off.

Analyzing the ECG rhythm. All of the AEDs analyze the patient's electrocardiogram for the presence of **ventricular fibrillation** and a **shockable ventricular tachycardia with a rate of 120 to 200 or greater** (the rate depending on the model of AED used). These two life-threatening dysrhythmias are considered to be **shockable.** All other rhythms and dysrhythmias, regardless of their origin, rate, and rhythm, are considered **nonshockable.** The ECG rhythm analysis system is activated either by **turning on** the AED or activating the **ECG analyze switch,** depending on the AED model.

Charging of the defibrillator. All of the AEDs have a charging circuit which charges the defibrillator capacitor from the battery to one of two energy levels: **200** or **360 joules (or watt-seconds).*** The first two shocks are usually delivered at the level of 200 joules, the third shock, at 360 joules. These energy levels are based on the 1988 recommendations of the American Heart Association. Subsequent shocks are usually delivered in a sequence of 360, 360, and 360 joules. In some

AEDs, the current energy level can be switched between 200 and 360 joules at the discretion of the operator by the activation of an **energy level switch** while the AED is charging. The defibrillator charging circuit is turned on either automatically following the completion of ECG analysis or by the rescuer activating the **charge switch.**

Delivering the shock. If the rhythm analysis determines that a **shockable rhythm** is present, i.e., **ventricular fibrillation** or a **shockable ventricular tachycardia with a rate of 120 to 200 or greater,** the AED will either automatically deliver a shock or instruct the operator audibly and visually that a **"SHOCK"** is indicated. If an organized ECG rhythm, such as normal sinus rhythm, or a dysrhythmia other than ventricular fibrillation or a shockable ventricular tachycardia is present, the AEDs will indicate that **"NO SHOCK"** is required.

It is *extremely important* that cardiac arrest is verified by the EMT/FR-D by checking the patient's level of consciousness, respirations, and pulse before any shock is delivered by an AED. **A pulse indicates that a perfusing rhythm is present and that a shock *should not be delivered!***

When using an SAED, the ECG rhythm is reanalyzed by the SAED and the EMT/FR-D after the delivery of each shock. The patient's level of consciousness and pulse are usually checked by the EMT/FR-D after the delivery of each or every third shock according to local protocol and at any time when **"NO SHOCK"** is indicated. **When using a fully automatic external defibrillator,** the ECG rhythm is reanalyzed by the defibrillator after each

---

*Most of the AEDs can be reprogrammed to deliver an additional energy level of 300 joules if required by local protocol.

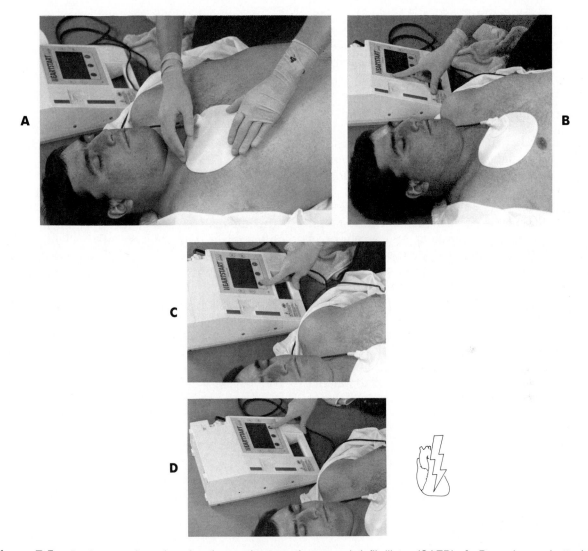

Figure 7-5. Basic procedures in using the semi-automatic external defibrillator (SAED). **A,** Preparing and attaching the defibrillator electrodes. **B,** Turning on the SAED. **C,** Analyzing the ECG rhythm, and charging the SAED. **D,** Delivering the shock, and recording patient information and ECG.

Turning on the AED. The AEDs are turned on either by activating an **ON/OFF switch** or by shock, and the patient's consciousness and pulse are checked by the EMT/FR-D after a single or a series of shocks, as the case may be, whenever the fully automatic external defibrillator indicates that a shock is not indicated or instructs the EMT/FR-D to check the patient's "breathing and pulse."

NOTE: During the ECG rhythm analysis, charging of the defibrillator, and delivery of the shock, all of the AEDs warn the operator, other rescuers, and bystanders to stand clear of the patient by audible beeping signals or vocal commands or both and by visual messages on the screen. Any movement of the patient or performance of CPR during the ECG rhythm analysis could cause artifacts in the electrocardiogram. These could be misinterpreted as ventricular fibrillation waves by the ECG rhythm analysis circuit, if an organized ECG rhythm is present, triggering a **"SHOCK"** command; or as an organized ECG rhythm, if ventricular fibrillation is present, triggering a **"NO SHOCK"** command. Furthermore, any person touching the patient or any object in contact with the patient could short-circuit the DC current through the person's body, causing the person to receive the full discharge of the defibrillator. The result could be accidental ventricular fibrillation and cardiac arrest.

Recording patient information and the patient's electrocardiogram (ECG) (optional). Local protocol may require that a verbal narrative containing information about the patient's identity, condition, and management be recorded along with the patient's ECG on a dual channel tape recorder. When required, the EMT/FR-D who is in charge evaluates the situation and records the following information as soon as possible after arriving at the scene:

- The identity of the EMT/FR-D and the other rescuers at the scene and the first responder unit or EMT/FR-D ambulance.
- A brief narrative which includes the following information and whatever else is required by medical control:
  - Patient's age and sex
  - Brief description of the present illness
  - Time of the cardiac arrest
  - Management provided from the time of the cardiac arrest to the time of arrival of the EMT/FR-D unit
  - Patient's present condition

Following the initial recording, the EMT/FR-D provides a running narrative of the results of the rhythm analyses and patient assessments, main actions taken (i.e., delivery of shocks and their energy levels, restarting of CPR, decision to transport, and so forth), and the time when these events took place.

Algorithms and protocols using the basic procedures common to the AEDs in the management of **a persistent shockable rhythm, a nonshockable rhythm,** and **a shockable rhythm converting into a perfusing rhythm** are presented on the following pages.

Algorithm 7-1. Basic AED procedures in a persistent shockable rhythm: 1. Ventricular fibrillation (V-FIB)
2. Pulseless ventricular tachycardia (V-TACH)

	Semi-automatic external defibrillators (SAEDs)		Fully automatic external defibrillators
First Medic 510, 610 **Heartstart 2000, 3000** **Lifepak 200, 250, 300**	**Responder 1200**	**Heartstart 1000s** **Rapid Zap 1000s**	**Heartstart 1000** **Rapid Zap 1000**

1. Confirm cardiac arrest.

2. Start CPR if two rescuers on scene.

3. Attach defibrillator electrodes.

4. **M** Turn on AED.

5. Stop CPR, if being performed, and stand clear.

"ANALYZE"

6. Palpate patient's pulse before or during ECG rhythm analysis (**OPTIONAL**).

7. **M** Analyze ECG rhythm. | **A** Analyze ECG rhythm. | **A** Analyze ECG rhythm.

"CHARGE"

8. **A** Charge defibrillator. | **M** Charge defibrillator. | **A** Charge defibrillator.

"SHOCK"

9. Stand clear. | Stand clear. | Stand clear.

10. **M** Deliver first shock. | **M** Deliver first shock. | **M** Deliver first shock.

Fully automatic:
6. **A** Analyze ECG rhythm.
7. **A** Charge defibrillator.
8. **A** Deliver first shock.

11. Palpate patient's pulse before or during ECG rhythm analysis (**OPTIONAL**).

"ANALYZE"

12. **M** Analyze ECG rhythm. | **A** Analyze ECG rhythm. | **A** Analyze ECG rhythm.

"CHARGE"

13. **A** Charge defibrillator. | **M** Charge defibrillator. | **A** Charge defibrillator.

"SHOCK"

14. Stand clear. | Stand clear. | Stand clear.

15. **M** Deliver second shock. | **M** Deliver second shock. | **M** Deliver second shock.

Fully automatic:
9. **A** Analyze ECG rhythm.
10. **A** Charge defibrillator.
11. **A** Deliver second shock.

Continued.

M = Function is turned on by pushing the appropriate button or switch.

A = Function is turned on automatically.

Algorithm 7-1.   Basic AED procedures in a persistent shockable rhythm: 1. Ventricular fibrillation (V-FIB)
(cont'd)   2. Pulseless ventricular tachycardia
                                                                                                           (V-TACH)

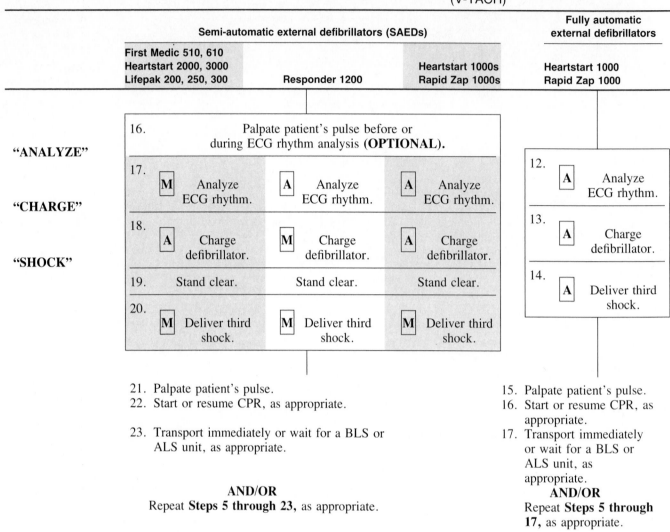

	Semi-automatic external defibrillators (SAEDs)			Fully automatic external defibrillators
	First Medic 510, 610 Heartstart 2000, 3000 Lifepak 200, 250, 300	Responder 1200	Heartstart 1000s Rapid Zap 1000s	Heartstart 1000 Rapid Zap 1000

"ANALYZE"

16.   Palpate patient's pulse before or during ECG rhythm analysis **(OPTIONAL).**

17.   **M** Analyze ECG rhythm.   **A** Analyze ECG rhythm.   **A** Analyze ECG rhythm.

"CHARGE"

12.   **A** Analyze ECG rhythm.

18.   **A** Charge defibrillator.   **M** Charge defibrillator.   **A** Charge defibrillator.

13.   **A** Charge defibrillator.

"SHOCK"

19.   Stand clear.   Stand clear.   Stand clear.

14.   **A** Deliver third shock.

20.   **M** Deliver third shock.   **M** Deliver third shock.   **M** Deliver third shock.

21. Palpate patient's pulse.
22. Start or resume CPR, as appropriate.

23. Transport immediately or wait for a BLS or ALS unit, as appropriate.

15. Palpate patient's pulse.
16. Start or resume CPR, as appropriate.
17. Transport immediately or wait for a BLS or ALS unit, as appropriate.

AND/OR
Repeat **Steps 5 through 23,** as appropriate.

AND/OR
Repeat **Steps 5 through 17,** as appropriate.

Protocol 7-1. Management of a persistent shockable rhythm using SAED: 1. Ventricular fibrillation (V-FIB)
2. Pulseless ventricular tachycardia (V-TACH)

EMT/FR-D activity	Patient's pulse and ECG	SAED interpretation and instructions
1. Confirm cardiac arrest. 2. Start CPR if two rescuers on scene. 3. Attach defibrillator electrodes. 4. Turn power on. 5. Begin recording patient information.* 6. Stand clear. 7. Stop CPR if being performed.	**No pulse**	
8. Assess patient's pulse before or during ECG rhythm analysis.* 9. Analyze ECG rhythm. 10. Charge defibrillator. 11. Stand clear. 12. Deliver first shock (200 J).	**No pulse** V-FIB **OR** V-TACH **Shockable rhythm**	"ANALYZE" "CHARGE" "SHOCK"
13. Reassess patient's pulse before or during ECG rhythm analysis.* 14. Reanalyze ECG rhythm. 15. Recharge defibrillator. 16. Stand clear. 17. Deliver second shock (200 J).	**No pulse** V-FIB **OR** V-TACH **Shockable rhythm**	"ANALYZE" "CHARGE" "SHOCK"
18. Reassess patient's pulse before or during ECG rhythm analysis* 19. Reanalyze ECG rhythm. 20. Recharge defibrillator. 21. Stand clear. 22. Deliver third shock (360 J).	**No pulse** V-FIB **OR** V-TACH **Shockable rhythm**	"ANALYZE" "CHARGE" "SHOCK"
23. Reassess patient's pulse. 24. Start or resume CPR, as appropriate. 25. Transport immediately or wait for a BLS or ALS unit, as appropriate.	**No pulse**	

AND/OR

Repeat steps 6 through 25, as appropriate, delivering 3 additional shocks in a sequence of 360, 360, and 360 J.

*Optional

Algorithm 7-2. Basic AED procedures in a nonshockable rhythm: 1. Ventricular asystole
2. Electromechanical dissociation (EMD)

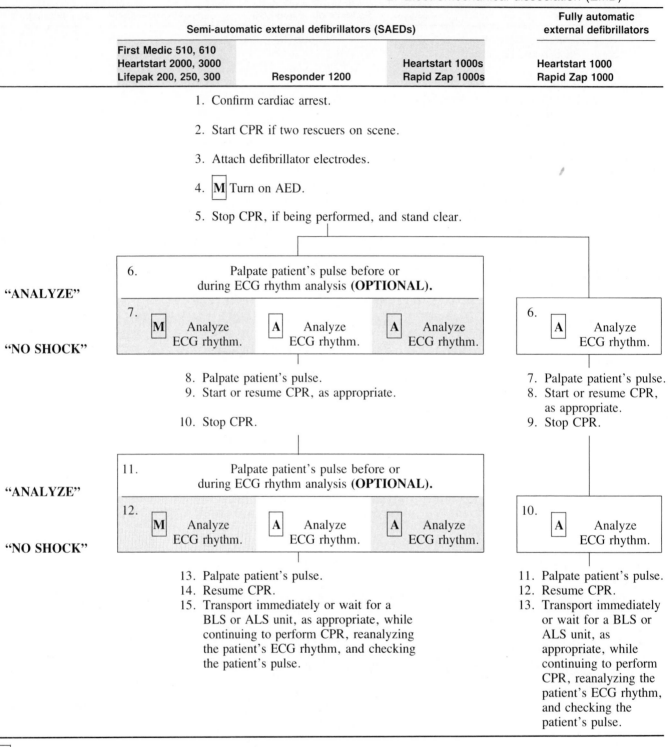

	Semi-automatic external defibrillators (SAEDs)			Fully automatic external defibrillators
First Medic 510, 610 Heartstart 2000, 3000 Lifepak 200, 250, 300	Responder 1200	Heartstart 1000s Rapid Zap 1000s	Heartstart 1000 Rapid Zap 1000	

1. Confirm cardiac arrest.

2. Start CPR if two rescuers on scene.

3. Attach defibrillator electrodes.

4. **M** Turn on AED.

5. Stop CPR, if being performed, and stand clear.

"ANALYZE"

6. Palpate patient's pulse before or during ECG rhythm analysis (**OPTIONAL**).

7. **M** Analyze ECG rhythm.   **A** Analyze ECG rhythm.   **A** Analyze ECG rhythm.

"NO SHOCK"

6. **A** Analyze ECG rhythm.

8. Palpate patient's pulse.
9. Start or resume CPR, as appropriate.

10. Stop CPR.

7. Palpate patient's pulse.
8. Start or resume CPR, as appropriate.
9. Stop CPR.

"ANALYZE"

11. Palpate patient's pulse before or during ECG rhythm analysis (**OPTIONAL**).

12. **M** Analyze ECG rhythm.   **A** Analyze ECG rhythm.   **A** Analyze ECG rhythm.

"NO SHOCK"

10. **A** Analyze ECG rhythm.

13. Palpate patient's pulse.
14. Resume CPR.
15. Transport immediately or wait for a BLS or ALS unit, as appropriate, while continuing to perform CPR, reanalyzing the patient's ECG rhythm, and checking the patient's pulse.

11. Palpate patient's pulse.
12. Resume CPR.
13. Transport immediately or wait for a BLS or ALS unit, as appropriate, while continuing to perform CPR, reanalyzing the patient's ECG rhythm, and checking the patient's pulse.

M = Function is turned on by pushing the appropriate button or switch.

A = Function is turned on automatically.

Protocol 7-2. Management of a nonshockable rhythm using SAED: 1. Ventricular asystole
2. Electromechanical dissociation (EMD)

EMT/FR-D activity	Patient's pulse and ECG	SAED interpretation and instructions
1. Confirm cardiac arrest. 2. Start CPR if two rescuers on scene. 3. Attach defibrillator electrodes. 4. Turn power on. 5. Begin recording patient information.* 6. Stand clear. 7. Stop CPR if being performed.	**No pulse**	
8. Assess patient's pulse before or during ECG rhythm analysis*	**No pulse**	
9. Analyze ECG rhythm.	Asystole	"ANALYZE"
10. Reassess patient's pulse.	OR	" NO SHOCK"
11. Start or resume CPR, as appropriate.	EMD **Nonshockable rhythm**	
12. Stop CPR.		
13. Reassess patient's pulse before or during ECG rhythm analysis*	**No pulse**	
14. Reanalyze ECG rhythm.	Asystole OR	"ANALYZE" "NO SHOCK"
	EMD **Nonshockable rhythm**	
15. Reassess patient's pulse. 16. Resume CPR. 17. Transport immediately or wait for a BLS or ALS unit, as appropriate, while continuing to perform CPR, reanalyzing the patient's ECG rhythm, and checking the patient's pulse.	**No pulse**	

*Optional

Algorithm 7-3.   Basic AED procedures in a shockable rhythm converting into a perfusing rhythm:
1. Ventricular fibrillation (V-FIB)
2. Pulseless ventricular tachycardia (V-TACH)

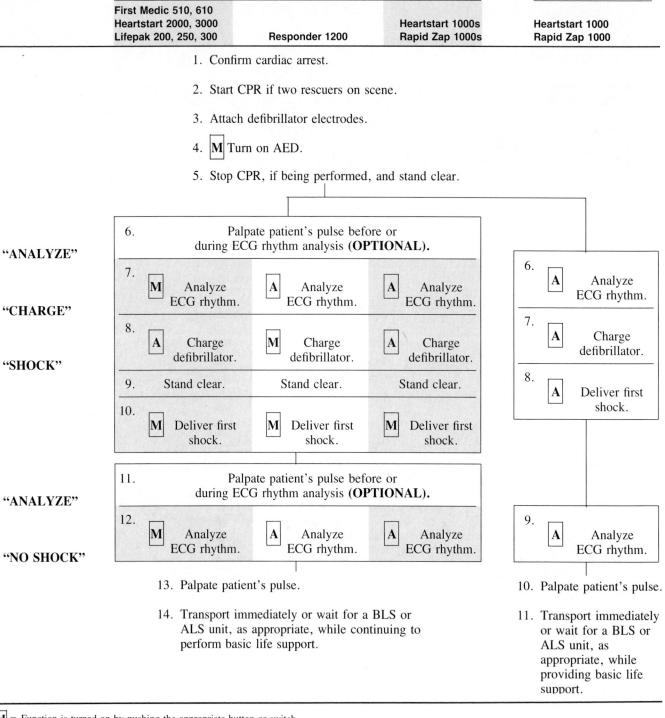

	Semi-automatic external defibrillators (SAEDs)			Fully automatic external defibrillators
First Medic 510, 610 Heartstart 2000, 3000 Lifepak 200, 250, 300	Responder 1200	Heartstart 1000s Rapid Zap 1000s		Heartstart 1000 Rapid Zap 1000

1. Confirm cardiac arrest.

2. Start CPR if two rescuers on scene.

3. Attach defibrillator electrodes.

4. |M| Turn on AED.

5. Stop CPR, if being performed, and stand clear.

"ANALYZE"

6. Palpate patient's pulse before or during ECG rhythm analysis (**OPTIONAL**).

7. |M| Analyze ECG rhythm. |A| Analyze ECG rhythm. |A| Analyze ECG rhythm.

"CHARGE"

8. |A| Charge defibrillator. |M| Charge defibrillator. |A| Charge defibrillator.

"SHOCK"

9. Stand clear.   Stand clear.   Stand clear.

10. |M| Deliver first shock. |M| Deliver first shock. |M| Deliver first shock.

"ANALYZE"

11. Palpate patient's pulse before or during ECG rhythm analysis (**OPTIONAL**).

12. |M| Analyze ECG rhythm. |A| Analyze ECG rhythm. |A| Analyze ECG rhythm.

"NO SHOCK"

13. Palpate patient's pulse.

14. Transport immediately or wait for a BLS or ALS unit, as appropriate, while continuing to perform basic life support.

6. |A| Analyze ECG rhythm.

7. |A| Charge defibrillator.

8. |A| Deliver first shock.

9. |A| Analyze ECG rhythm.

10. Palpate patient's pulse.

11. Transport immediately or wait for a BLS or ALS unit, as appropriate, while providing basic life support.

|M| = Function is turned on by pushing the appropriate button or switch.

|A| = Function is turned on automatically.

Protocol 7-3. Management of a shockable rhythm converting into a perfusing rhythm using SAED:
1. Ventricular fibrillation (V-FIB)
2. Pulseless ventricular tachycardia (V-TACH)

EMT/FR-D activity	Patient's pulse and ECG	SAED interpretation and instructions
1. Confirm cardiac arrest.	**No pulse**	
2. Start CPR if two rescuers on scene.		
3. Attach defibrillator electrodes.		
4. Turn power on.		
5. Begin recording patient information.*		
6. Stand clear.		
7. Stop CPR if being performed.		
8. Assess patient's pulse before or during ECG rhythm analysis.*	**No pulse**	
9. Analyze ECG rhythm.	V-FIB	"ANALYZE"
10. Charge defibrillator.		"CHARGE"
11. Stand clear.	V-TACH	
12. Deliver first shock (200 J).	**Shockable rhythm**	"SHOCK"
13. Reassess patient's pulse before or during ECG rhythm analysis.*	**Pulse present**	
14. Reanalyze ECG rhythm.	Organized ECG rhythm	"ANALYZE"
	Perfusing rhythm	"NO SHOCK"
15. Reassess patient's pulse.	**Pulse present**	
16. Transport immediately or wait for a BLS or ALS unit, as appropriate, while providing life support.		

*Optional

Chapter 8

Standard Automatic External Defibrillator Generic Protocols and Algorithms

OBJECTIVES

Upon completion of all or part of this chapter as required by your early defibrillation program, you should be able to complete the following objectives indicated by your instructor:

☐ Define a pre-arrival cardiac arrest.
☐ List the five major tasks in the initial management of a pre-arrival and EMT/FR-D-witnessed cardiac arrest and briefly describe them.
☐ List the order in which the five major tasks are performed according to the automated external defibrillator used in your early defibrillation program.
☐ Identify the automated external protocols and algorithms that will be followed in your early defibrillation program.
☐ Outline the following protocols as appropriate to your early defibrillation program:

- Initial management of pre-arrival cardiac arrest, without bystander CPR
  ☐ One rescuer
  ☐ Two rescuers
- Initial management of pre-arrival cardiac arrest, with bystander CPR
  ☐ One rescuer
  ☐ Two rescuers
- Management of EMT/FR-D-witnessed cardiac arrest on the scene or en route
  ☐ One rescuer
  ☐ Two rescuers
- Management of cardiac arrest following ECG rhythm analysis indicating "Shock"
  ☐ One rescuer
  ☐ Two rescuers
- Management of cardiac arrest following ECG rhythm analysis indicating "No shock"
  ☐ One rescuer
  ☐ Two rescuers
- Management of a perfusing rhythm
- Management of recurrent cardiac arrest

Upon arrival at the scene of a patient in cardiac arrest or one suspected of having an acute myocardial infarction, the EMT/FR-D will be faced with either:

- A patient already in cardiac arrest, unwitnessed by the EMT/FR-D. This will be referred to in this manual as a **pre-arrival arrest,**

OR

- A patient who is not in cardiac arrest.

The **pre-arrival cardiac arrest** may have been **witnessed** or **unwitnessed** by a bystander who may be a relative, a passerby, a fireman, a police officer, a prehospital emergency care provider, a nurse, or a doctor. Cardiopulmonary resuscitation may have been instituted immediately following cardiac arrest, some time later, or not at all. If CPR is being performed upon arrival of the EMT/FR-D at the scene, the cardiac arrest will be referred to as a **pre-arrival cardiac arrest with bystander CPR.** If CPR is not being performed, the cardiac arrest will be referred to as a **pre-arrival cardiac arrest without bystander CPR.**

If the patient is not in cardiac arrest when the EMT/FR-D arrives at the scene, the EMT/FR-D should be prepared to provide automated external

Types of Cardiac Arrests Encountered by EMT/FR-Ds

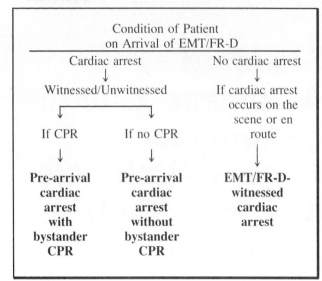

The Sequence of the MAJOR TASKS Performed by an EMT/FR-D in the Initial Management of Cardiac Arrest Following the Determination of Cardiac Arrest

1 Attach the defibrillator electrodes.
2 Turn on the **SAED** and begin the narrative if the **SAED** is equipped with a voice recorder and a narrative is required by local protocol.
3 Check the patient's pulse.*
4 Analyze the ECG rhythm.
5 Deliver the shock.

*The performance and sequence of this major task depends on local protocol.

The initial management of pre-arrival and EMT/FR-D-witnessed cardiac arrest, using the SAED after cardiac arrest has been verified, incorporates the following **five major tasks:***
1. **Preparing the patient's skin, and attaching the defibrillator electrodes**
2. **Turning on the SAED, and narrating the pertinent facts (if the SAED is equipped with a voice recorder and a narrative is required by local protocol)**
3. **Analyzing the patient's ECG**
4. **Checking the patient's pulse**
5. **Delivering the shock**

The sequence of the five major tasks performed by the EMT/FR-D except for the checking of the patient's pulse, which will be explained in the next paragraph, is essentially the same for all the SAEDs of the major defibrillator manufacturers (see the box above). The steps in performing the five major tasks are shown in **Scans 8-1 and 8-2,** one for **one-rescuer early defibrillation** and the other for **two-rescuer early defibrillation.** For the sake of brevity, these steps are not repeated each time the major tasks are presented in the protocols and algorithms that follow in this chapter. Steps in how to perform a narrative are included in **Task 2.** These steps may be omitted if the SAED used in the prehospital defibrillation program is not equipped with a voice recorder and the local protocol does not require a recorded narrative.

Because some local prehospital defibrillation protocols require **checking the patient's pulse** before or during every analysis of the ECG rhythm, contrary to the minimum standards for early defibrillation recommended by the American Heart

Text continued on p. 92.

*These tasks are based on the basic procedures common to the automated external defibrillators described in Chapter 7.

defibrillation at a moment's notice should the patient go into cardiac arrest. A cardiac arrest that occurs after the arrival of the EMT/FR-D at the scene, thereby being witnessed, will be referred to as an **EMT/FR-D-witnessed cardiac arrest.**

After the patient has been treated, the EMT/FR-D has two options, depending on the configuration of the EMS system within which the EMT/FR-D is operating. The EMT/FR-D may:
- Interface with a basic life support (BLS) unit or an advanced life support (ALS) unit at the scene or en route and hand off the patient to a higher level prehospital emergency care provider,

OR

- transport the patient directly to the nearest appropriate medical facility if the EMT/FR-D also provides basic life support as part of a BLS system.

The automated external defibrillator (AED) used by the EMT/FR-D may be a **semi-automatic external defibrillator (SAED)** or a **fully automatic external defibrillator.**

The **prehospital defibrillation protocols** and **algorithms** presented in this chapter detail the management of **pre-arrival cardiac arrest** with or without **bystander CPR** and **EMT/FR-D-witnessed cardiac arrest** by two rescuers—one trained in CPR and the other as an EMT/FR-D—and by a single EMT/FR-D rescuer. These protocols and algorithms are presented as guidelines for prehospital defibrillation programs and systems and may be modified according to local standards and protocols.

TASK 1 | ATTACH THE DEFIBRILLATOR ELECTRODES.

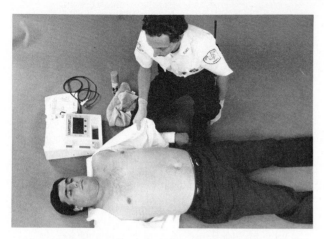

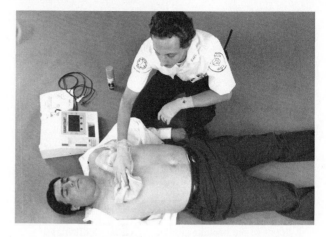

1. Prepare the patient and defibrillator electrode sites.
   a. Bare the patient's chest, using large bandage scissors to remove the clothing if necessary.
   b. Identify the two defibrillator electrode sites:
      (1) The **upper right anterior chest wall** (the area bordered by the right edge of the sternum and the lower border of the right clavicle)
      (2) The **left lower anterior chest wall** (the area over the left anterior axillary line)

c. Prepare the skin over the electrode sites by wiping the skin vigorously with a rough-textured towel if the skin is moist from sweating. If the skin is extremely sweaty, spray an antiperspirant aerosol, such as **Arrid Extra Dry,** on the electrode sites and wipe off the antiperspirant powder 20 to 30 seconds later with a dry towel.

If Nitropaste is present, wipe the substance off with a rough-textured towel, wiping in a direction away from the midline and downward.

NOTE: Occasionally, excessive hair may have to be quickly shaved or trimmed in the areas of defibrillator electrode placement, otherwise the electrodes will not adhere properly.

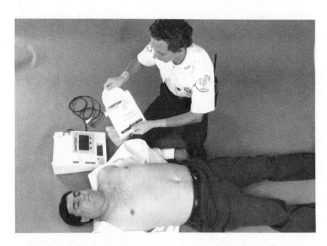

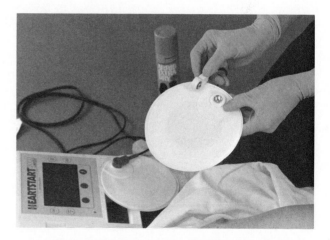

2. Assure that the electrode cables are attached to the SAED.
3. Prepare the defibrillator electrodes and attach them to the patient.
   a. Remove the defibrillator electrodes from their packaging.
   b. Identify the negative and positive electrodes, if appropriate.

c. Attach the electrode cables to the defibrillator electrodes, if they are supplied separately, making sure that the appropriate cables are attached to the appropriate electrodes, **i.e., the positive cable is attached to the positive electrode; the negative cable, to the negative electrode** (if the electrodes are so identified).

Continued.

Scan 8-1: One-Rescuer Early Defibrillation—Without Bystander CPR, cont'd

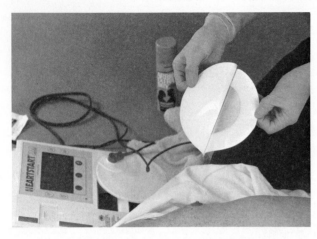

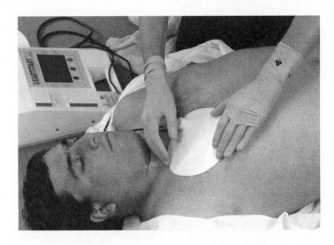

d. Remove the backing from the **negative defibrillator electrode**, and

attach the electrode to the **upper right anterior chest wall.**

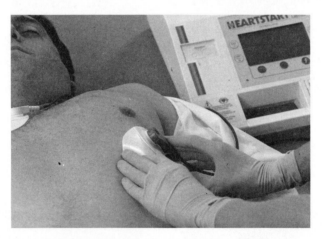

e. Remove the backing from the **positive defibrillator electrode,** and attach the electrode to the **left lower anterior chest wall.**

f. Ensure that the electrodes are firmly attached to the patient's chest by gently pressing down on the edges of the electrodes.

Scan 8-1: One-Rescuer Early Defibrillation—Without Bystander CPR, cont'd

TASK 2 | **TURN ON THE SAED AND BEGIN THE NARRATIVE.***

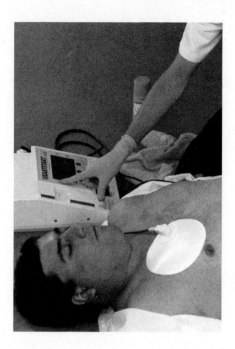

1. Turn on the SAED, and, if appropriate, make sure that the voice recorder is on and a cassette has been inserted into the tape recorder.
2. Begin narrating the case, if appropriate, identifying the **rescuer by name and identification number** and the **EMT/FR-D unit** responding, if appropriate, and noting the **time** and the **patient's age, sex,** and **condition,** including the **patient's pulse.** Other information may include the kind of cardiac arrest (medical or trauma), the onset of the cardiac arrest, whether the cardiac arrest was witnessed or not, whether bystander CPR was provided or not, the time of arrival of the EMT/FR-D unit, and so forth, as required by medical control.
3. Continue the narration, as appropriate, whenever the ECG rhythm is analyzed, a SAED advisory is given, a shock is delivered, the decision to transport is made, and so forth, and the time of the events, as required by medical control.

NOTE: **The information included in the narratives may be modified in accordance with the local prehospital defibrillation protocols and guidelines.**

***Omit the voice recording of the narrative if not required by local protocol.**

TASK 3 | **CHECK THE PATIENT'S PULSE.**

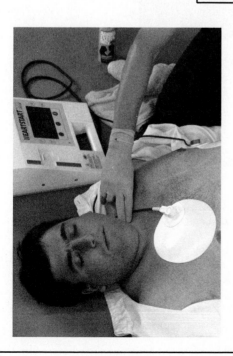

Palpate the patient's carotid artery for a spontaneous pulse, taking about 5 to 10 seconds before or during the analysis of the ECG rhythm, as appropriate, according to local protocol. **(This task is optional.)**

Continued.

Scan 8-1: One-Rescuer Early Defibrillation—Without Bystander CPR, cont'd

TASK 4   ANALYZE THE ECG RHYTHM.*

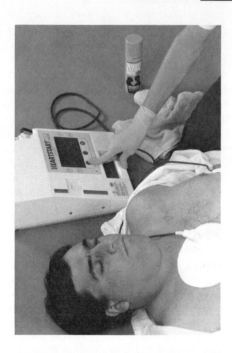

1. Initiate ECG rhythm analysis (if appropriate for model), assuring that no one is touching the patient.
   AND
2. Begin to count aloud, **"One thousand and one! One thousand and two! One thousand and three! . . "** to monitor the time it takes the SAED to analyze the ECG rhythm. (**This step is optional.**)

*****The patient's pulse may be checked during the analysis of the ECG rhythm if required by local protocol.**

TASK 5   DELIVER THE SHOCK.

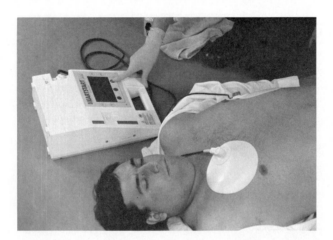

After warning everyone to **"STAND CLEAR!"**, press the **"SHOCK" BUTTON** to deliver the **SHOCK.**

TASK 1 | ATTACH THE DEFIBRILLATOR ELECTRODES.

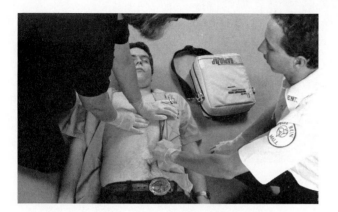

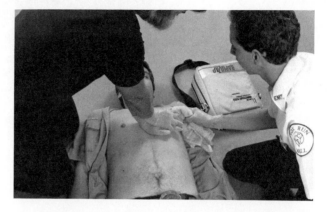

1. Prepare the patient and defibrillator electrode sites.

> **NOTE!**
> **DO NOT INTERRUPT CPR WHILE PREPARING THE PATIENT AND ELECTRODE SITES AND ATTACHING THE DEFIBRILLATOR ELECTRODES!**

  a. Bare the patient's chest, using large bandage scissors to remove the clothing if necessary.
  b. Identify the two defibrillator electrode sites:
    (1) The **upper right anterior chest wall** (the area bordered by the right edge of the sternum and the lower border of the right clavicle)
    (2) The **left lower anteior chest wall** (the area over the intersection of the left fourth intercostal space and the left anterior axillary line below the level of the nipple).

  c. Prepare the skin over the electrode sites by wiping the skin vigorously with a rough-textured towel if the skin is moist from sweating. If the skin is extremely sweaty, spray an antiperspirant aerosol, such as **Arrid Extra Dry,** on the electrode sites and wipe off the antiperspirant powder 20 to 30 seconds later with a dry towel.

If Nitropaste is present, wipe the substance off with a rough-textured towel, wiping in a direction away from the midline and downward.

NOTE: Occasionally, excessive hair may have to be quickly shaved or trimmed in the areas of defibrillator electrode placement, otherwise, the electrodes will not adhere properly.

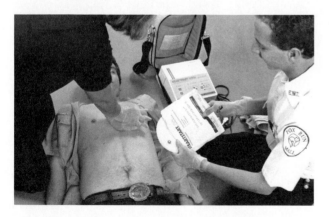

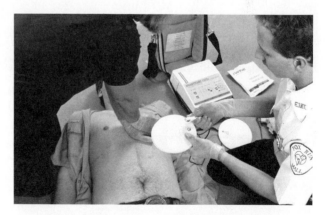

2. Assure that the electrode cables are attached to the SAED.
3. Prepare the defibrillator electrodes and attach them to the patient **while assuring that the other rescuer or the bystander is performing adequate CPR.**
  a. Remove the defibrillator electrodes from their packaging.
  b. Identify the negative and positive electrodes, if appropriate.

  c. Attach the electrode cables to the defibrillator electrodes, if they are supplied separately, making sure that the appropriate cables are attached to the appropriate electrodes, **i.e., the positive cable is attached to the positive electrode; the negative cable, to the negative electrode** (if the electrodes are so identified).

Continued.

Scan 8-2: Two-Rescuer Early Defibrillation/One-Rescuer Early Defibrillation—With Bystander CPR, cont'd

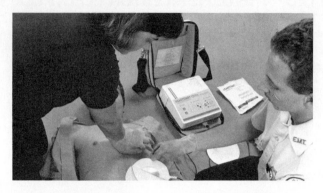

d. Remove the backing from the **negative defibrillator electrode,** and

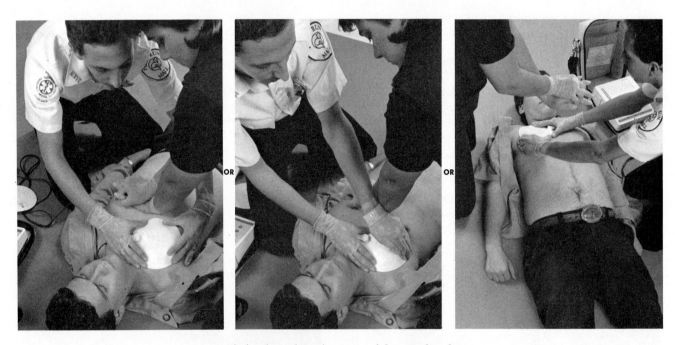

attach the electrode to the **upper right anterior chest wall using one of the alternate ways shown.**

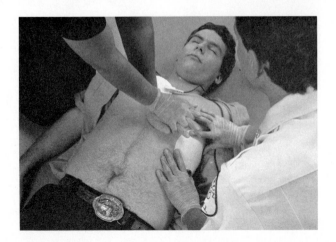

e. Remove the backing from the **positive defibrillator electrode,** and attach the electrode to the **left lower anterior chest wall.**

f. Ensure that the electrodes are firmly attached to the patient's chest by gently pressing down on the edges of the electrodes.

Scan 8-2: Two-Rescuer Early Defibrillation/One-Rescuer Early Defibrillation—With Bystander CPR, cont'd

TASK 2   **TURN ON THE SAED AND BEGIN THE NARRATIVE.***

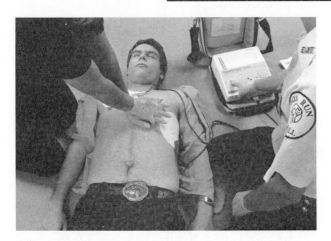

1. Turn on the SAED, and, if appropriate, make sure that the voice recorder is on and a cassette has been inserted into the tape recorder.

2. Begin narrating the case, if appropriate, identifying the **rescuer(s) by name and identification number** and the **EMT/FR-D unit** responding, as appropriate, and noting the **time** and the **patient's age, sex,** and **condition,** including the **patient's pulse.** Other information may include the kind of cardiac arrest (medical or trauma), the onset of the cardiac arrest, whether the cardiac arrest was witnessed or not, whether bystander CPR was provided or not, the time of arrival of the EMT/FR-D unit, and so forth, as required by medical control.

3. Continue the narration, as appropriate, whenever the ECG rhythm is analyzed, a SAED advisory is given, a shock is delivered, the decision to transport is made, and so forth, and the time of the events, as required by medical control.

NOTE: **The information included in the narratives may be modified in accordance with the local prehospital defibrillation protocols and guidelines.**

*Omit the voice recording of the narrative if not required by local protocol.

TASK 3   **CHECK THE PATIENT'S PULSE.**

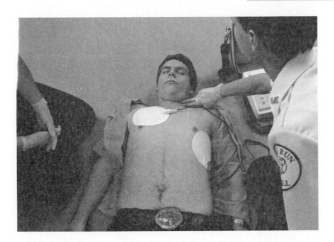

Palpate the patient's carotid artery for a spontaneous pulse, taking about 5 to 10 seconds before or during the analysis of the ECG rhythm, as appropriate, according to local protocol. **(This task is optional.)**

Continued.

Scan 8-2: Two-Rescuer Early Defibrillation/One-Rescuer Early Defibrillation—With Bystander CPR, cont'd

TASK 4 | ANALYZE THE ECG RHYTHM.*

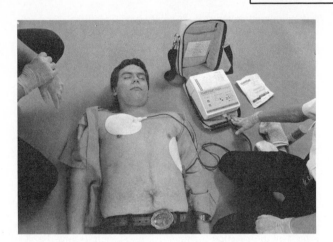

1. Initiate ECG rhythm analysis (if appropriate for model), assuring that no one is touching the patient.

AND

2. Begin to count aloud, **"One thousand and one! One thousand and two! One thousand and three! . . "** to monitor the time it takes the SAED to analyze the ECG rhythm. **(This step is optional.)**

*The patient's pulse may be checked during the analysis of the ECG rhythm if required by local protocol.**

TASK 5 | DELIVER THE SHOCK.

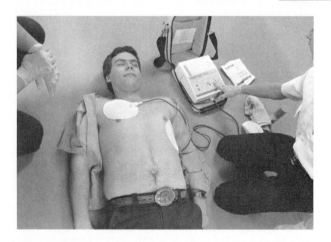

After warning everyone to **"STAND CLEAR!"** press the **"SHOCK" BUTTON** to deliver the **SHOCK.**

Preparation of the SAED

Prior to Responding to the Call or While En Route to the Scene

Check the **SAED** for the following:
- The **battery** is fully charged
- An **extra battery** is available
- The **defibrillator electrodes** and **cables** are present
- The **tape cassette** has been inserted, if appropriate
- The **computer module** has been inserted, if appropriate

Association, the protocols and algorithms in this book have been designed to reflect these minimum standards as well as any anticipated modifications in the organization and sequence of the major tasks. **For these reasons, the generic algorithms and protocols for prehospital defibrillation are presented in two formats: one based on the recommendations of the American Heart Association (Section 1) and the other, on a pulse check before or during every analysis of the ECG rhythm (Section 2).**

Generic SAED Protocols

The following generic protocols using a **SAED** in the management of cardiac arrest under a variety of conditions by one and two rescuers, with and without bystander CPR, are presented in Sections 1 and 2.

Protocol 1: Initial management of pre-arrival cardiac arrest—two rescuers, without bystander CPR. This protocol details the standard operating procedure used in providing **semi-automatic external defibrillation** by a team consisting of a rescuer certified in CPR **(rescuer one)** and an EMT/FR-D **(rescuer two)** upon arrival at the scene of a cardiac arrest **with no bystander CPR being performed.** Two variations of this protocol are provided, depending on whether one- or two-rescuer CPR is performed initially.

Protocol 1a This protocol is based on the initial CPR being performed by one rescuer—the CPR-trained rescuer accompanying the EMT/FR-D.

Protocol 1b This protocol is based on the initial CPR being performed by both the EMT/FR-D and the accompanying CPR-trained rescuer.

Protocol 2: Initial management of pre-arrival cardiac arrest—two rescuers, with bystander CPR. This protocol details the standard operating procedure used in providing **semi-automatic external defibrillation** by a team consisting of a rescuer certified in CPR **(rescuer one)** and an EMT/FR-D **(rescuer two)** upon arrival at the scene of a cardiac arrest **with bystander CPR being performed.**

Protocol 3: Initial management of EMT/FR-D-witnessed cardiac arrest on the scene or en route—two rescuers. This protocol details the standard operating procedure used in providing **semi-automatic external defibrillation** by a team consisting of a rescuer certified in CPR **(rescuer one)** and an EMT/FR-D **(rescuer two)** when the patient's cardiac arrest is witnessed by the team while on the scene or en route. As in **PROTOCOL 1** above, two variations are provided, depending on whether one- or two-rescuer CPR is performed initially.

Protocol 3a This protocol is based on the initial CPR being performed by one rescuer—the CPR-trained rescuer accompanying the EMT/FR-D.

Protocol 3b This protocol is based on the initial CPR being performed by both the EMT/FR-D and the accompanying CPR-trained rescuer.

Protocol 4: Management of cardiac arrest following ECG rhythm analysis indicating "SHOCK"—two rescuers. This protocol details the standard operating procedure used in continuing the management of cardiac arrest initiated in **PROTOCOL 1, 2,** or **3** after the SAED has analyzed the patient's ECG rhythm and determined that **"SHOCK"** is indicated.

Protocol 5: Management of cardiac arrest following ECG rhythm analysis indicating "NO SHOCK"—two rescuers. This protocol details the standard operating procedure used in continuing the management of cardiac arrest initiated in **PROTOCOL 1, 2,** or **3** after the SAED has analyzed the patient's ECG rhythm and determined that **"NO SHOCK"** is indicated.

Protocol 6: Initial management of pre-arrival cardiac arrest or EMT/FR-D-witnessed cardiac arrest while on the scene—one rescuer, without bystander CPR. This protocol details the standard operating procedure used in providing **semi-automatic external defibrillation** by a single rescuer—**the EMT/FR-D**—upon arrival at the scene of a cardiac arrest **with bystander CPR not being performed** or when the patient's cardiac arrest is witnessed by the EMT/FR-D while on the scene.

Protocol 7: Initial management of pre-arrival cardiac arrest—one rescuer, with bystander CPR. This protocol details the standard operating procedure used in providing **semi-automatic external defibrillation** by a single rescuer—**the EMT/FR-D**—upon arrival at the scene of a cardiac arrest **with bystander CPR being performed.**

Protocol 8: Management of cardiac arrest following ECG rhythm analysis indicating "SHOCK"—one rescuer. This protocol details the standard operating procedure used in continuing the management of cardiac arrest initiated in **PROTOCOL 6** or **7** after the SAED has analyzed the patient's ECG rhythm and determined that **"SHOCK"** is indicated.

Protocol 9: Management of cardiac arrest following ECG rhythm analysis indicating "NO SHOCK"—one rescuer. This protocol details the standard operating procedure used in continuing the management of cardiac arrest initiated in **PROTOCOL 6 OR 7** after the SAED has analyzed the patient's ECG rhythm and determined that **"NO SHOCK"** is indicated.

Pre-arrival and EMT/FR-D-witnessed Cardiac Arrest SAED Protocols for Two Rescuers

Initial Management of Cardiac Arrest: Two Rescuers

Pre-arrival Cardiac Arrest

If bystander CPR **IS NOT** being performed:
- Proceed to **PROTOCOL 1: Intial Management of Pre-arrival Cardiac Arrest—Two Rescuers, without Bystander CPR.**

If bystander CPR **IS** being performed:
- Proceed to **PROTOCOL 2: Initial Management of Pre-arrival Cardiac Arrest—Two Rescuers, with Bystander CPR.**

EMT/FR-D-witnessed Cardiac Arrest

- Proceed to **PROTOCOL 3: Initial Management of EMT/FR-D-Witnessed Cardiac Arrest while on the Scene or en Route—Two Rescuers.**

Continuing Management of Cardiac Arrest: Two Rescuers

If "**SHOCK**" is indicated:
- Proceed to **PROTOCOL 4: Management of Cardiac Arrest Following ECG Rhythm Analysis Indicating "SHOCK"—Two Rescuers.**

If "**NO SHOCK**" is indicated:
- Proceed to **PROTOCOL 5: Management of Cardiac Arrest Following ECG Rhythm Analysis Indicating "NO SHOCK"—Two Rescuers.**

Pre-arrival and EMT/FR-D-witnessed Cardiac Arrest SAED Protocols for One Rescuer

Initial Management of Cardiac Arrest: One Rescuer

Pre-arrival Cardiac Arrest

If bystander CPR **IS NOT** being performed:
- Proceed to **PROTOCOL 6: Initial Management of Pre-arrival Cardiac Arrest or EMT/FR-D-Witnessed Cardiac Arrest while on the Scene—One Rescuer, without Bystander CPR.**

If bystander CPR **IS** being performed:
- Proceed to **PROTOCOL 7: Initial Management of Pre-arrival Cardiac Arrest—One Rescuer, with Bystander CPR.**

EMT/FR-D-witnessed Cardiac Arrest

- Proceed to **PROTOCOL 6: Initial Management of Pre-arrival Cardiac Arrest or EMT/FR-D-Witnessed Cardiac Arrest while on the Scene—One Rescuer, without Bystander CPR.**

Continuing Management of Cardiac Arrest: One Rescuer

If "**SHOCK**" is indicated:
- Proceed to **PROTOCOL 8: Management of Cardiac Arrest Following ECG Rhythm Analysis Indicating "SHOCK"—One Rescuer.**

If "**NO SHOCK**" is indicated:
- Proceed to **PROTOCOL 9: Management of Cardiac Arrest Following ECG Rhythm Analysis Indicating "NO SHOCK"—One Rescuer.**

Protocol 10: Management of a perfusing rhythm—one or two rescuers. This protocol details the standard operating procedure used in continuing the management of cardiac arrest after successful defibrillation of a shockable rhythm and conversion to a perfusing rhythm accomplished in **PROTOCOL 4** or **8.**

Protocol 11: Management of recurrent cardiac arrest—one or two rescuers. This protocol details the standard operating procedure used in the management of a cardiac arrest **recurring** after the successful defibrillation of a shockable rhythm and conversion to a perfusing rhythm.

Generic SAED Algorithms

Algorithm 8-1: Two Rescuers, Based on the Recommendations of the American Heart Association

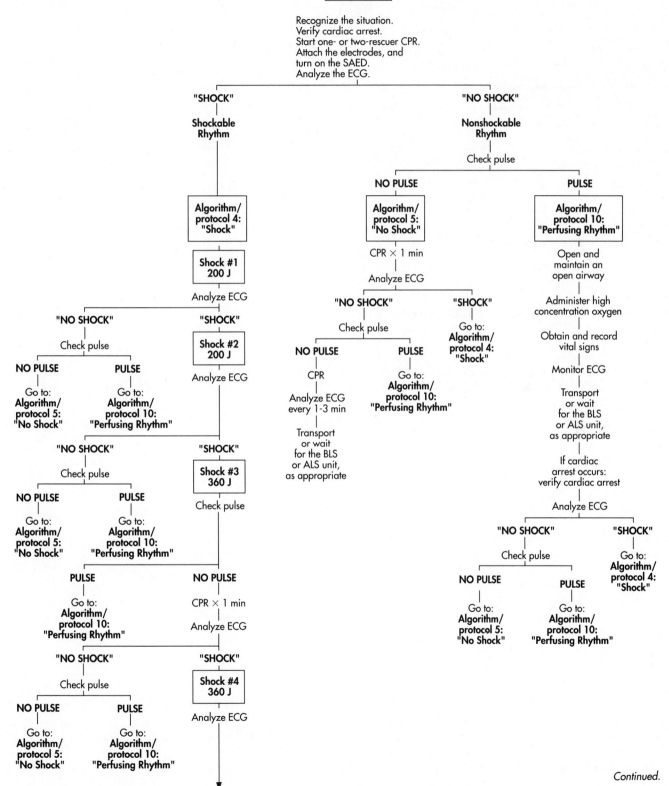

Continued.

Algorithm 8-1: Two Rescuers, Based on the Recommendations of the American Heart Association, cont'd

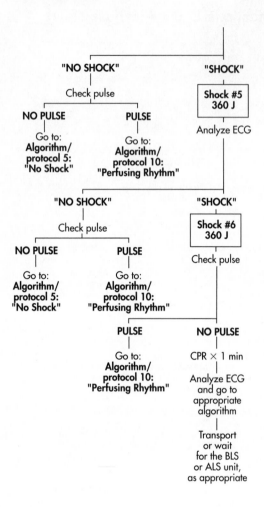

Algorithm 8-2: One Rescuer, Based on the Recommendations of the American Heart Association

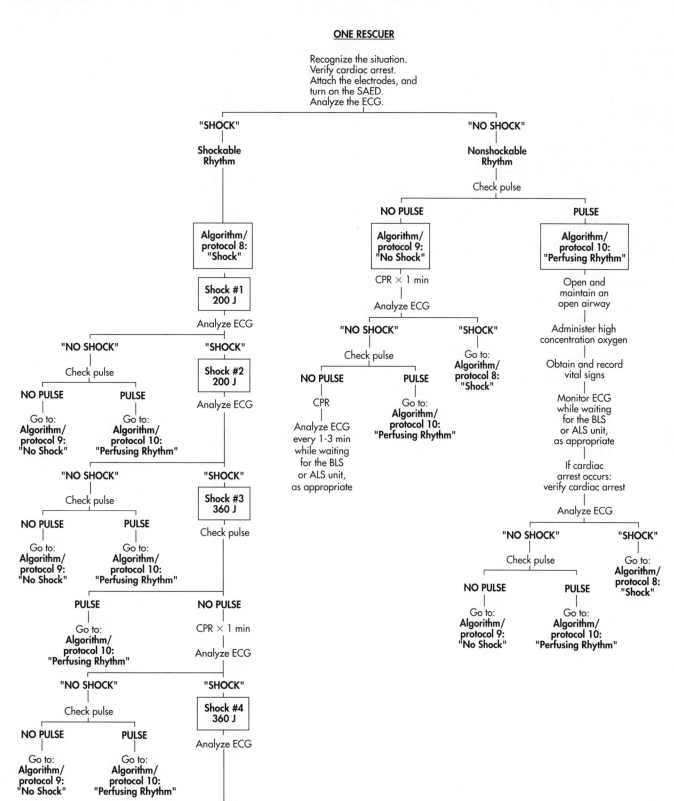

Continued.

Algorithm 8-2: One Rescuer, Based on the Recommendations of the American Heart Association, cont'd

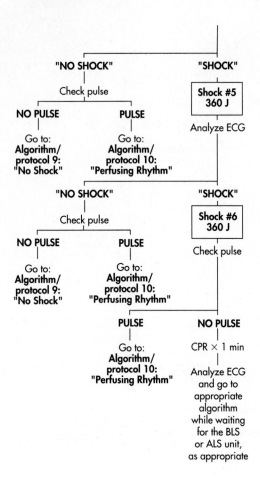

Algorithm 8-3: Two Rescuers, Based on a Pulse Check Before or During Every Analysis of the ECG Rhythm

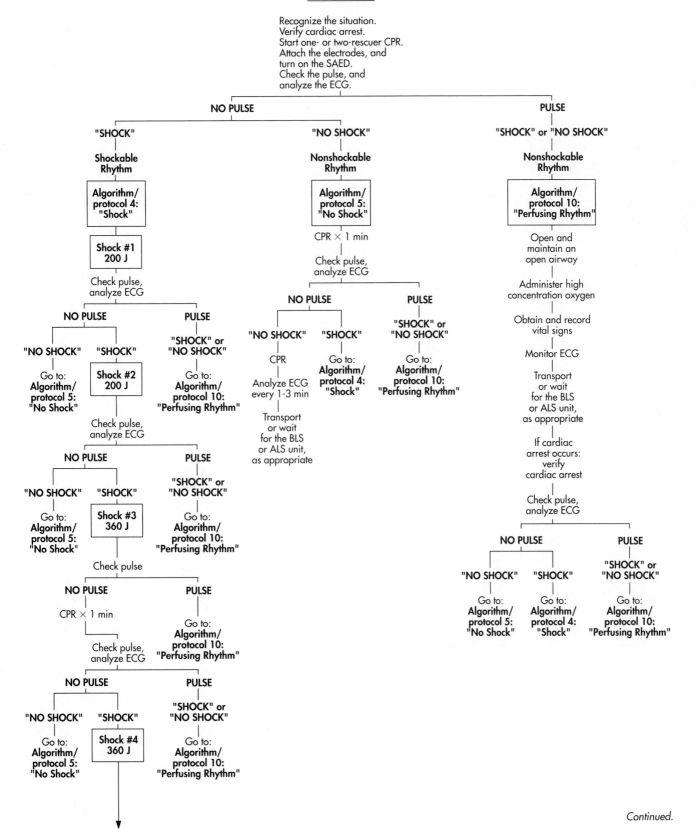

TWO RESCUERS

Recognize the situation.
Verify cardiac arrest.
Start one- or two-rescuer CPR.
Attach the electrodes, and turn on the SAED.
Check the pulse, and analyze the ECG.

Continued.

Algorithm 8-3: Two Rescuers, Based on a Pulse Check Before or During Every Analysis of the ECG Rhythm, cont'd

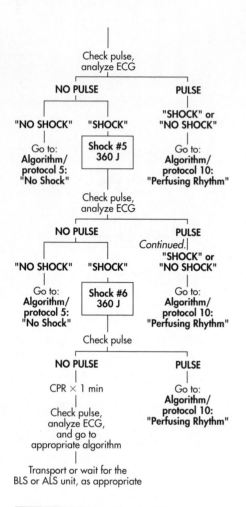

Algorithm 8-4: One Rescuer, Based on a Pulse Check Before or During Every Analysis of the ECG Rhythm

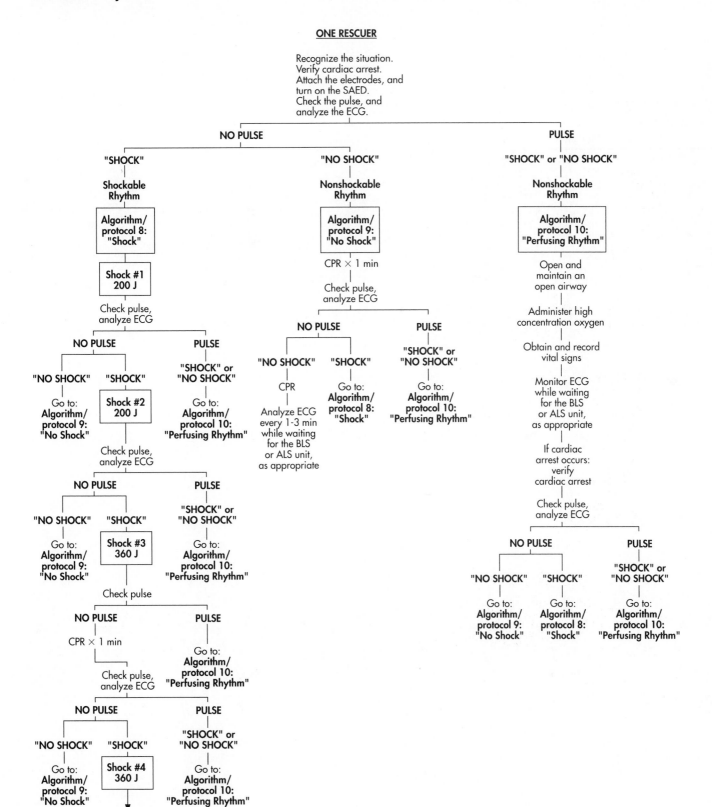

Continued.

Algorithm 8-4: One Rescuer, Based on a Pulse Check Before or During Every Analysis of the ECG Rhythm, cont'd

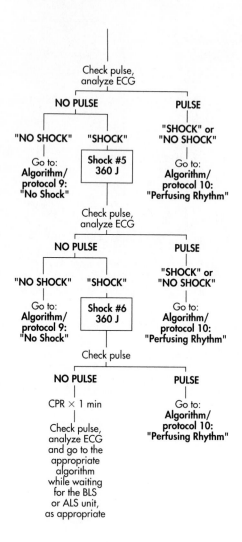

Section 1

Generic SAED Algorithms and Protocols, Based on the Recommendations of the American Heart Association

1. Initial Management of Pre-arrival Cardiac Arrest—Two Rescuers, without Bystander CPR

   ALGORITHM 1. One/two-rescuer CPR
   PROTOCOL 1a. One-rescuer CPR
   PROTOCOL 1b. Two-rescuer CPR

2. Initial Management of Pre-arrival Cardiac Arrest—Two Rescuers, with Bystander CPR

   ALGORITHM 2
   PROTOCOL 2

3. Initial Management of EMT/FR-D-witnessed Cardiac Arrest while on the Scene or en Route—Two Rescuers

   ALGORITHM 3. One/two-rescuer CPR
   PROTOCOL 3a. One-rescuer CPR
   PROTOCOL 3b. Two-rescuer CPR

4. Management of Cardiac Arrest Following ECG Rhythm Analysis Indicating "**SHOCK**"—Two Rescuers

   ALGORITHM 4
   PROTOCOL 4

5. Management of Cardiac Arrest Following ECG Rhythm Analysis Indicating "**NO SHOCK**"—Two Rescuers

   ALGORITHM 5
   PROTOCOL 5

6. Initial Management of Pre-arrival Cardiac Arrest or EMT/FR-D-witnessed Cardiac Arrest while on the Scene—One Rescuer, without Bystander CPR

   ALGORITHM 6
   PROTOCOL 6

7. Initial Management of Pre-arrival Cardiac Arrest—One Rescuer, with Bystander CPR

   ALGORITHM 7
   PROTOCOL 7

8. Management of Cardiac Arrest Following ECG Rhythm Analysis Indicating "**SHOCK**"—One Rescuer

   ALGORITHM 8
   PROTOCOL 8

9. Management of Cardiac Arrest Following ECG Rhythm Analysis Indicating "**NO SHOCK**"—One Rescuer

   ALGORITHM 9
   PROTOCOL 9

10. Management of a Perfusing Rhythm—One or Two Rescuers

    ALGORITHM 10
    PROTOCOL 10

11. Management of a Recurrent Cardiac Arrest—One or Two Rescuers

    ALGORITHM 11
    PROTOCOL 11

Initial Management of Pre-arrival Cardiac Arrest—Two Rescuers, without Bystander CPR

ALGORITHM 1 One/Two-Rescuer CPR
PROTOCOL 1a One-Rescuer CPR
PROTOCOL 1b Two-Rescuer CPR

ALGORITHM 1: Initial Management of Pre-arrival Cardiac Arrest—Two Rescuers, without Bystander CPR

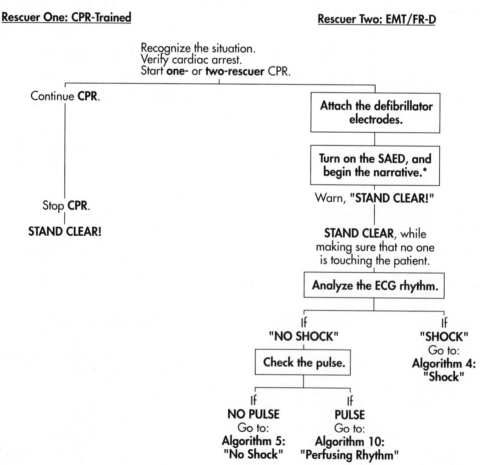

<u>Rescuer One: CPR-Trained</u>   <u>Rescuer Two: EMT/FR-D</u>

Recognize the situation.
Verify cardiac arrest.
Start **one-** or **two-rescuer** CPR.

Continue **CPR.**

Attach the defibrillator electrodes.

Turn on the SAED, and begin the narrative.*

Warn, **"STAND CLEAR!"**

Stop **CPR.**

STAND CLEAR!

STAND CLEAR, while making sure that no one is touching the patient.

Analyze the ECG rhythm.

If
"NO SHOCK"

If
"SHOCK"
Go to:
**Algorithm 4:
"Shock"**

Check the pulse.

If
NO PULSE
Go to:
**Algorithm 5:
"No Shock"**

If
PULSE
Go to:
**Algorithm 10:
"Perfusing Rhythm"**

---

* Omit the voice recording of the narrative if not required by local protocol.

PROTOCOL 1b: Initial Management of Pre-arrival Cardiac Arrest—Two Rescuers, without Bystander CPR, cont'd

Two-rescuer CPR	
Rescuer one: CPR-trained	Rescuer two: EMT/FR-D

	6. **TURN ON THE SAED, AND BEGIN THE NARRATIVE.***
	NOTE: Defibrillation takes precedence over CPR! The first shock is delivered as soon as the defibrillator electrodes have been attached, the ECG rhythm analyzed, and "SHOCK" indicated.
5. Stop **CPR** so that the patient is motionless **while** the ECG rhythm is being analyzed.	7. Warn, "STAND CLEAR!"
6. **STAND CLEAR!**	8. **STAND CLEAR WHILE MAKING SURE THAT NO ONE, INCLUDING ANY BY-STANDER AND BOTH RESCUERS, IS TOUCHING THE PATIENT OR ANYTHING IS IN CONTACT WITH THE PATIENT.**
	9. **ANALYZE THE ECG RHYTHM.**
	If "SHOCK" is indicated and the PATIENT'S PULSE IS ABSENT:
	10. Proceed to **PROTOCOL 4: Management of Cardiac Arrest Following ECG Rhythm Analysis Indicating "SHOCK"—Two Rescuers.**
	If "NO SHOCK" is indicated:
	11. **CHECK THE PATIENT'S PULSE.**
	If the patient's PULSE is absent:
	12. Proceed to **PROTOCOL 5: Management of Cardiac Arrest Following ECG Rhythm Analysis Indicating "NO SHOCK"—Two Rescuers.**
	If the patient's PULSE is present:
	13. Proceed to **PROTOCOL 10: Management of a Perfusing Rhythm—One or Two Rescuers.**

*Omit the voice recording of the narrative if it is not required by local protocol.

Initial Management of Pre-arrival Cardiac Arrest—Two Rescuers, with Bystander CPR

ALGORITHM 2
PROTOCOL 2

ALGORITHM 2: Initial Management of Pre-arrival Cardiac Arrest—Two Rescuers, with Bystander CPR

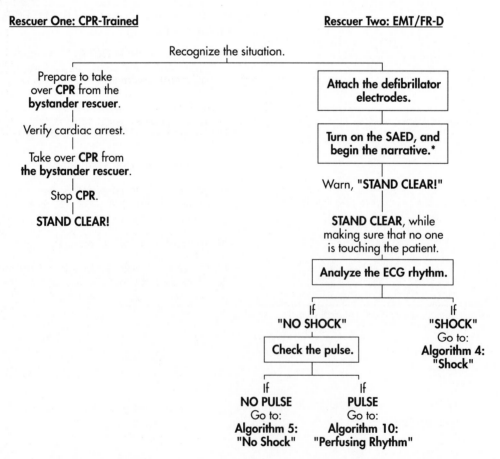

Rescuer One: CPR-Trained   **Rescuer Two: EMT/FR-D**

Recognize the situation.

Prepare to take over **CPR** from the **bystander rescuer**.

Verify cardiac arrest.

Take over **CPR** from the **bystander rescuer**.

Stop **CPR**.

STAND CLEAR!

Attach the defibrillator electrodes.

Turn on the SAED, and begin the narrative.*

Warn, "STAND CLEAR!"

STAND CLEAR, while making sure that no one is touching the patient.

Analyze the ECG rhythm.

If "NO SHOCK"   If "SHOCK"
                       Go to:
Check the pulse.   Algorithm 4: "Shock"

If NO PULSE   If PULSE
Go to: Go to:
Algorithm 5:   Algorithm 10:
"No Shock"   "Perfusing Rhythm"

* Omit the voice recording of the narrative if not required by local protocol.

PROTOCOL 2: Initial Management of Pre-arrival Cardiac Arrest—Two Rescuers, with Bystander CPR

Rescuer one: CPR-trained	Rescuer two: EMT/FR-D
1. Recognize the situation.	1. Recognize the situation and assume control.
2. Introduce yourself to the **bystander rescuer** performing **CPR.**	2. Explain the **SAED** procedure briefly to the bystanders, if appropriate.
3. Request the **bystander rescuer** to continue **CPR** through the next cycle of ventilations and then stop **CPR.**	3. Place the **SAED** next to the patient's head opposite the **bystander rescuer** while noting the time.
4. Take a position beside the patient's shoulder as the **bystander rescuer** completes the ventilations and moves away.	4. Take a position beside the patient's chest opposite the **bystander rescuer.**
5. Palpate the patient's carotid artery for a **spontaneous pulse,** taking 5 to 10 seconds.	5. ☐ **ATTACH THE DEFIBRILLATOR ELECTRODES.**

If the pulse is absent:

6. Announce, **"NO PULSE!"**

7. CONTINUE **one-rescuer CPR.**

   a. Deliver 2 breaths, taking 3 to 5 seconds.
   b. Clear the patient's airway if necessary.
   c. Locate the compression site on the patient's sternum.
   d. Compress the patient's sternum 15 times at a rate of 80 to 100 per minute.
   e. Ventilate 2 times, taking 3 to 5 seconds, between the fifteenth compression and the first one of the next series of compressions.

8. Continue **CPR** at a ratio of 15 chest compressions to 2 rescue breaths until told to **"STAND CLEAR,"** usually within 1 minute.

Rescuer two (continued):

6. ☐ **TURN ON THE SAED, AND BEGIN THE NARRATIVE.***

> **NOTE: Defibrillation takes precedence over CPR! The first shock is delivered as soon as the defibrillator electrodes have been attached, the ECG rhythm analyzed, and "SHOCK" indicated.**

9. Stop **CPR** so that the patient is motionless **while** the ECG rhythm is being analyzed.

10. **STAND CLEAR!**

Rescuer two (continued):

7. Warn, **"STAND CLEAR!"**

8. **STAND CLEAR WHILE MAKING SURE THAT NO ONE, INCLUDING THE BYSTANDER RESCUER AND ANY OTHER BYSTANDER AND BOTH RESCUERS, IS TOUCHING THE PATIENT OR ANYTHING IS IN CONTACT WITH THE PATIENT.**

9. ☐ **ANALYZE THE ECG RHYTHM.**

If **"SHOCK"** is indicated and the PATIENT'S PULSE IS ABSENT:

10. Proceed to **PROTOCOL 4: Management of Cardiac Arrest Following ECG Rhythm Analysis Indicating "SHOCK"—Two Rescuers.**

---

*Omit the voice recording of the narrative if it is not required by local protocol.

Continued.

PROTOCOL 2: Initial Management of Pre-arrival Cardiac Arrest—Two Rescuers, with Bystander CPR, cont'd

Rescuer one: CPR-trained	Rescuer two: EMT/FR-D
	If "NO SHOCK" is indicated:
	11. CHECK THE PATIENT'S PULSE.
	If the patient's PULSE is absent:
	12. Proceed to **PROTOCOL 5: Management of Cardiac Arrest Following ECG Rhythm Analysis Indicating "NO SHOCK"—Two Rescuers.**
	If the patient's PULSE is present:
	13. Proceed to **PROTOCOL 10: Management of a Perfusing Rhythm—One or Two Rescuers.**

Algorithm/Protocol 3

Initial Management of EMT/FR-D-witnessed Cardiac Arrest while on the Scene or en Route—Two Rescuers

ALGORITHM 3 One/Two-Rescuer CPR
PROTOCOL 3a One-Rescuer CPR
PROTOCOL 3b Two-Rescuer CPR

ALGORITHM 3: Initial Management of EMT/FR-D-witnessed Cardiac Arrest while on the Scene or en Route—Two Rescuers

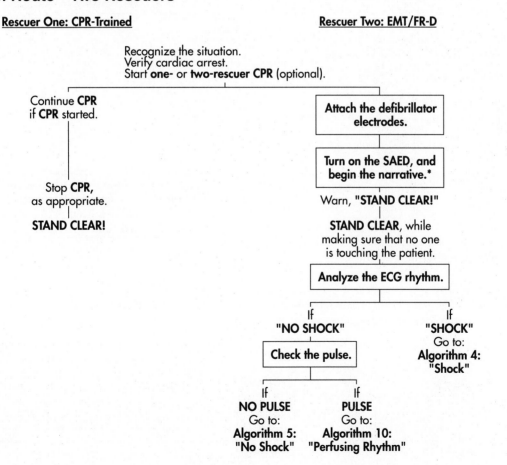

Rescuer One: CPR-Trained   **Rescuer Two: EMT/FR-D**

Recognize the situation.
Verify cardiac arrest.
Start **one-** or **two-rescuer CPR** (optional).

Continue **CPR**
if **CPR** started.

Stop **CPR,**
as appropriate.

STAND CLEAR!

Attach the defibrillator electrodes.

Turn on the SAED, and begin the narrative.*

Warn, "**STAND CLEAR!**"

STAND CLEAR, while making sure that no one is touching the patient.

Analyze the ECG rhythm.

If
"**NO SHOCK**"

Check the pulse.

If
"**SHOCK**"
Go to:
Algorithm 4:
"**Shock**"

If
NO PULSE
Go to:
Algorithm 5:
"**No Shock**"

If
PULSE
Go to:
Algorithm 10:
"**Perfusing Rhythm**"

---

* Omit the voice recording of the narrative if not required by local protocol.

PROTOCOL 3a: Initial Management of EMT/FR-D-witnessed Cardiac Arrest while on the Scene or en Route—Two Rescuers

One-rescuer CPR

Rescuer one: CPR-trained	Rescuer two: EMT/FR-D

Rescuer one: CPR-trained

1. Recognize the situation.

2. Verify cardiac arrest by determining **unresponsiveness**—by shaking the patient and shouting **"ARE YOU OK?"**

If the patient is unresponsive:

3. Start **one-rescuer CPR (optional).**

   a. Make sure that the patient is on a firm flat surface.
   b. Take a position beside the patient's shoulder opposite **rescuer two** (or as appropriate in the ambulance).
   c. Open the patient's airway.
   d. Look, feel, and listen for breathing, taking 3 to 5 seconds.

If breathing is absent:

   e. Announce, **"NO BREATHING!"**
   f. Deliver 2 initial breaths, taking 3 to 5 seconds.
   g. Clear the patient's airway if necessary.
   h. Palpate the patient's carotid artery for a **spontaneous pulse,** taking 5 to 10 seconds.

If the pulse is absent:

   i. Announce, **"NO PULSE!"**
   j. Locate the compression site on the patient's sternum.
   k. Compress the patient's sternum 15 times at a rate of 80 to 100 per minute.
   l. Ventilate 2 times, taking 3 to 5 seconds, between the fifteenth compression and the first one of the next series of compressions.

4. Continue **CPR** at a ratio of 15 chest compressions to 2 rescue breaths until told to **"STAND CLEAR,"** usually within 1 minute.

5. Stop **CPR** so that the patient is motionless **while** the ECG rhythm is being analyzed.

6. **STAND CLEAR!**

Rescuer two: EMT/FR-D

1. Recognize the situation and assume control.

> **NOTE: If cardiac arrest occurs in the ambulance en route to the hospital, request the driver to pull over to the side of the road and stop.**

2. Explain the **SAED** procedure briefly to the bystanders, if appropriate.

3. Place the **SAED** next to the patient's head while noting the time.

4. Take a position beside the patient's chest (or as appropriate in the ambulance).

5. **ATTACH THE DEFIBRILLATOR ELECTRODES.**

6. **TURN ON THE SAED, AND BEGIN THE NARRATIVE.***

> **NOTE: Defibrillation takes precedence over CPR! The first shock is delivered as soon as the defibrillator electrodes have been attached, the ECG rhythm analyzed, and "SHOCK" indicated.**

7. Warn, **"STAND CLEAR!"**

8. **STAND CLEAR WHILE MAKING SURE THAT NO ONE IS TOUCHING THE PATIENT OR ANYTHING IS IN CONTACT WITH THE PATIENT.**

9. **ANALYZE THE ECG RHYTHM.**

---

*Omit the voice recording of the narrative if it is not required by local protocol.   *Continued.*

PROTOCOL 3a: Initial Management of EMT/FR-D-witnessed Cardiac Arrest while on the Scene or en Route—Two Rescuers, cont'd

One-rescuer CPR	
Rescuer one: CPR-trained	**Rescuer two: EMT/FR-D**
	If "SHOCK" is indicated and the PATIENT'S PULSE IS ABSENT:
	10. Proceed to **PROTOCOL 4: Management of Cardiac Arrest Following ECG Rhythm Analysis Indicating "SHOCK"—Two Rescuers.**
	If "NO SHOCK" is indicated:
	11. | **CHECK THE PATIENT'S PULSE.** |
	If the patient's PULSE is absent:
	12. Proceed to **PROTOCOL 5: Management of Cardiac Arrest Following ECG Rhythm Analysis Indicating "NO SHOCK"—Two Rescuers.**
	If the patient's PULSE is present:
	13. Proceed to **PROTOCOL 10: Management of a Perfusing Rhythm—One or Two Rescuers.**

PROTOCOL 3b: Initial Management of EMT/FR-D-witnessed Cardiac Arrest while on the Scene or en Route—Two Rescuers

Two-rescuer CPR	
Rescuer one: CPR-trained	**Rescuer two: EMT/FR-D**
1. Recognize the situation.	1. Recognize the situation and assume control.
2. Verify cardiac arrest by determining **unresponsiveness**—by shaking the patient and shouting **"ARE YOU OK?"**	**NOTE: If cardiac arrest occurs in the ambulance en route to the hospital, request the driver to pull over to the side of the road and stop.**
	2. Explain the **SAED** procedure briefly to the bystanders, if appropriate.
	3. Place the **SAED** next to the patient's head while noting the time.
If the patient is unresponsive:	
3. Start **two-rescuer CPR (optional).**	4. Start **two-rescuer CPR (optional).**
a. Make sure that the patient is on a firm flat surface.	a. Take a position above the patient's head.
b. Take a position beside the patient's chest.	b. Open the patient's airway.
c. Locate the compression site on the patient's sternum.	c. Look, feel, and listen for breathing, taking 3 to 5 seconds.

Continued.

PROTOCOL 3b: Initial Management of EMT/FR-D-witnessed Cardiac Arrest while on the Scene or en Route—Two Rescuers, cont'd

Two-rescuer CPR	
Rescuer one: CPR-trained	**Rescuer two: EMT/FR-D**

Rescuer two: EMT/FR-D

If breathing is absent:

    d. Announce, **"NO BREATHING!"**

    e. Deliver 2 initial breaths, taking 3 to 5 seconds.

    f. Clear the patient's airway if necessary.

    g. Palpate the patient's carotid artery for a **spontaneous pulse,** taking 5 to 10 seconds.

If the pulse is absent:

    h. Announce, **"NO PULSE!"**

Rescuer one:

d. Compress the patient's sternum at a rate of 80 to 100 per minute.

4. CONTINUE CPR until told to **"STAND CLEAR,"** usually within 1 minute.

Rescuer two:

5. | **ATTACH THE DEFIBRILLATOR ELECTRODES.** |

6. | **TURN ON THE SAED, AND BEGIN THE NARRATIVE.*** |

> **NOTE: Defibrillation takes precedence over CPR!** The first shock is delivered as soon as the defibrillator electrodes have been attached, the ECG rhythm analyzed, and "SHOCK" indicated.

Rescuer one:

5. Stop **CPR** so that the patient is motionless **while** the ECG rhythm is being analyzed.

6. STAND CLEAR!

Rescuer two:

7. Warn, **"STAND CLEAR!"**

8. **STAND CLEAR WHILE MAKING SURE THAT NO ONE IS TOUCHING THE PATIENT OR ANYTHING IS IN CONTACT WITH THE PATIENT.**

9. | **ANALYZE THE ECG RHYTHM.** |

If "SHOCK" is indicated and the PATIENT'S PULSE IS ABSENT:

10. Proceed to **PROTOCOL 4: Management of Cardiac Arrest Following ECG Rhythm Analysis Indicating "SHOCK"—Two Rescuers.**

If "NO SHOCK" is indicated:

11. | **CHECK THE PATIENT'S PULSE.** |

If the patient's PULSE is absent:

12. Proceed to **PROTOCOL 5: Management of Cardiac Arrest Following ECG Rhythm Analysis Indicating "NO SHOCK"—Two Rescuers.**

If the patient's PULSE is present:

13. Proceed to **PROTOCOL 10: Management of a Perfusing Rhythm—One or Two Rescuers.**

---

*Omit the voice recording of the narrative if it is not required by local protocol.

Algorithm/Protocol 4

Management of Cardiac Arrest Following ECG Rhythm Analysis Indicating "SHOCK"—Two Rescuers

ALGORITHM 4
PROTOCOL 4

ALGORITHM 4: Management of Cardiac Arrest Following ECG Rhythm Analysis Indicating "SHOCK"—Two Rescuers

If "SHOCK" is indicated **THE FIRST TIME** and the patient's pulse is absent:

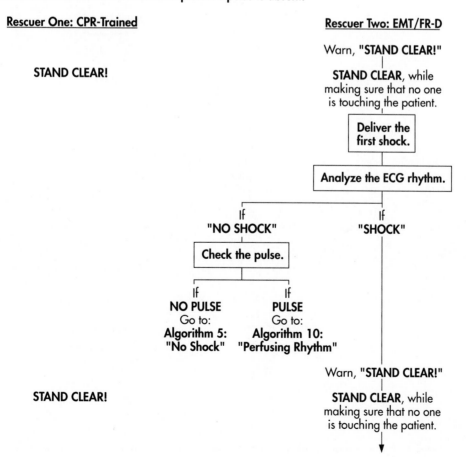

Rescuer One: CPR-Trained

STAND CLEAR!

STAND CLEAR!

Rescuer Two: EMT/FR-D

Warn, **"STAND CLEAR!"**

STAND CLEAR, while making sure that no one is touching the patient.

Deliver the first shock.

Analyze the ECG rhythm.

If "NO SHOCK"

Check the pulse.

If **NO PULSE**
Go to:
Algorithm 5:
"No Shock"

If **PULSE**
Go to:
Algorithm 10:
"Perfusing Rhythm"

If "SHOCK"

Warn, **"STAND CLEAR!"**

STAND CLEAR, while making sure that no one is touching the patient.

Continued.

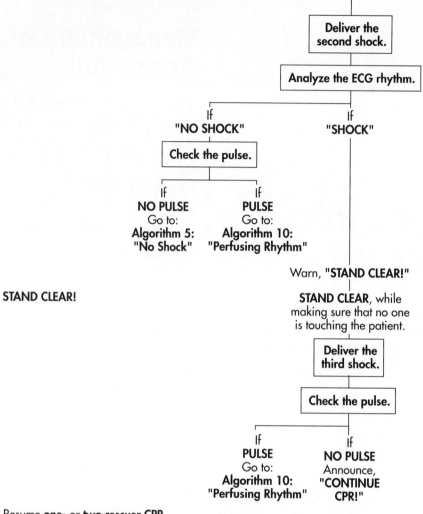

Resume **one-** or **two-rescuer CPR**.

Transport immediately or wait for the BLS or ALS unit, as appropriate, while continuing to perform **CPR**, reanalyzing the patient's ECG rhythm, delivering shocks, and checking the patient's pulse, according to local protocol, as follows:

Continue **one-** or **two-rescuer CPR** for 1 minute.

If en route, stop the ambulance.

Stop **CPR**.

STAND CLEAR!

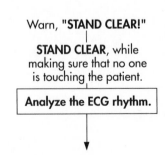

ALGORITHM 4: Management of Cardiac Arrest Following ECG Rhythm Analysis Indicating "SHOCK"—Two Rescuers, cont'd

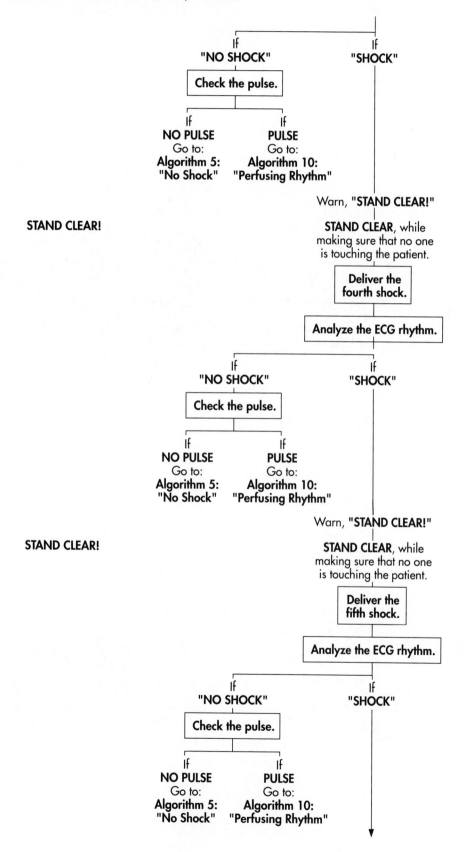

Continued.

ALGORITHM 4: Management of Cardiac Arrest Following ECG Rhythm Analysis Indicating "SHOCK"—Two Rescuers, cont'd

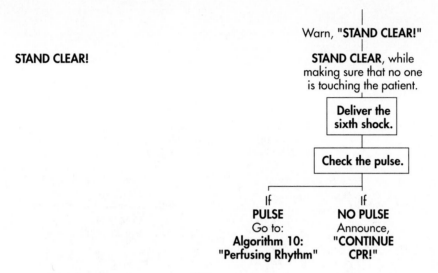

STAND CLEAR!

Warn, **"STAND CLEAR!"**

STAND CLEAR, while making sure that no one is touching the patient.

| Deliver the sixth shock. |

| Check the pulse. |

If
PULSE
Go to:
Algorithm 10:
"Perfusing Rhythm"

If
NO PULSE
Announce,
"CONTINUE CPR!"

Resume **one-** or **two- rescuer CPR.**

Transport immediately or wait for the BLS or ALS unit, as appropriate, while continuing to perform CPR, reanalyzing the patient's ECG rhythm, delivering shocks, and checking the patient's pulse, according to local protocol, as follows:

Continue **one-** or **two-** rescuer CPR for 1 minute.

If en route, stop the ambulance.

Stop **CPR.**

Analyze the ECG rhythm, and go to the appropriate algorithm.

PROTOCOL 4: Management of Cardiac Arrest Following ECG Rhythm Analysis Indicating "SHOCK"—Two Rescuers

If "SHOCK" is indicated THE FIRST TIME and the patient's pulse is absent:

Rescuer one: CPR-trained	Rescuer two:EMT/FR-D
	1. Warn "STAND CLEAR!"
1. STAND CLEAR!	2. STAND CLEAR WHILE MAKING SURE THAT NO ONE IS TOUCHING THE PATIENT OR ANYTHING IN CONTACT WITH THE PATIENT.

NOTE!

If "NO SHOCK" is indicated at any time:

- CHECK THE PATIENT'S PULSE.

If the patient's PULSE is present:
- Proceed to **PROTOCOL 10: Management of a Perfusing Rhythm—One or Two Rescuers.**

If the patient's PULSE is absent:
- Proceed to **PROTOCOL 5: Management of Cardiac Arrest following ECG Rhythm Analysis Indicating "NO SHOCK"—Two Rescuers.**

3. TURN ON THE CHARGING CIRCUIT, IF APPROPRIATE.

When the defibrillator is charged:

4. DELIVER THE FIRST SHOCK.

5. ANALYZE THE ECG RHYTHM.

If "SHOCK" is indicated and the PATIENT'S PULSE IS ABSENT:

6. Warn, "STAND CLEAR!"

2. STAND CLEAR!

7. STAND CLEAR WHILE MAKING SURE THAT NO ONE IS TOUCHING THE PATIENT OR ANYTHING IN CONTACT WITH THE PATIENT.

8. TURN ON THE CHARGING CIRCUIT, IF APPROPRIATE.

When the defibrillator is charged:

9. DELIVER THE SECOND SHOCK.

10. ANALYZE THE ECG RHYTHM.

If "SHOCK" is indicated and the PATIENT'S PULSE IS ABSENT:

11. Warn, "STAND CLEAR!"

3. STAND CLEAR!

12. STAND CLEAR WHILE MAKING SURE THAT NO ONE IS TOUCHING THE PATIENT OR ANYTHING IN CONTACT WITH THE PATIENT.

13. TURN ON THE CHARGING CIRCUIT, IF APPROPRIATE.

Continued.

PROTOCOL 4: Management of Cardiac Arrest Following ECG Rhythm Analysis Indicating "SHOCK"—Two Rescuers, cont'd

Rescuer one: CPR-trained	Rescuer two:EMT/FR-D

When the defibrillator is charged:

14. DELIVER THE THIRD SHOCK.

15. CHECK THE PATIENT'S PULSE.

If the patient's PULSE is absent:

16. Announce, "CONTINUE CPR!"

> **NOTE!**
>
> If a spontaneous pulse appears at any time:
>
> • Proceed to **PROTOCOL 10: Management of a Perfusing Rhythm.**

> **NOTE!**
>
> The total number of shocks delivered depends on the local protocol.

• Resume **one-** or **two-rescuer CPR,** proceed with one of the following options, as appropriate, and continue with the protocol.

A. **If the two rescuers are part of the crew of a BLS ambulance already at the scene AND an ALS unit is en route to the scene with an ESTIMATED TIME OF ARRIVAL GREATER THAN 8 MINUTES:**

OR

If an ALS unit is not available:

OR

If the BLS ambulance is to connect up with an ALS unit en route:

   • **TRANSPORT IMMEDIATELY, WHILE CONTINUING TO PERFORM CPR, REANALYZING THE PATIENT'S ECG RHYTHM, DELIVERING SHOCKS, AND CHECKING THE PATIENT'S PULSE EN ROUTE, ACCORDING TO LOCAL PROTOCOL.**

B. **If the two rescuers are part of the crew of a BLS ambulance already at the scene AND and ALS unit is en route to the scene with an ESTIMATED TIME OF ARRIVAL LESS THAN 8 MINUTES:**

   • **WAIT FOR THE ARRIVAL OF THE ALS UNIT, WHILE CONTINUING TO PERFORM CPR, REANALYZING THE PATIENT'S ECG RHYTHM, DELIVERING SHOCKS, AND CHECKING THE PATIENT'S PULSE, ACCORDING TO LOCAL PROTOCOL.**

C. **If the two rescuers are part of a first responder unit:**

   • **WAIT FOR THE ARRIVAL OF THE BLS OR ALS UNIT, AS APPROPRIATE, WHILE CONTINUING TO PERFORM CPR, REANALYZING THE PATIENT'S ECG RHYTHM, DELIVERING SHOCKS, AND CHECKING THE PATIENT'S PULSE, ACCORDING TO LOCAL PROTOCOL.**

Continued.

PROTOCOL 4: Management of Cardiac Arrest Following ECG Rhythm Analysis Indicating "SHOCK"—Two Rescuers, cont'd

If "SHOCK" is indicated THE FIRST TIME and the patient's pulse is absent:

Rescuer one: CPR-trained	Rescuer two:EMT/FR-D

> **D. If the two rescuers and the patient are already en route to the hospital:**
> - **RESUME TRANSPORT IMMEDIATELY, WHILE CONTINUING TO PERFORM CPR, REAN-ALYZING THE PATIENT'S ECG RHYTHM, DELIVERING SHOCKS, AND CHECKING THE PATIENT'S PULSE EN ROUTE, ACCORDING TO LOCAL PROTOCOL.**

- Continue **CPR** for 1 minute.

17. If en route to the hospital, request the driver to pull over to the side of the road and stop.

- Stop **CPR.**

18. Warn, **"STAND CLEAR!"**

4. STAND CLEAR!

19. STAND CLEAR WHILE MAKING SURE THAT NO ONE IS TOUCHING THE PATIENT OR ANYTHING IS IN CONTACT WITH THE PATIENT.

20. ANALYZE THE ECG RHYTHM.

If "SHOCK" is indicated and the PATIENT'S PULSE IS ABSENT:

21. Warn, **"STAND CLEAR!"**

5. STAND CLEAR!

22. STAND CLEAR WHILE MAKING SURE THAT NO ONE IS TOUCHING THE PATIENT OR ANYTHING IN CONTACT WITH THE PATIENT.

23. TURN ON THE CHARGING CIRCUIT, IF APPROPRIATE.

> **NOTE!**
>
> **If "NO SHOCK" is indicated at any time:**
>
> - CHECK THE PATIENT'S PULSE.
>
> **If the patient's PULSE is present:**
> - Proceed to **PROTOCOL 10: Management of a Perfusing Rhythm—One or Two Rescuers.**
>
> **If the patient's PULSE is absent:**
> - Proceed to **PROTOCOL 5: Management of Cardiac Arrest Following ECG Rhythm Analysis Indicating "NO SHOCK"—Two Rescuers.**

When the defibrillator is charged:

24. DELIVER THE FOURTH SHOCK.

25. ANALYZE THE ECG RHYTHM.

If "SHOCK" is indicated and the PATIENT'S PULSE IS ABSENT:

26. Warn, **"STAND CLEAR!"**

6. STAND CLEAR!

27. STAND CLEAR WHILE MAKING SURE THAT NO ONE IS TOUCHING THE PATIENT OR ANYTHING IS IN CONTACT WITH THE PATIENT.

28. TURN ON THE CHARGING CIRCUIT, IF APPROPRIATE.

Continued.

PROTOCOL 4: Management of Cardiac Arrest Following ECG Rhythm Analysis Indicating "SHOCK"—Two Rescuers, cont'd

Rescuer one: CPR-trained   **Rescuer two: EMT/FR-D**

When the defibrillator is charged:

29. | **DELIVER THE FIFTH SHOCK.** |

30. | **ANALYZE THE ECG RHYTHM.** |

If "SHOCK" is indicated and the PATIENT'S PULSE IS ABSENT:

31. Warn, "STAND CLEAR!"

7. STAND CLEAR!

32. **STAND CLEAR WHILE MAKING SURE THAT NO ONE IS TOUCHING THE PATIENT OR ANYTHING IS IN CONTACT WITH THE PATIENT.**

33. | **TURN ON THE CHARGING CIRCUIT, IF APPROPRIATE.** |

When the defibrillator is charged:

34. | **DELIVER THE SIXTH SHOCK.** |

35. | **CHECK THE PATIENT'S PULSE.** |

If the patient's PULSE is absent:

36. Announce, "CONTINUE CPR!"

NOTE!
If a spontaneous pulse appears at any time: • Proceed to **PROTOCOL 10: Management of a Perfusing Rhythm.**

NOTE!
The total number of shocks delivered depends on the local protocol.

• Resume **one-** or **two-rescuer CPR,** and proceed with **OPTION A, B, C,** or **D** outlined above, as appropriate, and continue with the protocol.

Algorithm/Protocol 5

Management of Cardiac Arrest Following ECG Rhythm Analysis Indicating "NO SHOCK"—Two Rescuers

ALGORITHM 5
PROTOCOL 5

ALGORITHM 5: Management of Cardiac Arrest Following ECG Rhythm Analysis Indicating "NO SHOCK"—Two Rescuers

If "NO SHOCK" is indicated THE FIRST TIME and the patient's pulse is absent:

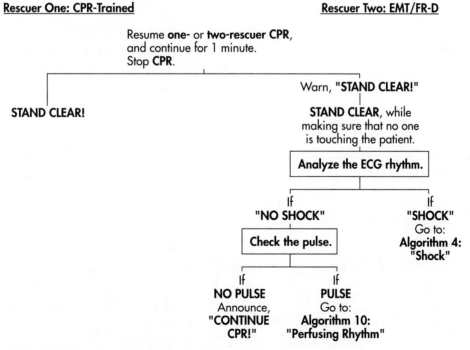

Rescuer One: CPR-Trained   **Rescuer Two: EMT/FR-D**

Resume **one-** or **two-rescuer CPR**, and continue for 1 minute. Stop **CPR**.

STAND CLEAR!

Warn, **"STAND CLEAR!"**

STAND CLEAR, while making sure that no one is touching the patient.

Analyze the ECG rhythm.

If "NO SHOCK" — Check the pulse.

If "SHOCK" Go to: **Algorithm 4: "Shock"**

If NO PULSE Announce, **"CONTINUE CPR!"**

If PULSE Go to: **Algorithm 10: "Perfusing Rhythm"**

Resume **one-** or **two-rescuer CPR**.

Transport immediately or wait for the BLS or ALS unit, as appropriate, while continuing to perform **CPR**, reanalyzing the ECG rhythm, every 1 to 3 minutes, and checking the patient's pulse, according to local protocol.

PROTOCOL 5: Management of Cardiac Arrest Following ECG Rhythm Analysis Indicating "NO SHOCK"—Two Rescuers

If "NO SHOCK" is indicated THE FIRST TIME and the patient's pulse is absent:

Rescuer one: CPR-trained	Rescuer two: EMT/FR-D
	• Resume **one-** or **two-rescuer CPR,** and continue for 1 minute.
	• Stop **CPR.**
	1. Warn, "STAND CLEAR!"
1. STAND CLEAR!	2. **STAND CLEAR WHILE MAKING SURE THAT NO ONE IS TOUCHING THE PATIENT OR ANYTHING IN CONTACT WITH THE PATIENT.**
	3. ANALYZE THE ECG RHYTHM.
	If "SHOCK" is indicated and the PATIENT'S PULSE IS ABSENT:
	4. Proceed to **PROTOCOL 4: Management of Cardiac Arrest Following ECG Rhythm Analysis Indicating "SHOCK"—Two Rescuers.**
	If "NO SHOCK" is indicated:
	5. CHECK THE PATIENT'S PULSE.
	If the patient's PULSE is present:
	6. Proceed to **PROTOCOL 10: Management of a Perfusing Rhythm—One or Two Rescuers.**
	If the patient's PULSE is absent:
	7. Announce, "CONTINUE CPR!"

• Resume **one-** or **two-rescuer CPR,** and proceed with one of the following options, as appropriate:

A. **If the two rescuers are part of the crew of a BLS ambulance already at the scene AND an ALS unit is en route to the scene with an ESTIMATED TIME OF ARRIVAL GREATER THAN 8 MINUTES:**

OR

If an ALS unit is not available:

OR

If the BLS ambulance is to connect up with an ALS unit en route:

• **TRANSPORT IMMEDIATELY, WHILE CONTINUING TO PERFORM CPR, REANALYZING THE ECG RHYTHM EVERY 1 TO 3 MINUTES, AND CHECKING THE PATIENT'S PULSE EN ROUTE, ACCORDING TO LOCAL PROTOCOL.**

Continued.

PROTOCOL 5: Management of Cardiac Arrest Following ECG Rhythm Analysis Indicating "NO SHOCK"—Two Rescuers, cont'd

Rescuer one: CPR-trained   Rescuer two: EMT/FR-

B. If the two rescuers are part of the crew of a BLS ambulance already at the scene AND an ALS unit is en route to the scene with an ESTIMATED TIME OF ARRIVAL LESS THAN 8 MINUTES:

- WAIT FOR THE ARRIVAL OF THE ALS UNIT, WHILE CONTINUING TO PERFORM CPR, REANALYZING THE ECG RHYTHM EVERY 1 TO 3 MINUTES, AND CHECKING THE PATIENT'S PULSE, ACCORDING TO LOCAL PROTOCOL.

C. If the two rescuers are part of a first responder unit:

- WAIT FOR THE ARRIVAL OF THE BLS OR ALS UNIT, AS APPROPRIATE, WHILE CONTINUING TO PERFORM CPR, REANALYZING THE ECG RHYTHM EVERY 1 TO 3 MINUTES, AND CHECKING THE PATIENT'S PULSE, ACCORDING TO LOCAL PROTOCOL.

D. If the two rescuers and the patient are already en route to the hospital:

- RESUME TRANSPORT IMMEDIATELY, WHILE CONTINUING TO PERFORM CPR, REANALYZING THE ECG RHYTHM EVERY 1 TO 3 MINUTES, AND CHECKING THE PATIENT'S PULSE EN ROUTE, ACCORDING TO LOCAL PROTOCOL.

Algorithm/Protocol 6

Initial Management of Pre-arrival Cardiac Arrest or EMT/FR-D-witnessed Cardiac Arrest While on the Scene—One Rescuer, Without Bystander CPR

ALGORITHM 6
PROTOCOL 6

ALGORITHM 6: Initial Management of Pre-arrival Cardiac Arrest or EMT/FR-D-witnessed Cardiac Arrest while on the Scene—One Rescuer, without Bystander CPR

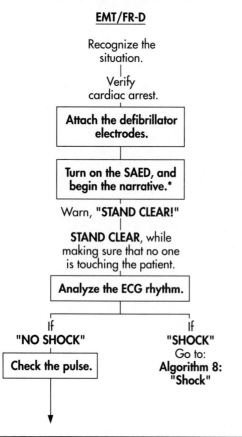

EMT/FR-D

Recognize the situation.
|
Verify cardiac arrest.

Attach the defibrillator electrodes.

Turn on the SAED, and begin the narrative.*

Warn, **"STAND CLEAR!"**
|
STAND CLEAR, while making sure that no one is touching the patient.

Analyze the ECG rhythm.

If **"NO SHOCK"**

Check the pulse.

If **"SHOCK"**
Go to:
Algorithm 8: "Shock"

NOTE!

Defibrillation takes precedence over CPR if the EMT/FR-D is alone and no other person trained in CPR is available!

---

* Omit the voice recording of the narrative if it is not required by local protocol.

Continued.

ALGORITHM 6: Initial Management of Pre-arrival Cardiac Arrest or EMT/FR-D-witnessed Cardiac Arrest while on the Scene—One Rescuer, without Bystander CPR, cont'd

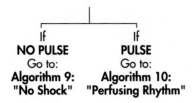

If	If
NO PULSE	**PULSE**
Go to:	Go to:
Algorithm 9:	**Algorithm 10:**
"No Shock"	**"Perfusing Rhythm"**

PROTOCOL 6: Initial Management of Pre-arrival Cardiac Arrest or EMT/FR-D-witnessed Cardiac Arrest while on the Scene—One Rescuer, Without Bystander CPR

EMT/FR-D

1. Recognize the situation and assume control.

2. Verify cardiac arrest by determining **unresponsiveness**—by shaking the patient and shouting **"ARE YOU OK?"**

If the patient is unresponsive:

3. Make sure that the patient is on a firm flat surface **while** explaining the **SAED** procedure briefly to the bystanders, if appropriate.

4. Determine **breathlessness and pulselessness.**

If the pulse and respirations are absent:

5. Place the **SAED** on the floor next to the patient's head while noting the time.

6. Take a position beside the patient's chest.

7. | **ATTACH THE DEFIBRILLATOR ELECTRODES.** |

8. | **TURN ON THE SAED, AND BEGIN THE NARRATIVE.*** |

9. Warn, **"STAND CLEAR!"**

10. **STAND CLEAR WHILE MAKING SURE THAT NO ONE IS TOUCHING THE PATIENT OR ANYTHING IN CONTACT WITH THE PATIENT.**

11. | **ANALYZE THE ECG RHYTHM.** |

> **NOTE!**
>
> **DEFIBRILLATION TAKES PRECEDENCE OVER CPR IF THE EMT/FR-D IS ALONE AND NO OTHER PERSON TRAINED IN CPR IS AVAILABLE!**

---

*Omit the voice recording of the narrative if it is not required by local protocol.   *Continued.*

PROTOCOL 6: Initial Management of Pre-arrival Cardiac Arrest or EMT/FR-D-witnessed Cardiac Arrest while on the Scene—One Rescuer, Without Bystander CPR, cont'd

---

EMT/FR-D

If "SHOCK" is indicated and the PATIENT'S PULSE IS ABSENT:

12. Proceed to **PROTOCOL 8: Management of Cardiac Arrest Following ECG Rhythm Analysis Indicating "SHOCK"—One Rescuer.**

If "NO SHOCK" is indicated:

13. | CHECK THE PATIENT'S PULSE. |

If the patient's PULSE is absent:

14. Proceed to **PROTOCOL 9: Management of Cardiac Arrest Following ECG Rhythm Analysis Indicating "NO SHOCK"—One Rescuer.**

If the patient's PULSE is present:

15. Proceed to **PROTOCOL 10: Management of a Perfusing Rhythm—One or Two Rescuers.**

Algorithm/Protocol 7

Initial Management of Pre-arrival Cardiac Arrest—One Rescuer, with Bystander CPR

ALGORITHM 7
PROTOCOL 7

ALGORITHM 7: Initial Management of Pre-arrival Cardiac Arrest—One Rescuer, with Bystander CPR

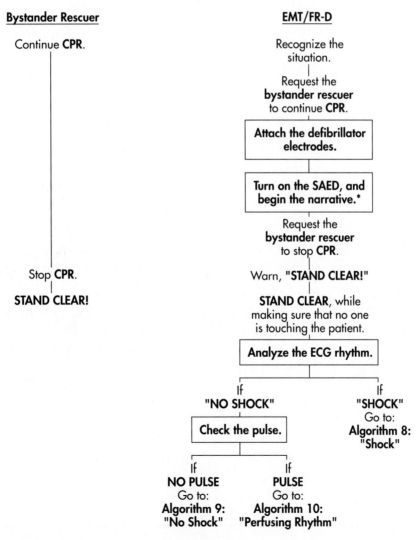

Bystander Rescuer | EMT/FR-D

Continue **CPR**.

Recognize the situation.

Request the **bystander rescuer** to continue **CPR**.

Attach the defibrillator electrodes.

Turn on the SAED, and begin the narrative.*

Request the **bystander rescuer** to stop **CPR**.

Stop **CPR**.
STAND CLEAR!

Warn, "**STAND CLEAR!**"

STAND CLEAR, while making sure that no one is touching the patient.

Analyze the ECG rhythm.

If "NO SHOCK"

If "SHOCK" Go to: Algorithm 8: "Shock"

Check the pulse.

If NO PULSE Go to: Algorithm 9: "No Shock"

If PULSE Go to: Algorithm 10: "Perfusing Rhythm"

---

* Omit the voice recording of the narrative if it is not required by local protocol.

PROTOCOL 7: Initial Management of Pre-arrival Cardiac Arrest—One Rescuer, with Bystander CPR

Bystander rescuer	EMT/FR-D
1. Continue **CPR.**	**1.** Recognize the situation and assume control.
	2. Introduce yourself to the **bystander rescuer** performing **CPR.**
	3. Request the **bystander rescuer** to continue **CPR.**
	4. Explain the **SAED** procedure briefly to the bystanders, if appropriate.
	5. Place the **SAED** next to the patient's head opposite the **bystander rescuer** while noting the time.
	6. Take a position beside the patient's chest opposite the **bystander rescuer.**
	7. ATTACH THE DEFIBRILLATOR ELECTRODES.
	8. TURN ON THE SAED, AND BEGIN THE NARRATIVE.*
	NOTE! Defibrillation takes precedence over CPR! The first shock is delivered as soon as the defibrillator electrodes have been attached, the ECG rhythm analyzed, and "SHOCK" indicated.
	9. Request the **bystander rescuer** to stop **CPR.**
2. Stop **CPR.**	**10.** Warn, "STAND CLEAR!"
3. STAND CLEAR!	**11.** STAND CLEAR WHILE MAKING SURE THAT NO ONE, INCLUDING THE BYSTANDER RESCUER AND ANY OTHER BYSTANDER, IS TOUCHING THE PATIENT OR ANYTHING IN CONTACT WITH THE PATIENT.
	12. ANALYZE THE ECG RHYTHM.
	If "SHOCK" is indicated and the PATIENT'S PULSE IS ABSENT:
	13. Proceed to **PROTOCOL 8: Management of Cardiac Arrest Following ECG Rhythm Analysis Indicating "SHOCK"—One Rescuer.**
	If "NO SHOCK" is indicated:
	14. CHECK THE PATIENT'S PULSE.

*Omit the voice recording of the narrative if it is not required by local protocol.   *Continued.*

PROTOCOL 7: Initial Management of Pre-arrival Cardiac Arrest—One Rescuer, with Bystander CPR, cont'd

Bystander rescuer	EMT/FR-D
	If the patient's PULSE is absent: 15. Proceed to **PROTOCOL 9: Management of Cardiac Arrest Following ECG Rhythm Analysis Indicating "NO SHOCK"—One Rescuer.** **If the patient's PULSE is present:** 16. Proceed to **PROTOCOL 10: Management of a Perfusing Rhythm—One or Two Rescuers.**

Management of Cardiac Arrest Following ECG Rhythm Analysis Indicating "SHOCK"—One Rescuer

ALGORITHM 8
PROTOCOL 8

ALGORITHM 8: Management of Cardiac Arrest Following ECG Rhythm Analysis Indicating "SHOCK"—One Rescuer

If "SHOCK" is indicated THE FIRST TIME and the patient's pulse is absent:

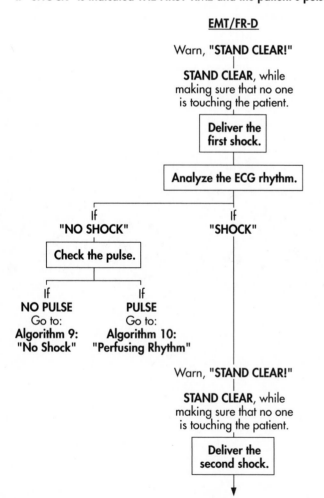

EMT/FR-D

Warn, "**STAND CLEAR!**"

STAND CLEAR, while making sure that no one is touching the patient.

| Deliver the first shock. |

| Analyze the ECG rhythm. |

If "NO SHOCK"

| Check the pulse. |

If NO PULSE
Go to:
Algorithm 9:
"No Shock"

If PULSE
Go to:
Algorithm 10:
"Perfusing Rhythm"

If "SHOCK"

Warn, "**STAND CLEAR!**"

STAND CLEAR, while making sure that no one is touching the patient.

| Deliver the second shock. |

Continued.

ALGORITHM 8: Management of Cardiac Arrest Following ECG Rhythm Analysis Indicating "SHOCK"—ONE Rescuer, cont'd

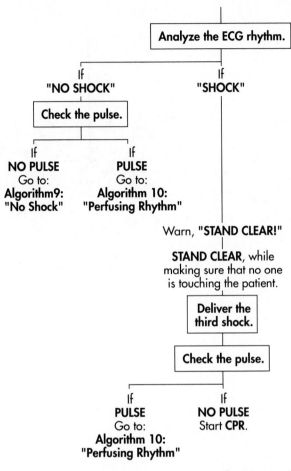

Analyze the ECG rhythm.

If **"NO SHOCK"**

Check the pulse.

If **NO PULSE**
Go to:
Algorithm9:
"No Shock"

If **PULSE**
Go to:
Algorithm 10:
"Perfusing Rhythm"

If **"SHOCK"**

Warn, **"STAND CLEAR!"**

STAND CLEAR, while making sure that no one is touching the patient.

Deliver the third shock.

Check the pulse.

If **PULSE**
Go to:
Algorithm 10:
"Perfusing Rhythm"

If **NO PULSE**
Start **CPR**.

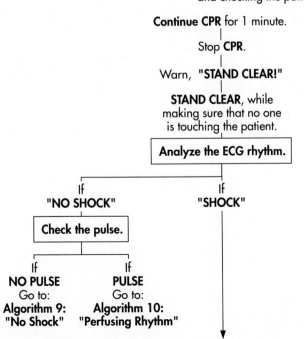

Wait for the arrival of the BLS or ALS unit, as appropriate, while continuing to perform **CPR**, reanalyzing the patient's ECG rhythm, delivering shocks, and checking the patient's pulse, according to local protocol, as follows:

Continue CPR for 1 minute.

Stop **CPR**.

Warn, **"STAND CLEAR!"**

STAND CLEAR, while making sure that no one is touching the patient.

Analyze the ECG rhythm.

If **"NO SHOCK"**

Check the pulse.

If **NO PULSE**
Go to:
Algorithm 9:
"No Shock"

If **PULSE**
Go to:
Algorithm 10:
"Perfusing Rhythm"

If **"SHOCK"**

Continued.

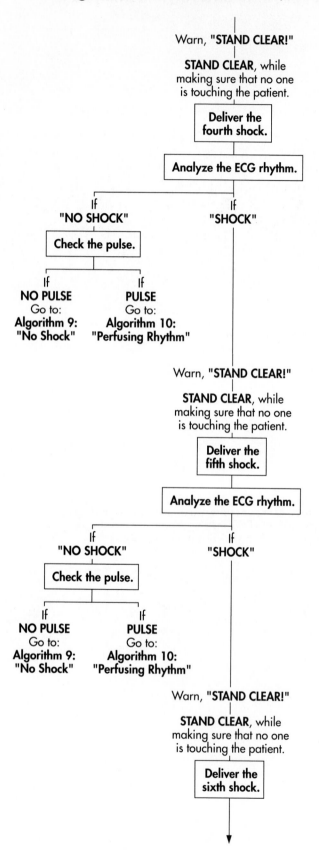

Warn, **"STAND CLEAR!"**

STAND CLEAR, while making sure that no one is touching the patient.

Deliver the fourth shock.

Analyze the ECG rhythm.

If **"NO SHOCK"**

Check the pulse.

If **NO PULSE**
Go to:
Algorithm 9: "No Shock"

If **PULSE**
Go to:
Algorithm 10: "Perfusing Rhythm"

If **"SHOCK"**

Warn, **"STAND CLEAR!"**

STAND CLEAR, while making sure that no one is touching the patient.

Deliver the fifth shock.

Analyze the ECG rhythm.

If **"NO SHOCK"**

Check the pulse.

If **NO PULSE**
Go to:
Algorithm 9: "No Shock"

If **PULSE**
Go to:
Algorithm 10: "Perfusing Rhythm"

If **"SHOCK"**

Warn, **"STAND CLEAR!"**

STAND CLEAR, while making sure that no one is touching the patient.

Deliver the sixth shock.

Continued.

ALGORITHM 8: Management of Cardiac Arrest Following ECG Rhythm Analysis Indicating "SHOCK"—ONE Rescuer, cont'd

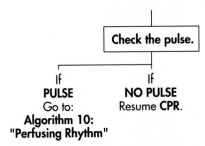

Check the pulse.

If
PULSE
Go to:
Algorithm 10:
"Perfusing Rhythm"

If
NO PULSE
Resume **CPR**.

Wait for the arrival of the BLS or ALS unit, as appropriate, while continuing to perform **CPR**, reanalyzing the patient's ECG rhythm, delivering shocks, and checking the patient's pulse, according to local protocol, as follows:

Continue **CPR** for 1 minute.

Stop **CPR**.

Analyze the ECG rhythm, and go to the appropriate algorithm.

PROTOCOL 8: Management of Cardiac Arrest Following ECG Rhythm Analysis Indicating "SHOCK"—One Rescuer

If "SHOCK" is indicated THE FIRST TIME and the patient's pulse is absent:

EMT/FR-D

1. Warn, "STAND CLEAR!"

2. STAND CLEAR WHILE MAKING SURE THAT NO ONE IS TOUCHING THE PATIENT OR ANYTHING IS IN CONTACT WITH THE PATIENT.

3. | TURN ON THE CHARGING CIRCUIT, IF APPROPRIATE. |

When the defibrillator is charged:

4. | DELIVER THE FIRST SHOCK. |

5. | ANALYZE THE ECG RHYTHM. |

If "SHOCK" is indicated and the PATIENT'S PULSE IS ABSENT:

6. Warn, "STAND CLEAR!"

7. STAND CLEAR WHILE MAKING SURE THAT NO ONE IS TOUCHING THE PATIENT OR ANYTHING IS IN CONTACT WITH THE PATIENT.

8. | TURN ON THE CHARGING CIRCUIT, IF APPROPRIATE. |

When the defibrillator is charged:

9. | DELIVER THE SECOND SHOCK. |

10. | ANALYZE THE ECG RHYTHM. |

If "SHOCK" is indicated and the PATIENT'S PULSE IS ABSENT:

11. Warn, "STAND CLEAR!"

12. STAND CLEAR WHILE MAKING SURE THAT NO ONE IS TOUCHING THE PATIENT OR ANYTHING IS IN CONTACT WITH THE PATIENT.

13. | TURN ON THE CHARGING CIRCUIT, IF APPROPRIATE. |

When the defibrillator is charged:

14. | DELIVER THE THIRD SHOCK. |

NOTE!

If "NO SHOCK" is indicated at any time:

- | CHECK THE PATIENT'S PULSE. |

If the patient's PULSE is present:

- Proceed to **PROTOCOL 10: Management of a Perfusing Rhythm—One or Two Rescuers.**

If the patient's PULSE is absent:

- Proceed to **PROTOCOL 9: Management of Cardiac Arrest Following ECG Rhythm Analysis Indicating "NO SHOCK"—One Rescuer.**

Continued.

PROTOCOL 8: Management of Cardiac Arrest Following ECG Rhythm Analysis Indicating "SHOCK"—One Rescuer, cont'd

EMT/FR-D

15. | **CHECK THE PATIENT'S PULSE.** |

If the patient's PULSE is absent:

16. Start **CPR,** and continue for 1 minute.

NOTE!

If a spontaneous pulse appears at any time:

- Proceed to **PROTOCOL 10: Management of a Perfusing Rhythm.**

NOTE!

The total number of shocks delivered depends on the local protocol.

---

17. Stop **CPR.**

18. Warn, **"STAND CLEAR!"**

19. **STAND CLEAR WHILE MAKING SURE THAT NO ONE IS TOUCHING THE PATIENT OR ANYTHING IN CONTACT WITH THE PATIENT.**

20. | **ANALYZE THE ECG RHYTHM.** |

If "SHOCK" is indicated and the PATIENT'S PULSE IS ABSENT:

21. Warn, **"STAND CLEAR!"**

22. **STAND CLEAR WHILE MAKING SURE THAT NO ONE IS TOUCHING THE PATIENT OR ANYTHING IS IN CONTACT WITH THE PATIENT.**

23. | **TURN ON THE CHARGING CIRCUIT, IF APPROPRIATE.** |

When the defibrillator is charged:

24. | **DELIVER THE FOURTH SHOCK.** |

25. | **ANALYZE THE ECG RHYTHM.** |

If "SHOCK" is indicated and the PATIENT'S PULSE IS ABSENT:

26. Warn, **"STAND CLEAR!"**

NOTE!

If "NO SHOCK" is indicated at any time:

- | **CHECK THE PATIENT'S PULSE.** |

  If the patient's PULSE is present:

  - Proceed to **PROTOCOL 10: Management of a Perfusing Rhythm—One or Two Rescuers.**

  If the patient's PULSE is absent:

  - Proceed to **PROTOCOL 9: Management of Cardiac Arrest Following ECG Rhythm Analysis Indicating "NO SHOCK"—One Rescuer.**

Continued.

PROTOCOL 8: Management of Cardiac Arrest Following ECG Rhythm Analysis Indicating "SHOCK"—One Rescuer, cont'd

EMT/FR-D

27. STAND CLEAR WHILE MAKING SURE THAT NO ONE IS TOUCHING THE PATIENT OR ANYTHING IS IN CONTACT WITH THE PATIENT.

28. | TURN ON THE CHARGING CIRCUIT, IF APPROPRIATE. |

When the defibrillator is charged:

29. | DELIVER THE FIFTH SHOCK. |

30. | ANALYZE THE ECG RHYTHM. |

If "SHOCK" is indicated and the PATIENT'S PULSE IS ABSENT:

31. Warn, "STAND CLEAR!"

32. STAND CLEAR WHILE MAKING SURE THAT NO ONE IS TOUCHING THE PATIENT OR ANYTHING IS IN CONTACT WITH THE PATIENT.

33. | TURN ON THE CHARGING CIRCUIT, IF APPROPRIATE. |

When the defibrillator is charged:

34. | DELIVER THE SIXTH SHOCK. |

35. | CHECK THE PATIENT'S PULSE. |

If the patient's PULSE is absent:

36. Resume **CPR**.

NOTE!

If a spontaneous pulse appears at any time:

- Proceed to **PROTOCOL 10: Management of a Perfusing Rhythm.**

NOTE!

The total number of shocks delivered depends on the local protocol.

---

37. Wait for the arrival of the BLS or ALS unit, as appropriate, while continuing to perform **CPR,** reanalyzing the patient's ECG rhythm, delivering shocks, and checking the patient's pulse, according to local protocol.

Algorithm/Protocol 9

Management of Cardiac Arrest Following ECG Rhythm Analysis Indicating "NO SHOCK"—One Rescuer

ALGORITHM 9
PROTOCOL 9

ALGORITHM 9: Management of Cardiac Arrest Following ECG Rhythm Analysis Indicating "NO SHOCK"—One Rescuer

If "NO SHOCK" is indicated THE FIRST TIME and the patient's pulse is absent:

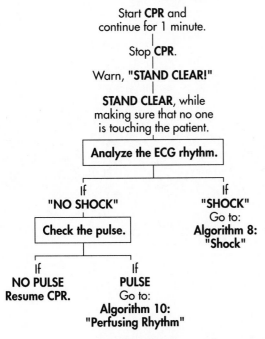

EMT/FR-D

Start **CPR** and
continue for 1 minute.

Stop **CPR**.

Warn, **"STAND CLEAR!"**

STAND CLEAR, while
making sure that no one
is touching the patient.

| Analyze the ECG rhythm. |

If
"NO SHOCK"

If
"SHOCK"
Go to:
**Algorithm 8:
"Shock"**

| Check the pulse. |

If
NO PULSE
Resume CPR.

If
PULSE
Go to:
**Algorithm 10:
"Perfusing Rhythm"**

Wait for the BLS or ALS unit, as appropriate, while continuing
to perform **CPR**, reanalyzing the ECG rhythm every 1 to 3 minutes,
and checking the patient's pulse at the scene, according to
local protocol.

PROTOCOL 9: Management of Cardiac Arrest Following ECG Rhythm Analysis Indicating "NO SHOCK"—One Rescuer

If "NO SHOCK" is indicated THE FIRST TIME and the patient's pulse is absent:

EMT/FR-D

1. Start **CPR,** and continue for 1 minute (i.e., 4 cycles of 15 external chest compressions and 2 ventilations).

2. Stop **CPR.**

3. Warn, **"STAND CLEAR!"**

4. **STAND CLEAR WHILE MAKING SURE THAT NO ONE IS TOUCHING THE PATIENT OR ANYTHING IS IN CONTACT WITH THE PATIENT.**

5. | **ANALYZE THE ECG RHYTHM.** |

If "SHOCK" is indicated and the PATIENT'S PULSE IS ABSENT:

6. Proceed to **PROTOCOL 8: Management of Cardiac Arrest Following ECG Rhythm Analysis Indicating "SHOCK"—One Rescuer.**

If "NO SHOCK" is indicated:

7. | **CHECK THE PATIENT'S PULSE.** |

If the patient's PULSE is present:

8. Proceed to **PROTOCOL 10: Management of a Perfusing Rhythm—One or Two Rescuers.**

If the patient's PULSE is absent:

9. Resume **CPR.**

10. Wait for the arrival of the BLS or ALS unit, as appropriate, while continuing to perform **CPR,** reanalyzing the patient's ECG rhythm every 1 to 3 minutes, and checking the patient's pulse, according to local protocol.

Algorithm/Protocol 10

Management of Perfusing Rhythm— One or Two Rescuers

ALGORITHM 10
PROTOCOL 10

ALGORITHM 10: Management of Prefusing Rhythm—One or Two Rescuers

Establish and maintain
an open airway.

Determine the adequacy
of the patient's
circulation.

Administer high
concentration oxygen.

Suction the airway
as necessary.

Obtain and record
the vital signs.

Transport or wait
for the BLS or ALS unit,
as appropriate,
Keeping the patient warm.

**If the patient's respiratory rate is or becomes less than 12 per minute or the respirations
are or become shallow:**

OR

If the patient is or becomes unconscious:

Insert an oropharygeal
or a nasopharyngeal
airway, as appropriate.

Provide ventilatory
assistance using high
concentration oxygen.

PROTOCOL 10: Management of a Perfusing Rhythm—One or Two Rescuers

1. Establish and maintain an **open airway.**

2. Suction the airway as necessary.

3. Determine if the patient's circulation is adequate.

4. Administer high concentration oxygen by a nonre-breathing mask with a reservoir bag at a flow rate of 10 to 15 liters per minutes. If a face mask is not tolerated, administer the oxygen by a nasal cannula at 6 liters per minute.

5. Obtain and record the vital signs, and repeat them at least every 5 minutes or as often as possible, circumstances permitting.

If the adult patient's respiratory rate is or becomes less than 12 per minute or the respirations become or are shallow and the patient is confused, restless, or cyanotic:

6. Insert an oropharyngeal airway if the gag reflex is absent or a nasopharyngeal airway if gag reflex is present.

7. Assist the patient's ventilation with high concentration oxygen using a bag-valve-mask (BVM) with an oxygen reservoir, a manually triggered oxygen-powered resuscitator, or an automatic ventilator.

NOTE!
ADEQUATE VENTILATION REQUIRES DISABLING THE POP-OFF VALVE IF THE BAG-VALVE-MASK IS SO EQUIPPED.

8. Evaluate the **effectiveness** of the ventilations.

If the patient is or becomes unconscious:

9. Insert an oropharyngeal airway if the gag reflex is absent or a nasopharyngeal airway if the gag reflex is present.

10. Ventilate the patient with high concentration oxygen using a bag-valve-mask (BVM) with an oxygen reservoir, a manually triggered oxygen-powered resuscitator, or an automatic ventilator.

11. **If cardiac arrest recurs** proceed to **PROTOCOL 11: Management of Recurrent Cardiac Arrest—One or Two Rescuers.**

12. Transport or resume transport immediately or wait for the BLS or ALS unit, as appropriate.

If two rescuers are present:

A. **If the two rescuers are part of the crew of a BLS ambulance already at the scene AND an ALS unit is en route to the scene with an ESTIMATED TIME OF ARRIVAL GREATER THAN 8 MINUTES:**

OR

If an ALS unit is not available:

OR

If the BLS ambulance is to connect up with an ALS unit en route:

- **TRANSPORT IMMEDIATELY.**

B. **If the two rescuers are part of the crew of a BLS ambulance already at the scene AND an ALS unit is en route to the scene with an ESTIMATED TIME OF ARRIVAL LESS THAN 8 MINUTES:**

- **WAIT FOR THE ARRIVAL OF THE ALS UNIT.**

C. **If the two rescuers are part of a first responder unit:**

- **WAIT FOR THE ARRIVAL OF THE BLS OR ALS UNIT, AS APPROPRIATE.**

D. **If the two rescuers and the patient are already en route to the hospital:**

- **RESUME TRANSPORT IMMEDIATELY.**

Continued.

PROTOCOL 10: Management of a Perfusing Rhythm—One or Two Rescuers, cont'd

If one rescuer is present:

E. If the rescuer is part of a first responder unit:

- **WAIT FOR THE ARRIVAL OF THE BLS OR ALS UNIT, AS APPROPRIATE.**

Management of a Recurrent Cardiac Arrest—One or Two Rescuers

ALGORITHM 11
PROTOCOL 11

ALGORITHM 11: Management of a Recurrent Cardiac Arrest—One or Two Rescuers

If
**RECURRENT
CARDIAC ARREST**

If
TWO RESCUERS
Go to:
Algorithm 3:
**"Initial Management
Witnessed Arrest—
Two Rescuers"**

If
ONE RESCUER
Go to:
Algorithm 6:
**"Initial Management
Pre-arrival/witnessed
Arrest —One Rescuer"**

PROTOCOL 11: Management of a Recurrent Cardiac Arrest—One or Two Rescuers

If two rescuers are present:

1. Proceed to **PROTOCOL 3: Initial Management of EMT/FR-D-witnessed Cardiac Arrest while on the Scene or en Route—Two Rescuers.**

If one rescuer is present:

2. Proceed to **PROTOCOL 6: Initial Management of Pre-arrival Cardiac Arrest or EMT/FR-D-witnessed Cardiac Arrest while on the Scene—One Rescuer, without Bystander CPR.**

Section 2

Generic SAED Algorithms and Protocols, Based on a Pulse Check Before or During Every Analysis of the ECG Rhythm

1. Initial Management of Pre-arrival Cardiac Arrest—Two Rescuers, without Bystander CPR

   ALGORITHM 1. One/Two-Rescuer CPR
   PROTOCOL 1a. One-Rescuer CPR
   PROTOCOL 1b. Two-Rescuer CPR

2. Initial Management of Pre-arrival Cardiac Arrest—Two Rescuers, with Bystander CPR

   ALGORITHM 2
   PROTOCOL 2

3. Initial Management of EMT/FR-D-witnessed Cardiac Arrest while on the Scene or en Route—Two Rescuers

   ALGORITHM 3. One/Two-Rescuer CPR
   PROTOCOL 3a. One-Rescuer CPR
   PROTOCOL 3b. Two-Rescuer CPR

4. Management of Cardiac Arrest Following ECG Rhythm Analysis Indicating **"SHOCK"**—Two Rescuers

   ALGORITHM 4
   PROTOCOL 4

5. Management of Cardiac Arrest Following ECG Rhythm Analysis Indicating **"NO SHOCK"**—Two Rescuers

   ALGORITHM 5
   PROTOCOL 5

6. Initial Management of Pre-arrival Cardiac Arrest or EMT/FR-D-witnessed Cardiac Arrest while on the Scene—One Rescuer, without Bystander CPR

   ALGORITHM 6
   PROTOCOL

7. Initial Management of Pre-arrival Cardiac Arrest—One Rescuer, with Bystander CPR

   ALGORITHM 7
   PROTOCOL 7

8. Management of Cardiac Arrest Following ECG Rhythm Analysis Indicating **"SHOCK"**—One Rescuer

   ALGORITHM 8
   PROTOCOL 8

9. Management of Cardiac Arrest Following ECG Rhythm Analysis Indicating **"NO SHOCK"**—One Rescuer

   ALGORITHM 9
   PROTOCOL 9

10. Management of a Perfusing Rhythm—One or Two Rescuers

    ALGORITHM 10
    PROTOCOL 10

11. Management of a Recurrent Cardiac Arrest—One or Two Rescuers

    ALGORITHM 11
    PROTOCOL 11

Algorithm/Protocol 1

Initial Management of Pre-arrival Cardiac Arrest—Two Rescuers, without Bystander CPR

ALGORITHM 1 One/Two-Rescuer CPR
PROTOCOL 1a One-Rescuer CPR
PROTOCOL 1b Two-Rescuer CPR

ALGORITHM 1: Initial Management of Pre-arrival Cardiac Arrest—Two Rescuers, without Bystander CPR

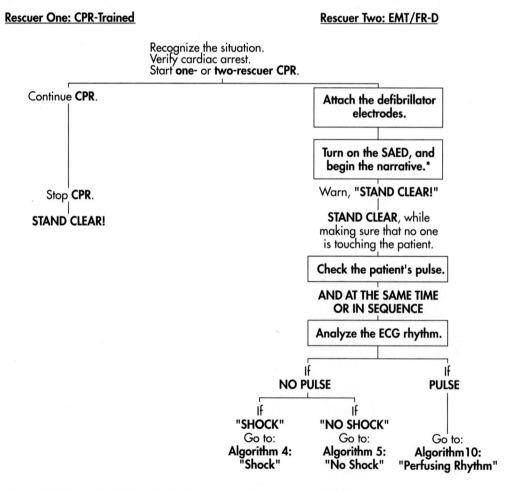

---

* Omit the voice recording of the narrative if not required by local protocol.

PROTOCOL 1a: Initial Management of Pre-arrival Cardiac Arrest—Two Rescuers, without Bystander CPR

One-rescuer CPR	
Rescuer one: CPR-trained	**Rescuer two: EMT/FR-D**

Rescuer one: CPR-trained

1. Recognize the situation.

2. Verify cardiac arrest by determining **unresponsiveness**—by shaking the patient and shouting **"ARE YOU OK?"**

If the patient is unresponsive:

3. Start **one-rescuer CPR.**

   a. Make sure that the patient is on a firm flat surface.
   b. Take a position beside the patient's shoulder opposite **rescuer two.**
   c. Open the patient's airway.
   d. Look, feel, and listen for breathing, taking 3 to 5 seconds.

If breathing is absent:

   e. Announce, **"NO BREATHING!"**
   f. Deliver 2 initial breaths, taking 3 to 5 seconds.
   g. Clear the patient's airway if necessary.
   h. Palpate the patient's carotid artery for a **spontaneous pulse,** taking 5 to 10 seconds.

If the pulse is absent:

   i. Announce, **"NO PULSE!"**
   j. Locate the compression site on the patient's sternum.
   k. Compress the patient's sternum 15 times at a rate of 80 to 100 per minute.
   l. Ventilate 2 times, taking 3 to 5 seconds, between the fifteenth compression and the first one of the next series of compressions.

4. Continue **CPR** at a ratio of 15 chest compressions to 2 rescue breaths until told to **"STAND CLEAR,"** usually within 1 minute.

5. Stop **CPR** so that the patient is motionless **while** the ECG rhythm is being analyzed.

6. **STAND CLEAR!**

Rescuer two: EMT/FR-D

1. Recognize the situation and assume control.

2. Explain the **SAED** procedure briefly to the bystanders, if appropriate.

3. Place the **SAED** next to the patient's head while noting the time.

4. Take a position beside the patient's chest.

5. | **ATTACH THE DEFIBRILLATOR ELECTRODES.** |

6. | **TURN ON THE SAED, AND BEGIN THE NARRATIVE.*** |

> **NOTE: Defibrillation takes precedence over CPR! The first shock is delivered as soon as the defibrillator electrodes have been attached, the ECG rhythm analyzed, and "SHOCK" indicated.**

7. Warn, **"STAND CLEAR!"**

8. **STAND CLEAR WHILE MAKING SURE THAT NO ONE, INCLUDING ANY BYSTANDER AND BOTH RESCUERS, IS TOUCHING THE PATIENT OR ANYTHING IS IN CONTACT WITH THE PATIENT.**

9. | **CHECK THE PATIENT'S PULSE.** |

**AND AT THE SAME TIME
OR IN SEQUENCE**

10. | **ANALYZE THE ECG RHYTHM.** |

---

*Omit the voice recording of the narrative if it is not required by local protocol.   *Continued.*

PROTOCOL 1a: Initial Management of Pre-arrival Cardiac Arrest—Two Rescuers, without Bystander CPR, cont'd

One-rescuer CPR	
Rescuer one: CPR-trained	**Rescuer two: EMT/FR-D**
	If "SHOCK" is indicated and the PATIENT'S PULSE IS ABSENT:
	11. Proceed to **PROTOCOL 4: Management of Cardiac Arrest Following ECG Rhythm Analysis Indicating "SHOCK"—Two Rescuers.**
	If "NO SHOCK" is indicated and the PATIENT'S PULSE IS ABSENT:
	12. Proceed to **PROTOCOL 5: Management of Cardiac Arrest Following ECG Rhythm Analysis Indicating "NO SHOCK"—Two Rescuers.**
	If the patient's PULSE is present:
	13. Proceed to **PROTOCOL 10: Management of a Perfusing Rhythm—One or Two Rescuers.**

PROTOCOL 1b: Initial Management of Pre-arrival Cardiac Arrest—Two Rescuers, without Bystander CPR

Two-rescuer CPR	
Rescuer one: CPR-trained	**Rescuer two: EMT/FR-D**
1. Recognize the situation.	1. Recognize the situation and assume control.
2. Verify cardiac arrest by determining **unresponsiveness**—by shaking the patient and shouting **"ARE YOU OK?"**	2. Explain the **SAED** procedure briefly to the bystanders, if appropriate.
If the patient is unresponsive:	3. Place the **SAED** next to the patient's head while noting the time.
3. Start **two-rescuer CPR.**	4. Start **two-rescuer CPR.**

a. Make sure that the patient is on a firm flat surface.
   b. Take a position beside the patient's chest.
   c. Locate the compression site on the patient's sternum.
	a. Take a position above the patient's head.
	   b. Open the patient's airway.
	   c. Look, feel, and listen for breathing, taking 3 to 5 seconds.

	If breathing is absent:

	d. Announce, **"NO BREATHING!"**
	   e. Deliver 2 initial breaths, taking 3 to 5 seconds.
	   f. Clear the patient's airway if necessary.
	   g. Palpate the patient's carotid artery for a **spontaneous pulse,** taking 5 to 10 seconds.

	If the pulse is absent:
d. Compress the patient's sternum at a rate of 80 to 100 per minute.	h. Announce, **"NO PULSE!"**

*Omit the voice recording of the narrative if it is not required by local protocol.

Continued.

PROTOCOL 1b: Initial Management of Pre-arrival Cardiac Arrest—Two Rescuers, without Bystander CPR, cont'd

Two-rescuer CPR	
Rescuer one: CPR-trained	**Rescuer two: EMT/FR-D**

4. Continue **CPR** until told to "STAND CLEAR," usually within 1 minute.

5. | ATTACH THE DEFIBRILLATOR ELECTRODES. |

6. | TURN ON THE SAED, AND BEGIN THE NARRATIVE.* |

> **NOTE: Defibrillation takes precedence over CPR! The first shock is delivered as soon as the defibrillator electrodes have been attached, the ECG rhythm analyzed, and "SHOCK" indicated.**

5. Stop **CPR** so that the patient is motionless **while** the ECG rhythm is being analyzed.

6. STAND CLEAR!

7. Warn, "STAND CLEAR!"

8. STAND CLEAR WHILE MAKING SURE THAT NO ONE, INCLUDING ANY BY-STANDER AND BOTH RESCUERS, IS TOUCHING THE PATIENT OR ANYTHING IS IN CONTACT WITH THE PATIENT.

9. | CHECK THE PATIENT'S PULSE. |

**AND AT THE SAME TIME
OR IN SEQUENCE**

10. | ANALYZE THE ECG RHYTHM. |

If "SHOCK" is indicated and the PATIENT'S PULSE IS ABSENT:

11. Proceed to **PROTOCOL 4: Management of Cardiac Arrest Following ECG Rhythm Analysis Indicating "SHOCK"—Two Rescuers.**

If "NO SHOCK" is indicated and the PATIENT'S PULSE IS ABSENT:

12. Proceed to **PROTOCOL 5: Management of Cardiac Arrest Following ECG Rhythm Analysis Indicating "NO SHOCK"—Two Rescuers.**

If the patient's PULSE is present:

13. Proceed to **PROTOCOL 10: Management of a Perfusing Rhythm—One or Two Rescuers.**

---

*Omit the voice recording of the narrative if it is not required by local protocol.

Algorithm/Protocol 2

Initial Management of Pre-arrival Cardiac Arrest—Two Rescuers, with Bystander CPR

ALGORITHM 2
PROTOCOL 2

ALGORITHM 2: Initial Management of Pre-arrival Cardiac Arrest—Two Rescuers, with Bystander CPR

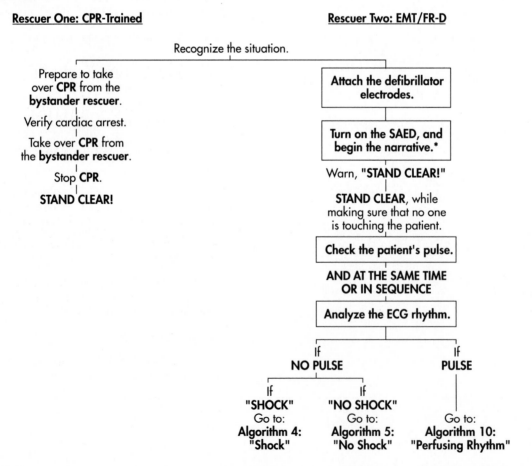

Rescuer One: CPR-Trained   Rescuer Two: EMT/FR-D

Recognize the situation.

Prepare to take over **CPR** from the **bystander rescuer**.

Verify cardiac arrest.

Take over **CPR** from the **bystander rescuer**.

Stop **CPR**.

STAND CLEAR!

Attach the defibrillator electrodes.

Turn on the SAED, and begin the narrative.*

Warn, **"STAND CLEAR!"**

STAND CLEAR, while making sure that no one is touching the patient.

Check the patient's pulse.

AND AT THE SAME TIME OR IN SEQUENCE

Analyze the ECG rhythm.

If **NO PULSE**   If **PULSE**

If **"SHOCK"**   If **"NO SHOCK"**

Go to: Go to: Go to:
Algorithm 4: "Shock"   **Algorithm 5: "No Shock"**   **Algorithm 10: "Perfusing Rhythm"**

---

* Omit the voice recording of the narrative if it is not required by local protocol.

PROTOCOL 2: Initial Management of Pre-arrival Cardiac Arrest—Two Rescuers, with Bystander CPR

Rescuer one: CPR-trained	Rescuer two: EMT/FR-D
1. Recognize the situation.	1. Recognize the situation and assume control.
2. Introduce yourself to the **bystander rescuer** performing **CPR.**	2. Explain the **SAED** procedure briefly to the bystanders, if appropriate.
3. Request the **bystander rescuer** to continue **CPR** through the next cycle of ventilations and then stop **CPR.**	3. Place the **SAED** next to the patient's head opposite the **bystander rescuer** while noting the time.
4. Take a position beside the patient's shoulder as the **bystander rescuer** completes the ventilations and moves away.	4. Take a position beside the patient's chest opposite the **bystander rescuer.**

Rescuer one (continued):

5. Palpate the patient's carotid artery for a **spontaneous pulse,** taking 5 to 10 seconds.

If the pulse is absent:

6. Announce, **"NO PULSE!"**

7. Continue **one-rescuer CPR.**

   a. Deliver 2 breaths, taking 3 to 5 seconds.
   b. Clear the patient's airway if necessary.
   c. Locate the compression site on the patient's sternum.
   d. Compress the patient's sternum 15 times at a rate of 80 to 100 per minute.
   e. Ventilate 2 times, taking 3 to 5 seconds, between the fifteenth compression and the first one of the next series of compressions.

8. Continue **CPR** at a ratio of 15 chest compressions to 2 rescue breaths until told to **"STAND CLEAR,"** usually within 1 minute.

9. Stop **CPR** so that the patient is motionless **while** the ECG rhythm is being analyzed.

10. **STAND CLEAR!**

Rescuer two (continued):

5. ┌─────────────────────────────────┐
   │ **ATTACH THE DEFIBRILLATOR**   │
   │ **ELECTRODES.**   │
   └─────────────────────────────────┘

6. ┌─────────────────────────────────┐
   │ **TURN ON THE SAED, AND**   │
   │ **BEGIN THE NARRATIVE.***   │
   └─────────────────────────────────┘

┌──┐
│ **NOTE: Defibrillation takes precedence over** │
│ **CPR! The first shock is delivered as soon as the** │
│ **defibrillator electrodes have been attached, the** │
│ **ECG rhythm analyzed, and "SHOCK" indi-** │
│ **cated.** │
└──┘

7. Warn, **"STAND CLEAR!"**

8. **STAND CLEAR WHILE MAKING SURE THAT NO ONE, INCLUDING THE BYSTANDER RESCUER AND ANY OTHER BYSTANDER AND BOTH RESCUERS, IS TOUCHING THE PATIENT OR ANYTHING IS IN CONTACT WITH THE PATIENT.**

9. ┌─────────────────────────────────┐
   │ **CHECK THE PATIENT'S PULSE.** │
   └─────────────────────────────────┘

   AND AT THE SAME TIME
   OR IN SEQUENCE

10. ┌─────────────────────────────────┐
    │ **ANALYZE THE ECG RHYTHM.**   │
    └─────────────────────────────────┘

---

*Omit the voice recording of the narrative if it is not required by local protocol.

Continued.

PROTOCOL 2: Initial Management of Pre-arrival Cardiac Arrest—Two Rescuers, with Bystander CPR, cont'd

Rescuer one: CPR-trained	Rescuer two: EMT/FR-D
	If "SHOCK" is indicated and the PATIENT'S PULSE IS ABSENT:
	11. Proceed to **PROTOCOL 4: Management of Cardiac Arrest Following ECG Rhythm Analysis Indicating "SHOCK"—Two Rescuers.**
	If "NO SHOCK" is indicated and the PATIENT'S PULSE IS ABSENT:
	12. Proceed to **PROTOCOL 5: Management of Cardiac Arrest Following ECG Rhythm Analysis Indicating "NO SHOCK"—Two Rescuers.**
	If the patient's PULSE is present:
	13. Proceed to **PROTOCOL 10: Management of a Perfusing Rhythm—One or Two Rescuers.**

Algorithm/Protocol 3

Initial Management of EMT/FR-D-witnessed Cardiac Arrest while on the Scene or en Route—Two Rescuers

ALGORITHM 3 One/Two-Rescuer CPR
PROTOCOL 3a One-Rescuer CPR
PROTOCOL 3b Two-Rescuer CPR

ALGORITHM 3: Initial Management of EMT/FR-D-witnessed Cardiac Arrest while on the Scene or en Route—Two Rescuers

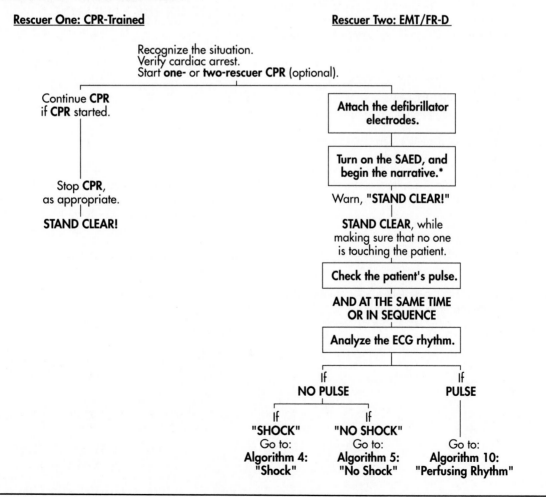

Rescuer One: CPR-Trained

Rescuer Two: EMT/FR-D

Recognize the situation.
Verify cardiac arrest.
Start **one-** or **two-rescuer CPR** (optional).

Continue **CPR**
if **CPR** started.

Stop **CPR**,
as appropriate.

STAND CLEAR!

Attach the defibrillator electrodes.

Turn on the SAED, and begin the narrative.*

Warn, "**STAND CLEAR!**"

STAND CLEAR, while making sure that no one is touching the patient.

Check the patient's pulse.

AND AT THE SAME TIME OR IN SEQUENCE

Analyze the ECG rhythm.

If
NO PULSE

If
PULSE

If
"SHOCK"
Go to:
**Algorithm 4:
"Shock"**

If
"NO SHOCK"
Go to:
**Algorithm 5:
"No Shock"**

Go to:
**Algorithm 10:
"Perfusing Rhythm"**

---

* Omit the voice recording of the narrative if it is not required by local protocol.

PROTOCOL 3a: Initial Management of EMT/FR-D-witnessed Cardiac Arrest while on the Scene or en Route—Two Rescuers

One-rescuer CPR

Rescuer one: CPR-trained	Rescuer two: EMT/FR-D
1. Recognize the situation.	1. Recognize the situation and assume control.

Rescuer one: CPR-trained

1. Recognize the situation.

2. Verify cardiac arrest by determining **unresponsive-ness**—by shaking the patient and shouting **"ARE YOU OK?"**

If the patient is unresponsive:

3. Start **one-rescuer CPR (optional).**

   a. Make sure that the patient is on a firm flat surface.
   b. Take a position beside the patient's shoulder opposite **rescuer two** (or as appropriate in the ambulance).
   c. Open the patient's airway.
   d. Look, feel, and listen for breathing, taking 3 to 5 seconds.

If breathing is absent:

   e. Announce, **"NO BREATHING!"**
   f. Deliver 2 initial breaths, taking 3 to 5 seconds.
   g. Clear the patient's airway if necessary.
   h. Palpate the patient's carotid artery for a **spontaneous pulse,** taking 5 to 10 seconds.

If the pulse is absent:

   i. Announce, **"NO PULSE!"**
   j. Locate the compression site on the patient's sternum.
   k. Compress the patient's sternum 15 times at a rate of 80 to 100 per minute.
   l. Ventilate 2 times, taking 3 to 5 seconds, between the fifteenth compression and the first one of the next series of compressions.

4. Continue **CPR** at a ratio of 15 chest compressions to 2 rescue breaths until told to **"STAND CLEAR,"** usually within 1 minute.

5. Stop **CPR** so that the patient is motionless **while** the ECG rhythm is being analyzed.

6. **STAND CLEAR!**

Rescuer two: EMT/FR-D

1. Recognize the situation and assume control.

> **NOTE: If cardiac arrest occurs in the ambulance en route to the hospital, request the driver to pull over to the side of the road and stop.**

2. Explain the **SAED** procedure briefly to the bystanders, if appropriate.

3. Place the **SAED** next to the patient's head while noting the time.

4. Take a position beside the patient's chest (or as appropriate in the ambulance).

5. **ATTACH THE DEFIBRILLATOR ELECTRODES.**

6. **TURN ON THE SAED, AND BEGIN THE NARRATIVE.***

> **NOTE: Defibrillation takes precedence over CPR! The first shock is delivered as soon as the defibrillator electrodes have been attached, the ECG rhythm analyzed, and "SHOCK" indicated.**

7. Warn, **"STAND CLEAR!"**

8. **STAND CLEAR WHILE MAKING SURE THAT NO ONE IS TOUCHING THE PATIENT OR ANYTHING IS IN CONTACT WITH THE PATIENT.**

9. **CHECK THE PATIENT'S PULSE.**

AND AT THE SAME TIME OR IN SEQUENCE

10. **ANALYZE THE ECG RHYTHM.**

---

*Omit the voice recording of the narrative if it is not required by local protocol.   *Continued.*

PROTOCOL 3a: Initial Management of EMT/FR-D-witnessed Cardiac Arrest while on the Scene or en Route—Two Rescuers, cont'd

One-rescuer CPR	
Rescuer one: CPR-trained	Rescuer two: EMT/FR-D
	If "SHOCK" is indicated and the PATIENT'S PULSE IS ABSENT:
	11. Proceed to **PROTOCOL 4: Management of Cardiac Arrest Following ECG Rhythm Analysis Indicating "SHOCK"**—Two Rescuers.
	If "NO SHOCK" is indicated and the PATIENT'S PULSE IS ABSENT:
	12. Proceed to **PROTOCOL 5: Management of Cardiac Arrest Following ECG Rhythm Analysis Indicating "NO SHOCK"**—Two Rescuers.
	If the patient's PULSE is present:
	13. Proceed to **PROTOCOL 10: Management of a Perfusing Rhythm**—One or Two Rescuers.

PROTOCOL 3b: Initial Management of EMT/FR-D-witnessed Cardiac Arrest while on the Scene or en Route—Two Rescuers

Two-rescuer CPR	
Rescuer one: CPR-trained	Rescuer two: EMT/FR-D
1. Recognize the situation.	1. Recognize the situation and assume control.
2. Verify cardiac arrest by determining **unresponsiveness**—by shaking the patient and shouting **"ARE YOU OK?"**	**NOTE: If cardiac arrest occurs in the ambulance en route to the hospital, request the driver to pull over to the side of the road and stop.**
	2. Explain the **SAED** procedure briefly to the bystanders, if appropriate.
	3. Place the **SAED** next to the patient's head while noting the time.
If the patient is unresponsive:	
3. Start **two-rescuer CPR (optional).**	4. Start **two-rescuer CPR (optional).**

a. Make sure that the patient is on a firm flat surface.
   b. Take a position beside the patient's chest.
   c. Locate the compression site on the patient's sternum.
	a. Take a position above the patient's head.
	   b. Open the patient's airway.
	   c. Look, feel, and listen for breathing, taking 3 to 5 seconds.

	If breathing is absent:

	d. Announce, **"NO BREATHING!"**
	   e. Deliver 2 initial breaths, taking 3 to 5 seconds.
	   f. Clear the patient's airway if necessary.
	   g. Palpate the patient's carotid artery for a **spontaneous pulse,** taking 5 to 10 seconds.

Continued.

PROTOCOL 3b: Initial Management of EMT/FR-D-witnessed Cardiac Arrest while on the Scene or en Route—Two Rescuers,cont'd

Two-rescuer CPR	
Rescuer one: CPR-trained	**Rescuer two: EMT/FR-D**

Rescuer one: CPR-trained

    d. Compress the patient's sternum at a rate of 80 to 100 per minute.

4. Continue **CPR** until told to **"STAND CLEAR,"** usually within 1 minute.

5. Stop **CPR** so that the patient is motionless **while** the ECG rhythm is being analyzed.

6. STAND CLEAR!

Rescuer two: EMT/FR-D

If the pulse is absent:

    h. Announce, **"NO PULSE!"**

5. | **ATTACH THE DEFIBRILLATOR ELECTRODES.** |

6. | **TURN ON THE SAED, AND BEGIN THE NARRATIVE.*** |

> **NOTE: Defibrillation takes precedence over CPR! The first shock is delivered as soon as the defibrillator electrodes have been attached, the ECG rhythm analyzed, and "SHOCK" indicated.**

7. Warn, **"STAND CLEAR!"**

8. STAND CLEAR WHILE MAKING SURE THAT NO ONE IS TOUCHING THE PATIENT OR ANYTHING IS IN CONTACT WITH THE PATIENT.

9. | **CHECK THE PATIENT'S PULSE.** |

**AND AT THE SAME TIME
OR IN SEQUENCE**

10. | **ANALYZE THE ECG RHYTHM.** |

If "SHOCK" is indicated and the PATIENT'S PULSE IS ABSENT:

11. Proceed to **PROTOCOL 4: Management of Cardiac Arrest Following ECG Rhythm Analysis Indicating "SHOCK"—Two Rescuers.**

If "NO SHOCK" is indicated and the PATIENT'S PULSE IS ABSENT:

12. Proceed to **PROTOCOL 5: Management of Cardiac Arrest Following ECG Rhythm Analysis Indicating "NO SHOCK"—Two Rescuers.**

If the patient's PULSE is present:

13. Proceed to **PROTOCOL 10: Management of a Perfusing Rhythm—One or Two Rescuers.**

---

*Omit the voice recording of the narrative if it is not required by local protocol.

Algorithm/Protocol 4

Management of Cardiac Arrest Following ECG Rhythm Analysis Indicating "SHOCK"—Two Rescuers

ALGORITHM 4
PROTOCOL 4

ALGORITHM 4: Management of Cardiac Arrest Following ECG Rhythm Analysis Indicating "SHOCK"—Two Rescuers

If "SHOCK" is indicated THE FIRST TIME and the patient's pulse is absent:

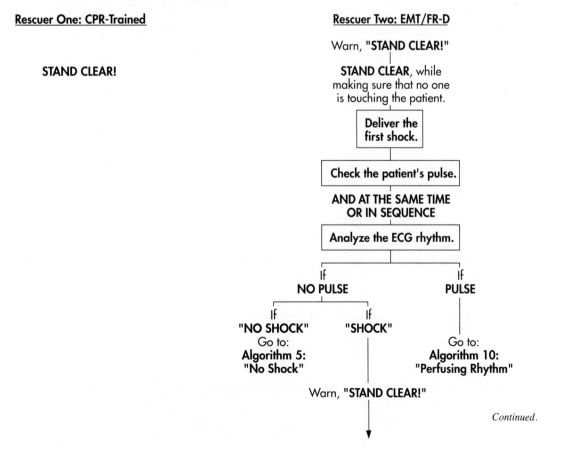

Rescuer One: CPR-Trained

STAND CLEAR!

Rescuer Two: EMT/FR-D

Warn, "STAND CLEAR!"

STAND CLEAR, while making sure that no one is touching the patient.

Deliver the first shock.

Check the patient's pulse.

AND AT THE SAME TIME OR IN SEQUENCE

Analyze the ECG rhythm.

If NO PULSE

If PULSE

If "NO SHOCK"
Go to:
Algorithm 5:
"No Shock"

If "SHOCK"

Go to:
Algorithm 10:
"Perfusing Rhythm"

Warn, "STAND CLEAR!"

Continued.

ALGORITHM 4: Management of Cardiac Arrest Following ECG Rhythm Analysis Indicating "SHOCK"—Two Rescuers, cont'd

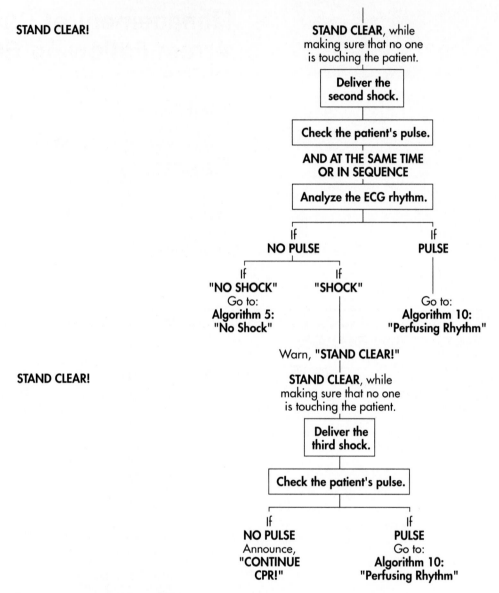

STAND CLEAR!

STAND CLEAR, while making sure that no one is touching the patient.

Deliver the second shock.

Check the patient's pulse.

AND AT THE SAME TIME OR IN SEQUENCE

Analyze the ECG rhythm.

If
NO PULSE

If
PULSE

If
"NO SHOCK"
Go to:
Algorithm 5:
"No Shock"

If
"SHOCK"

Go to:
Algorithm 10:
"Perfusing Rhythm"

Warn, "STAND CLEAR!"

STAND CLEAR!

STAND CLEAR, while making sure that no one is touching the patient.

Deliver the third shock.

Check the patient's pulse.

If
NO PULSE
Announce,
"CONTINUE CPR!"

If
PULSE
Go to:
Algorithm 10:
"Perfusing Rhythm"

Resume **one-** or **two-rescuer** CPR.

Transport immediately or wait for the BLS or ALS unit, as appropriate, while continuing to perform **CPR**, reanalyzing the patient's ECG rhythm, delivering shocks, and checking the patient's pulse, according to local protocol, as follows:

Continue **one-** or **two-rescuer** CPR for 1 minute.

If en route, stop the ambulance.

Stop **CPR**.

Continued

ALGORITHM 4: Management of Cardiac Arrest Following ECG Rhythm Analysis Indicating "SHOCK"—Two Rescuers, cont'd

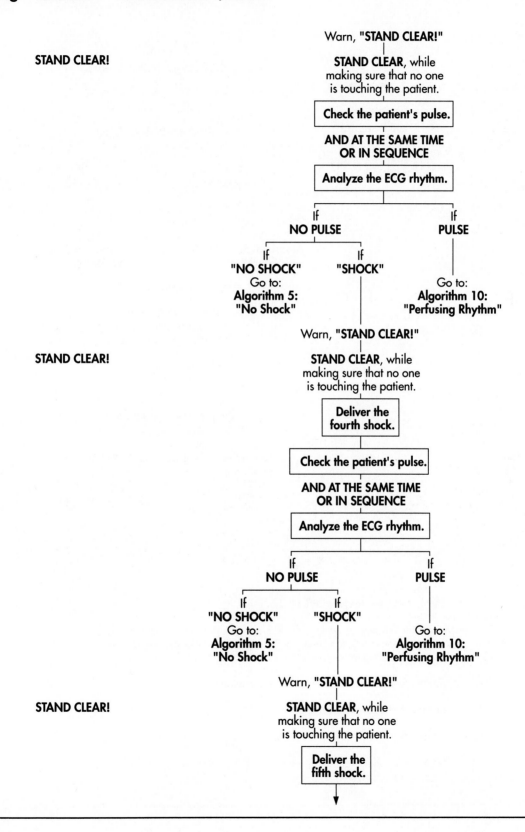

ALGORITHM 4: Management of Cardiac Arrest Following ECG Rhythm Analysis Indicating "SHOCK"—Two Rescuers, cont'd

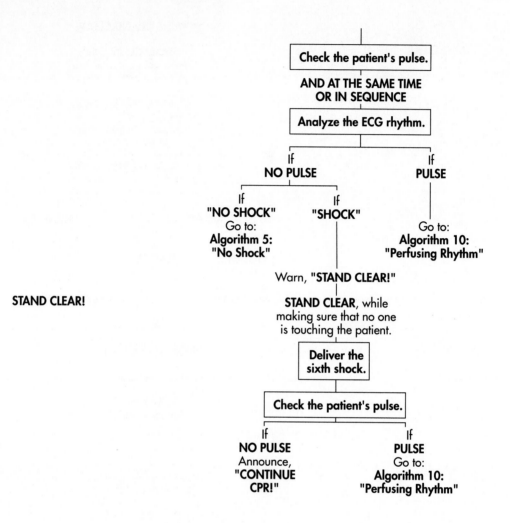

Resume **one-** or **two-rescuer CPR**.

Transport immediately or wait for the BLS or ALS unit, as appropriate, while continuing to perform **CPR**, reanalyzing the patient's ECG rhythm, delivering shocks, and checking the patient's pulse, according to local protocol, as follows:

Continue **one-** or **two-rescuer CPR** for 1 minute.

If en route, stop the ambulance.

Stop **CPR**.

Check the patient's pulse, analyze the ECG rhythm, and go to the appropriate algorithm.

PROTOCOL 4: Management of Cardiac Arrest Following ECG Rhythm Analysis Indicating "SHOCK"—Two Rescuers

If "SHOCK" is indicated THE FIRST TIME and the patient's pulse is absent:

Rescuer one: CPR-trained	Rescuer two: EMT/FR-D

Rescuer two: EMT/FR-D

1. Warn, "STAND CLEAR!"

Rescuer one: CPR-trained

1. STAND CLEAR!

2. STAND CLEAR WHILE MAKING SURE THAT NO ONE IS TOUCHING THE PATIENT OR ANYTHING IN CONTACT WITH THE PATIENT.

> **NOTE!**
>
> If "NO SHOCK" is indicated at any time:
>
> If the patient's PULSE is present:
>
> - Proceed to **PROTOCOL 10: Management of a Perfusing Rhythm—One or Two Rescuers.**
>
> If the patient's PULSE is absent:
>
> - Proceed to **PROTOCOL 5: Management of Cardiac Arrest Following ECG Rhythm Analysis Indicating "No Shock"—Two Rescuers.**

3. TURN ON THE CHARGING CIRCUIT, IF APPROPRIATE.

When the defibrillator is charged:

4. DELIVER THE FIRST SHOCK.

5. CHECK THE PATIENT'S PULSE.

AND AT THE SAME TIME OR IN SEQUENCE

6. ANALYZE THE ECG RHYTHM.

If "SHOCK" is indicated and the PATIENT'S PULSE IS ABSENT:

7. Warn, "STAND CLEAR!"

2. STAND CLEAR!

8. STAND CLEAR WHILE MAKING SURE THAT NO ONE IS TOUCHING THE PATIENT OR ANYTHING IS IN CONTACT WITH THE PATIENT.

9. TURN ON THE CHARGING CIRCUIT, IF APPROPRIATE.

When the defibrillator is charged:

10. DELIVER THE SECOND SHOCK.

11. CHECK THE PATIENT'S PULSE.

AND AT THE SAME TIME OR IN SEQUENCE

12. ANALYZE THE ECG RHYTHM.

If "SHOCK" is indicated and the PATIENT'S PULSE IS ABSENT:

13. Warn, "STAND CLEAR!"

Continued.

PROTOCOL 4: Management of Cardiac Arrest Following ECG Rhythm Analysis Indicating "SHOCK"—Two Rescuers, cont'd

Rescuer one: CPR-trained	Rescuer two: EMT/FR-D
3. STAND CLEAR!	14. STAND CLEAR WHILE MAKING SURE THAT NO ONE IS TOUCHING THE PATIENT OR ANYTHING IS IN CONTACT WITH THE PATIENT.

14. STAND CLEAR WHILE MAKING SURE THAT NO ONE IS TOUCHING THE PATIENT OR ANYTHING IS IN CONTACT WITH THE PATIENT.

15. TURN ON THE CHARGING CIRCUIT, IF APPROPRIATE.

When the defibrillator is charged:

16. DELIVER THE THIRD SHOCK.

17. CHECK THE PATIENT'S PULSE.

If the patient's PULSE is absent:

18. Announce, "CONTINUE CPR!"

NOTE!

If a spontaneous pulse appears at any time:

- Proceed to **PROTOCOL 10: Management of a Perfusing Rhythm.**

NOTE!

The total number of shocks delivered depends on the local protocol.

- Resume **one-** or **two-rescuer CPR,** proceed with one of the following options, as appropriate, and continue with the protocol:

A. If the two rescuers are part of the crew of the BLS ambulance already at the scene AND an ALS unit is en route to the scene with an **ESTIMATED TIME OF ARRIVAL GREATER THAN 8 MINUTES:**

OR

If an ALS unit is not available:

OR

If the BLS ambulance is to connect up with an ALS unit en route:

- **TRANSPORT IMMEDIATELY, WHILE CONTINUING TO PERFORM CPR, REANALYZING THE PATIENT'S ECG RHYTHM, DELIVERING SHOCKS, AND CHECKING THE PATIENT'S PULSE EN ROUTE, ACCORDING TO LOCAL PROTOCOL.**

Continued.

PROTOCOL 4: Management of Cardiac Arrest Following ECG Rhythm Analysis Indicating "SHOCK"—Two Rescuers, cont'd

Rescuer one: CPR-trained	Rescuer two: EMT/FR-D

B. If the two rescuers are part of the crew of a BLS ambulance already at the scene and an ALS unit is en route to the scene with an ESTIMATED TIME OF ARRIVAL LESS THAN 8 MINUTES:

- **WAIT FOR THE ARRIVAL OF THE ALS UNIT, WHILE CONTINUING TO PERFORM CPR, REANALYZING THE PATIENT'S ECG RHYTHM, DELIVERING SHOCKS, AND CHECKING THE PATIENT'S PULSE, ACCORDING TO LOCAL PROTOCOL.**

C. If the two rescuers are part of a first responder unit:

- **WAIT FOR THE ARRIVAL OF THE BLS OR ALS UNIT, AS APPROPRIATE, WHILE CONTINUING TO PERFORM CPR, REANALYZING THE PATIENT'S ECG RHYTHM, DELIVERING SHOCKS, AND CHECKING THE PATIENT'S PULSE, ACCORDING TO LOCAL PROTOCOL.**

D. If the two rescuers and the patient are already en route to the hospital:

- **RESUME TRANSPORT IMMEDIATELY, WHILE CONTINUING TO PERFORM CPR, REANALYZING THE PATIENT'S ECG RHYTHM, DELIVERING SHOCKS, AND CHECKING THE PATIENT'S PULSE EN ROUTE, ACCORDING TO LOCAL PROTOCOL.**

- Continue **CPR** for 1 minute.

        19. If en route to the hospital, request the driver to pull over to the side of the road and stop.

        20. Warn, **"STAND CLEAR!"**

- Stop **CPR.**

4. STAND CLEAR!

        21. STAND CLEAR WHILE MAKING SURE THAT NO ONE IS TOUCHING THE PATIENT OR ANYTHING IS IN CONTACT WITH THE PATIENT.

        22. | **CHECK THE PATIENT'S PULSE.** |

        AND AT THE SAME TIME OR IN SEQUENCE

        23. | **ANALYZE THE ECG RHYTHM.** |

        If "SHOCK" is indicated and the PATIENT'S PULSE IS ABSENT:

        24. Warn, **"STAND CLEAR!"**

Continued.

PROTOCOL 4: Management of Cardiac Arrest Following ECG Rhythm Analysis Indicating "SHOCK"—Two Rescuers, cont'd

Rescuer one: CPR-trained	Rescuer two: EMT/FR-D

Rescuer one: CPR-trained

5. STAND CLEAR!

NOTE!

If "NO SHOCK" is indicated at any time:

If the patient's PULSE is present:

- Proceed to **PROTOCOL 10: Management of a Perfusing Rhythm—One or Two rescuers.**

If the patient's PULSE is absent:

- Proceed to **PROTOCOL 5: Management of Cardiac Arrest Following ECG Rhythm Analysis Indicating "No Shock"—Two Rescuers.**

---

6. STAND CLEAR!

Rescuer two: EMT/FR-D

25. STAND CLEAR WHILE MAKING SURE THAT NO ONE IS TOUCHING THE PATIENT OR ANYTHING IS IN CONTACT WITH THE PATIENT.

26. TURN ON THE CHARGING CIRCUIT, IF APPROPRIATE.

When the defibrillator is charged:

27. DELIVER THE FOURTH SHOCK.

28. CHECK THE PATIENT'S PULSE.

AND AT THE SAME TIME OR IN SEQUENCE

29. ANALYZE THE ECG RHYTHM.

If "SHOCK" is indicated and the PATIENT'S PULSE IS ABSENT:

30. Warn, "STAND CLEAR"

31. STAND CLEAR WHILE MAKING SURE THAT NO ONE IS TOUCHING THE PATIENT OR ANYTHING IS IN CONTACT WITH THE PATIENT.

32. TURN ON THE CHARGING CIRCUIT, IF APPROPRIATE.

When the defibrillator is charged:

33. DELIVER THE FIFTH SHOCK.

34. CHECK THE PATIENT'S PULSE.

AND AT THE SAME TIME OR IN SEQUENCE

35. ANALYZE THE ECG RHYTHM.

If "SHOCK" is indicated and the PATIENT'S PULSE IS ABSENT:

36. Warn, "STAND CLEAR!"

Continued.

PROTOCOL 4: Management of Cardiac Arrest Following ECG Rhythm Analysis Indicating "SHOCK"—Two Rescuers, cont'd

Rescuer one: CPR-trained	Rescuer two: EMT/FR-D
7. STAND CLEAR!	37. STAND CLEAR WHILE MAKING SURE THAT NO ONE IS TOUCHING THE PATIENT OR ANYTHING IS IN CONTACT WITH THE PATIENT.

38. TURN ON THE CHARGING CIRCUIT, IF APPROPRIATE.

When the defibrillator is charged.

39. DELIVER THE SIXTH SHOCK.

40. CHECK THE PATIENT'S PULSE.

If the patient's PULSE is absent:

41. Announce, "CONTINUE CPR!"

NOTE!

If a spontaneous pulse appears at any time:
- Proceed to **PROTOCOL 10: Management of a Perfusing Rhythm.**

NOTE!

The total number of shocks delivered depends on the local protocol.

- Resume **one-** or **two-rescuer CPR,** and proceed with **OPTION A, B, C,** or **D,** outlined above, as appropriate, and continue with the protocol.

Management of Cardiac Arrest Following ECG Rhythm Analysis Indicating "NO SHOCK"—Two Rescuers

ALGORITHM 5
PROTOCOL 5

ALGORITHM 5: Management of Cardiac Arrest Following ECG Rhythm Analysis Indicating "NO SHOCK"—Two Rescuers

If "NO SHOCK" is indicated THE FIRST TIME and the patient's pulse is absent:

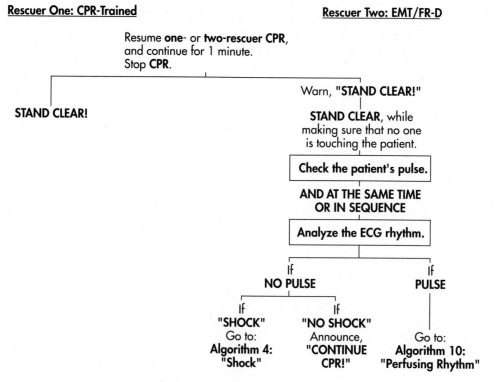

Rescuer One: CPR-Trained

Rescuer Two: EMT/FR-D

Resume **one-** or **two-rescuer CPR,**
and continue for 1 minute.
Stop **CPR.**

STAND CLEAR!

Warn, **"STAND CLEAR!"**

STAND CLEAR, while
making sure that no one
is touching the patient.

Check the patient's pulse.

**AND AT THE SAME TIME
OR IN SEQUENCE**

Analyze the ECG rhythm.

If
NO PULSE

If
PULSE

If
"SHOCK"
Go to:
**Algorithm 4:
"Shock"**

If
"NO SHOCK"
Announce,
**"CONTINUE
CPR!"**

Go to:
**Algorithm 10:
"Perfusing Rhythm"**

Resume **one-** or **two-rescuer CPR.**

Transport immediately or wait for the BLS or ALS unit, as appropriate, while
continuing to perform **CPR,** reanalyzing the ECG rhythm every 1 to 3 minutes,
and checking the patient's pulse, according to local protocol.

PROTOCOL 5: Management of Cardiac Arrest Following ECG Rhythm Analysis Indicating "NO SHOCK"—Two Rescuers

If "NO SHOCK" is indicated THE FIRST TIME and the patient's pulse is absent:

Rescuer one: CPR-trained	Rescuer two: EMT/FR-D

- Resume **one- or two-rescuer CPR, and** continue for 1 minute.
- Stop **CPR.**

    1. Warn, "STAND CLEAR!"

1. STAND CLEAR!

    2. STAND CLEAR WHILE MAKING SURE THAT NO ONE IS TOUCHING THE PATIENT OR ANYTHING IN CONTACT WITH THE PATIENT.

    3. CHECK THE PATIENT'S PULSE.

        AND AT THE SAME TIME OR IN SEQUENCE

    4. ANALYZE THE ECG RHYTHM.

If "SHOCK" is indicated and the PATIENT'S PULSE IS ABSENT:

    5. Proceed to **PROTOCOL 4: Management of Cardiac Arrest Following ECG Rhythm Analysis Indicating "SHOCK"—Two Rescuers.**

If the patient's PULSE is present:

    6. Proceed to **PROTOCOL 10: Management of a Perfusing Rhythm—One or Two Rescuers.**

If "NO SHOCK" is indicated and the PATIENT'S PULSE IS ABSENT:

    7. Announce, "CONTINUE CPR!"

- Resume **one-** or **two-rescuer CPR,** and proceed with one of the following options, as appropriate:

A. **If the two rescuers are part of the crew of a BLS ambulance already at the scene AND an ALS unit is en route to the scene with an ESTIMATED TIME OF ARRIVAL GREATER THAN 8 MINUTES:**

OR

If an ALS unit is not available:

OR

If the BLS ambulance is to connect up with an ALS unit en route:

- **TRANSPORT IMMEDIATELY, WHILE CONTINUING TO PERFORM CPR, REANALYZING THE ECG RHYTHM EVERY 1 TO 3 MINUTES, AND CHECKING THE PATIENT'S PULSE EN ROUTE, ACCORDING TO LOCAL PROTOCOL.**

Continued.

PROTOCOL 5: Management of Cardiac Arrest Following ECG Rhythm Analysis Indicating "NO SHOCK"—Two Rescuers, cont'd

Rescuer one: CPR-trained   **Rescuer two: EMT/FR-D**

B. If the two rescuers are part of the crew of a BLS ambulance already at the scene AND an ALS unit is en route to the scene with an ESTIMATED TIME OF ARRIVAL LESS THAN 8 MINUTES:

- **WAIT FOR THE ARRIVAL OF THE ALS UNIT, WHILE CONTINUING TO PERFORM CPR, REANALYZING THE ECG RHYTHM EVERY 1 TO 3 MINUTES, AND CHECKING THE PATIENT'S PULSE, ACCORDING TO LOCAL PROTOCOL.**

C. If the two rescuers are part of a first responder unit:

- **WAIT FOR THE ARRIVAL OF THE BLS OR ALS UNIT, AS APPROPRIATE, WHILE CONTINUING TO PERFORM CPR, REANALYZING THE ECG RHYTHM EVERY 1 TO 3 MINUTES, AND CHECKING THE PATIENT'S PULSE, ACCORDING TO LOCAL PROTOCOL.**

D. If the two rescuers and the patient are already en route to the hospital:

- **RESUME TRANSPORT IMMEDIATELY, WHILE CONTINUING TO PERFORM CPR, REANALYZING THE ECG RHYTHM EVERY 1 TO 3 MINUTES, AND CHECKING THE PATIENT'S PULSE EN ROUTE, ACCORDING TO LOCAL PROTOCOL.**

Initial Management of Pre-arrival Cardiac Arrest or EMT/FR-D-witnessed Cardiac Arrest while on the Scene—One Rescuer, without Bystander CPR

ALGORITHM 6
PROTOCOL 6

ALGORITHM 6: Initial Management of Pre-arrival Cardiac Arrest or EMT/FR-D-witnessed Cardiac Arrest while on the Scene—One Rescuer, without Bystander CPR

EMT/FR-D

Recognize the
situation.

Verify
cardiac arrest.

Attach the defibrillator electrodes.

Turn on the SAED, and begin the narrative.*

Warn, "**STAND CLEAR!**"

STAND CLEAR, while
making sure that no one
is touching the patient.

Check the patient's pulse.

**AND AT THE SAME TIME
OR IN SEQUENCE**

Analyze the ECG rhythm.

> **NOTE!**
>
> **Defibrillation takes precedence over CPR if the EMT/FR-D is alone and no other person trained in CPR is available!**

---

*Omit the voice recording of the narrative if it is not required by local protocol.

Continued.

ALGORITHM 6: Initial Management of Pre-arrival Cardiac Arrest or EMT/FR-D-witnessed Cardiac Arrest while on the Scene—One Rescuer, without Bystander CPR, cont'd

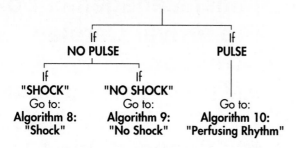

If
NO PULSE

If
PULSE

If
"SHOCK"
Go to:
Algorithm 8:
"Shock"

If
"NO SHOCK"
Go to:
Algorithm 9:
"No Shock"

Go to:
Algorithm 10:
"Perfusing Rhythm"

PROTOCOL 6: Initial Management of Pre-arrival Cardiac Arrest or EMT/FR-D-witnessed Cardiac Arrest while on the Scene—One Rescuer, without Bystander CPR

EMT/FR-D

1. Recognize the situation and assume control.

2. Verify cardiac arrest by determining **unresponsiveness**—by shaking the patient and shouting **"ARE YOU OK?"**

If the patient is unresponsive:

3. Make sure that the patient is on a firm flat surface **while** explaining the **SAED** procedure briefly to the bystanders, if appropriate.

4. Determine **breathlessness and pulselessness**.

If the pulse and respirations are absent:

5. Place the **SAED** on the floor next to the patient's head while noting the time.

6. Take a position beside the patient's chest.

7. | **ATTACH THE DEFIBRILLATOR ELECTRODES.** |

8. | **TURN ON THE SAED, AND BEGIN THE NARRATIVE.*** |

9. Warn, **"STAND CLEAR!"**

10. **STAND CLEAR WHILE MAKING SURE THAT NO ONE IS TOUCHING THE PATIENT OR ANYTHING IN CONTACT WITH THE PATIENT.**

> **NOTE!**
>
> **DEFIBRILLATION TAKES PRECEDENCE OVER CPR IF THE EMT/FR-D IS ALONE AND NO OTHER PERSON TRAINED IN CPR IS AVAILABLE!**

*Omit the voice recording of the narrative if it is not required by local protocol.

Continued.

PROTOCOL 6: Initial Management of Pre-arrival Cardiac Arrest or EMT/FR-D-witnessed Cardiac Arrest while on the Scene—One Rescuer, without Bystander CPR, cont'd

EMT/FR-D

11. | CHECK THE PATIENT'S PULSE. |

   AND AT THE SAME TIME
   OR IN SEQUENCE

12. | ANALYZE THE ECG RHYTHM. |

If "SHOCK" is indicated and the PATIENT'S PULSE IS ABSENT:

13. Proceed to **PROTOCOL 8: Management of Cardiac Arrest Following ECG Rhythm Analysis Indicating "SHOCK"—One Rescuer.**

If "NO SHOCK" is indicated and the PATIENT'S PULSE IS ABSENT:

14. Proceed to **PROTOCOL 9: Management of Cardiac Arrest Following ECG Rhythm Analysis Indicating "NO SHOCK"—One Rescuer.**

If the patient's PULSE is present:

15. Proceed to **PROTOCOL 10: Management of a Perfusing Rhythm—One or Two Rescuers.**

Initial Management of Pre-arrival Cardiac Arrest—One Rescuer, with Bystander CPR

ALGORITHM 7
PROTOCOL 7

ALGORITHM 7: Initial Management of Pre-arrival Cardiac Arrest—One Rescuer, with Bystander CPR

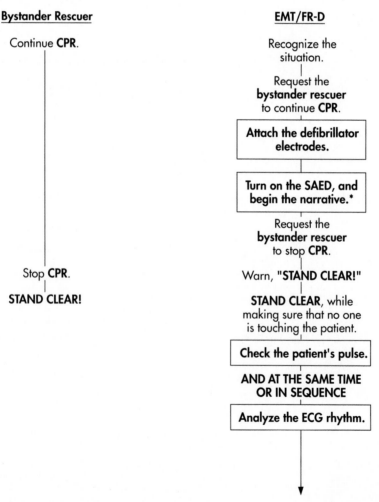

ALGORITHM 7: Initial Management of Pre-arrival Cardiac Arrest—One Rescuer, with Bystander CPR, cont'd

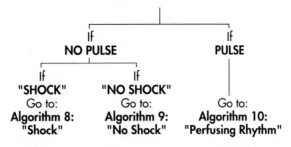

PROTOCOL 7: Initial Management of Pre-arrival Cardiac Arrest—One Rescuer, with Bystander CPR

Bystander rescuer	EMT/FR-D
1. Continue **CPR**.	1. Recognize the situation and assume control.
	2. Introduce yourself to the **bystander rescuer** performing **CPR**.
	3. Request the **bystander rescuer** to contiue **CPR**.
	4. Explain the **SAED** procedure briefly to the bystanders, if apporpriate.
	5. Place the **SAED** next to the patient's head opposite the **bystander rescuer** while noting the time.
	6. Take a position beside the patient's chest opposite the **bystander rescuer.**
	7. ATTACH THE DEFIBRILLATOR ELECTRODES.
	8. TURN ON THE SAED, AND BEGIN THE NARRATIVE.*
	NOTE! Defibrillation takes precedence over CPR! The first shock is delivered as soon as the defibrillator electrodes have been attached, the ECG rhythm analyzed, and "SHOCK" indicated.
	9. Request the **bystander rescuer** to stop **CPR**.
2. Stop **CPR**.	10. Warn, "STAND CLEAR!"
3. STAND CLEAR!	11. STAND CLEAR WHILE MAKING SURE THAT NO ONE, INCLUDING THE BYSTANDER RESCUER AND ANY OTHER BYSTANDER, IS TOUCHING THE PATIENT OR ANYTHING IS IN CONTACT WITH THE PATIENT

*Omit the voice recording of the narrative if it is not required by local protocol.   *Continued.*

PROTOCOL 7: Initial Management of Pre-arrival Cardiac Arrest—One Rescuer, with Bystander CPR, cont'd

Bystander rescuer	EMT/FR-D
	12. CHECK THE PATIENT'S PULSE.

**AND AT THE SAME TIME
OR IN SEQUENCE**

13. ANALYZE THE ECG RHYTHM.

If "SHOCK" is indicated and the PATIENT'S PULSE IS ABSENT:

14. Proceed to **PROTOCOL 8: Management of Cardiac Arrest Following ECG Rhythm Analysis Indicating "SHOCK"—One Rescuer.**

If "NO SHOCK" is indicated and the PATIENT'S PULSE IS ABSENT:

15. Proceed to **PROTOCOL 9: Management of Cardiac Arrest Following ECG Rhythm Analysis Indicating "NO SHOCK"—One Rescuer.**

If the patient's PULSE is present:

16. Proceed to **PROTOCOL 10: Management of a Perfusing Rhythm—One or Two Rescuers.**

Algorithm/Protocol 8

Management of Cardiac Arrest Following ECG Rhythm Analysis Indicating "SHOCK"— One Rescuer

ALGORITHM 8
PROTOCOL 8

ALGORITHM 8: Management of Cardiac Arrest Following ECG Rhythm Analysis Indicating "SHOCK"—One Rescuer

If "SHOCK" is indicated THE FIRST TIME and the patient's pulse is absent:

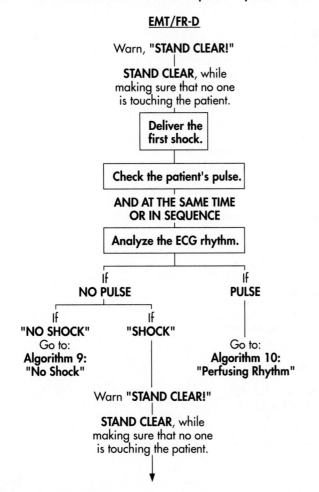

EMT/FR-D

Warn, **"STAND CLEAR!"**

STAND CLEAR, while making sure that no one is touching the patient.

Deliver the first shock.

Check the patient's pulse.

AND AT THE SAME TIME OR IN SEQUENCE

Analyze the ECG rhythm.

If **NO PULSE**

If **PULSE**

If **"NO SHOCK"**
Go to:
Algorithm 9:
"No Shock"

If **"SHOCK"**

Go to:
Algorithm 10:
"Perfusing Rhythm"

Warn **"STAND CLEAR!"**

STAND CLEAR, while making sure that no one is touching the patient.

Continued.

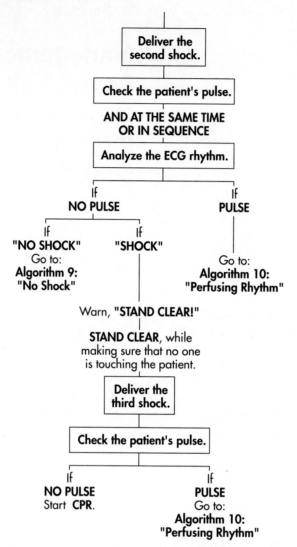

Deliver the second shock.

Check the patient's pulse.

AND AT THE SAME TIME OR IN SEQUENCE

Analyze the ECG rhythm.

If
NO PULSE

If
PULSE

If
"NO SHOCK"
Go to:
**Algorithm 9:
"No Shock"**

If
"SHOCK"

Go to:
**Algorithm 10:
"Perfusing Rhythm"**

Warn, **"STAND CLEAR!"**

STAND CLEAR, while making sure that no one is touching the patient.

Deliver the third shock.

Check the patient's pulse.

If
NO PULSE
Start **CPR.**

If
PULSE
Go to:
**Algorithm 10:
"Perfusing Rhythm"**

Wait for the arrival of the BLS or ALS unit, as appropriate, while continuing to perform **CPR**, reanalyzing the patient's ECG rhythm, delivering shocks, and checking the patient's pulse, according to local protocol, as follows:

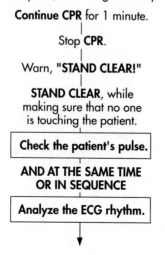

Continue CPR for 1 minute.

Stop **CPR.**

Warn, **"STAND CLEAR!"**

STAND CLEAR, while making sure that no one is touching the patient.

Check the patient's pulse.

AND AT THE SAME TIME OR IN SEQUENCE

Analyze the ECG rhythm.

Continued.

ALGORITHM 8: Management of Cardiac Arrest Following ECG Rhythm Analysis Indicating "SHOCK"—One Rescuer, cont'd

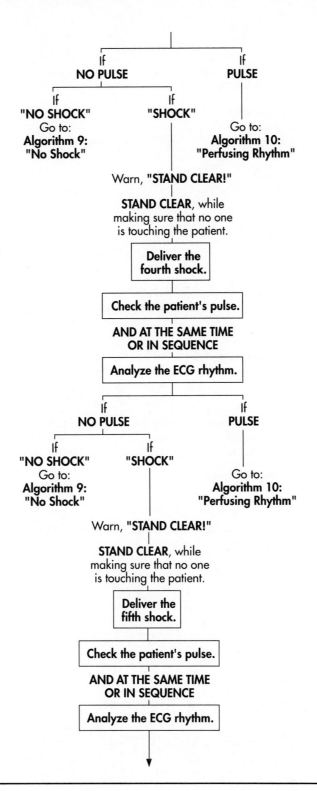

ALGORITHM 8: Management of Cardiac Arrest Following ECG Rhythm Analysis Indicating "SHOCK"—One Rescuer, cont'd

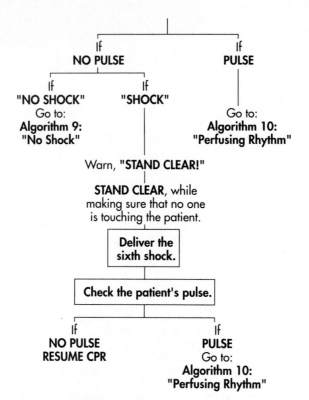

Wait for the arrival of the BLS or ALS unit, as appropriate, while continuing to perform **CPR**, reanalyzing the patient's ECG rhythm, delivering shocks, and checking the patient's pulse, according to local protocol, as follows:

Continue **CPR** for 1 minute.

Stop **CPR**.

Check the patient's pulse, analyze the ECG rhythm, and go to the appropriate protocol.

PROTOCOL 8: Management of Cardiac Arrest Following ECG Rhythm Analysis Indicating "SHOCK"—One Rescuer

If "SHOCK" is indicated THE FIRST TIME and the patient's pulse is absent:

EMT/FR-D

1. Warn, "STAND CLEAR!"

2. **STAND CLEAR WHILE MAKING SURE THAT NO ONE IS TOUCHING THE PATIENT OR ANYTHING IN CONTACT WITH THE PATIENT**

3. TURN ON THE CHARGING CIRCUIT, IF APPROPRIATE.

When the defibrillator is charged:

4. DELIVER THE FIRST SHOCK.

5. CHECK THE PATIENT'S PULSE.

AND AT THE SAME TIME
OR IN SEQUENCE

6. ANALYZE THE ECG RHYTHM.

If "SHOCK" is indicated and the PATIENT'S PULSE IS ABSENT:

7. Warn, "STAND CLEAR!"

8. **STAND CLEAR WHILE MAKING SURE THAT NO ONE IS TOUCHING THE PATIENT OR ANYTHING IS IN CONTACT WITH THE PATIENT.**

9. TURN ON THE CHARGING CIRCUIT, IF APPROPRIATE.

When the defibrillator is charged:

10. DELIVER THE SECOND SHOCK.

11. CHECK THE PATIENT'S PULSE.

AND AT THE SAME TIME
OR IN SEQUENCE

12. ANALYZE THE ECG RHYTHM.

If "SHOCK" is indicated and the PATIENT'S PULSE IS ABSENT:

13. Warn, "STAND CLEAR!"

14. **STAND CLEAR WHILE MAKING SURE THAT NO ONE IS TOUCHING THE PATIENT OR ANYTHING IN CONTACT WITH THE PATIENT.**

NOTE!

If "NO SHOCK" is indicated at any time:

If the patient's PULSE is present:

- Proceed to **PROTOCOL 10: Management of a Perfusing Rhythm—One or Two Rescuers.**

If the patient's PULSE is absent:

- Proceed to **PROTOCOL 9: Management of Cardiac Arrest Following ECG Rhythm Analysis Indicating "No Shock"—One Rescuer.**

Continued.

PROTOCOL 8: Management of Cardiac Arrest Following ECG Rhythm Analysis Indicating "SHOCK"—One Rescuer, cont'd

EMT/FR-D

15. | TURN ON THE CHARGING CIRCUIT, IF APPROPRIATE. |

When the defibrillator is charged:

16. | DELIVER THE THIRD SHOCK. |

17. | CHECK THE PATIENT'S PULSE. |

If the patient's PULSE is absent:

18. Start **CPR,** and continue for 1 minute.

NOTE!

If a spontaneous pulse appears at any time:

- Proceed to **PROTOCOL 10. Management of a Perfusing Rhythm.**

NOTE!

The total number of shocks delivered depends on the local protocol.

---

19. Stop **CPR.**

20. Warn, "STAND CLEAR!"

21. STAND CLEAR WHILE MAKING SURE THAT NO ONE IS TOUCHING THE PATIENT OR ANYTHING IN CONTACT WITH THE PATIENT.

22. | CHECK THE PATIENT'S PULSE. |

AND AT THE SAME TIME OR IN SEQUENCE

23. | ANALYZE THE ECG RHYTHM. |

If "SHOCK" is indicated and the PATIENT'S PULSE IS ABSENT:

24. Warn, "STAND CLEAR!"

25. STAND CLEAR WHILE MAKING SURE THAT NO ONE IS TOUCHING THE PATIENT OR ANYTHING IS IN CONTACT WITH THE PATIENT.

NOTE!

If "NO SHOCK" is indicated at any time:

If the patient's PULSE is present:

- Proceed to **PROTOCOL 10: Management of a Perfusing Rhythm—One or Two Rescuers.**

If the patient's PULSE is absent:

- Proceed to **PROTOCOL 9: Management of Cardiac Arrest Following ECG Rhythm Analysis Indicating "No Shock"—One Rescuer.**

Continued.

PROTOCOL 8: Management of Cardiac Arrest Following ECG Rhythm Analysis Indicating "SHOCK"—One Rescuer, cont'd

EMT/FR-D

26. | TURN ON THE CHARGING CIRCUIT, IF APPROPRIATE.

When the defibrillator is charged:

27. | DELIVER THE FOURTH SHOCK.

28. | CHECK THE PATIENT'S PULSE.

    AND AT THE SAME TIME
    OR IN SEQUENCE

29. | ANALYZE THE ECG RHYTHM.

If "SHOCK" is indicated and the PATIENT'S PULSE IS ABSENT:

30. Warn, "STAND CLEAR!"

31. STAND CLEAR WHILE MAKING SURE THAT NO ONE IS TOUCHING THE PATIENT OR ANYTHING IS IN CONTACT WITH THE PATIENT.

32. | TURN ON THE CHARGING CIRCUIT, IF APPROPRIATE.

When the defibrillator is charged:

33. | DELIVER THE FIFTH SHOCK.

34. | CHECK THE PATIENT'S PULSE.

    AND AT THE SAME TIME
    OR IN SEQUENCE

35. | ANALYZE THE ECG RHYTHM.

If "SHOCK" is indicated and the PATIENT'S PULSE IS ABSENT:

36. Warn, "STAND CLEAR!"

37. STAND CLEAR WHILE MAKING SURE THAT NO ONE IS TOUCHING THE PATIENT OR ANYTHING IS IN CONTACT WITH THE PATIENT

Continued.

PROTOCOL 8: Management of Cardiac Arrest Following ECG Rhythm Analysis Indicating "SHOCK"—One Rescuer, cont'd

EMT/FR-D

38. | TURN ON THE CHARGING CIRCUIT, IF APPROPRIATE. |

When the defibrillator is charged:

39. | DELIVER THE SIXTH SHOCK. |

40. | CHECK THE PATIENT'S PULSE. |

If the patient's PULSE is absent:

41. Resume **CPR**.

NOTE!
If a spontaneous pulse appears at any time: • Proceed to **PROTOCOL 10: Management of a Perfusing Rhythm.**

NOTE!
The total number of shocks delivered depends on the local protocol.

42. Wait for the arrival of the BLS or ALS unit, as appropriate, while continuing to perform **CPR**, reanalyzing the patient's ECG rhythm, delivering shocks, and checking the patient's pulse, according to local protocol.

Algorithm/Protocol 9

Management of Cardiac Arrest Following ECG Rhythm Analysis Indicating "NO SHOCK"—One Rescuer

ALGORITHM 9
PROTOCOL 9

ALGORITHM 9: Management of Cardiac Arrest Following ECG Rhythm Analysis Indicating "NO SHOCK"—One Rescuer

If "NO SHOCK" is indicated THE FIRST TIME and the patient's pulse is absent:

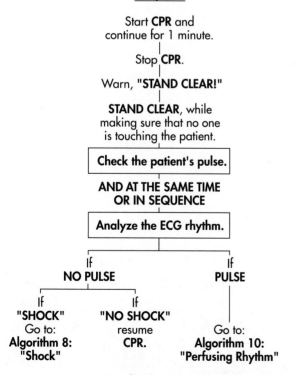

EMT/FR-D

Start **CPR** and
continue for 1 minute.

Stop **CPR**.

Warn, **"STAND CLEAR!"**

STAND CLEAR, while
making sure that no one
is touching the patient.

| Check the patient's pulse. |

**AND AT THE SAME TIME
OR IN SEQUENCE**

| Analyze the ECG rhythm. |

If **NO PULSE**   If **PULSE**

If   If
"SHOCK"   **"NO SHOCK"**
Go to: resume   Go to:
Algorithm 8:   **CPR.**   **Algorithm 10:**
"Shock"   **"Perfusing Rhythm"**

Wait for the BLS or ALS unit, as appropriate, while continuing
to perform **CPR**, reanalyzing the ECG every 1 to 3 minutes,
and checking the patient's pulse at the scene, according to
local protocol.

PROTOCOL 9: Management of Cardiac Arrest Following ECG Rhythm Analysis Indicating "NO SHOCK"—One Rescuer

If "NO SHOCK" is indicated THE FIRST TIME and the patient's pulse is absent:

EMT/FR-D

1. Start **CPR,** and continue for 1 minute (i.e., 4 cycles of 15 external chest compressions and 2 ventilations).

2. Stop **CPR.**

3. Warn, "STAND CLEAR!"

4. **STAND CLEAR WHILE MAKING SURE THAT NO ONE IS TOUCHING THE PATIENT OR ANYTHING IS IN CONTACT WITH THE PATIENT.**

5. CHECK THE PATIENT'S PULSE.

   **AND AT THE SAME TIME
   OR IN SEQUENCE**

6. ANALYZE THE ECG RHYTHM.

If "SHOCK" is indicated and the PATIENT'S PULSE IS ABSENT:

7. Proceed to **PROTOCOL 8: Management of Cardiac Arrest Following ECG Rhythm Analysis Indicating "SHOCK"—One Rescuer.**

If the patient's PULSE is present:

8. Proceed to **PROTOCOL 10: Management of a Perfusing Rhythm—One or Two Rescuers.**

If "NO SHOCK" is indicated and the PATIENT'S PULSE IS ABSENT:

9. Resume **CPR.**

10. Wait for the arrival of the BLS or ALS unit, as appropriate, while continuing to perform **CPR,** reanalyzing the patient's ECG rhythm every 1 to 3 minutes, and checking the patient's pulse, according to local protocol.

Algorithm/Protocol 10

Management of a Perfusing Rhythm— One or Two Rescuers

ALGORITHM 10
PROTOCOL 10

ALGORITHM 10: Management of Prefusing Rhythm—One or Two Rescuers

Establish and maintain
an open airway.
|
Determine the adequacy
of the patient's
circulation.
|
Administer high
concentration oxygen.
|
Suction the airway
as necessary.
|
Obtain and record
the vital signs.
|
Transport or wait
for the BLS or ALS unit,
as appropriate,
Keeping the patient warm.

**If the patient's respiratory rate is or becomes less than 12 per minute or the respirations
are or become shallow:**

OR

If the patient is or becomes unconscious:

Insert an oropharyngeal
or a nasopharyngeal
airway, as appropriate.
|
Provide ventilatory
assistance using high
concentration oxygen.

PROTOCOL 10: Management of a Perfusing Rhythm—One or Two Rescuers

1. Establish and maintain an open airway.

2. Suction the airway as necessary.

3. Determine if the patient's circulation is adequate.

4. Administer high concentration oxygen by a nonrebreathing mask with a reservoir bag at a flow rate of 10 to 15 liters per minute. If a face mask is not tolerated, administer the oxygen by a nasal cannula at 6 liters per minute.

5. Obtain and record the vital signs, and repeat them at least every 5 minutes or as often as possible, circumstances permitting.

If the adult patient's respiratory rate is or becomes less than 12 per minute or the respirations are or become shallow and the patient is confused, restless, or cyanotic:

6. Insert an oropharyngeal airway if the gag reflex is absent or a nasopharyngeal airway if the gag reflex is present.

7. Assist the patient's ventilation with high concentration oxygen using a bag-valve-mask (BVM) with an oxygen reservoir, a manually triggered oxygen-powered resuscitator, or an automatic ventilator.

NOTE!

ADEQUATE VENTILATION REQUIRES DISABLING THE POP-OFF VALVE IF THE BAG-VALVE-MASK IS SO EQUIPPED.

---

8. Evaluate the effectiveness of the ventilations.

If the patient is or becomes unconscious:

9. Insert an oropharyngeal airway if the gag reflex is absent or a nasopharyngeal airway if the gag reflex is present.

10. Ventilate the patient with high concentration oxygen using a bag-valve-mask (BVM) with an oxygen reservoir, a manually triggered oxygen-powered resuscitator, or an automatic ventilator.

11. **If cardiac arrest recurs,** proceed to **PROTOCOL 11: Management of Recurrent Cardiac Arrest—One or Two Rescuers.**

12. Transport or resume transport immediately or wait for the BLS or ALS unit as appropriate.

PROTOCOL 10: Management of a Perfusing Rhythm—One or Two Rescuers, cont'd

If two rescuers are present:

A. If the two rescuers are part of the crew of a BLS ambulance already at the scene AND an ALS unit is en route to the scene with an ESTIMATED TIME OF ARRIVAL GREATER THAN 8 MINUTES:

OR

If an ALS unit is not available:

OR

If the BLS ambulance is to connect up with an ALS unit en route:

- **TRANSPORT IMMEDIATELY.**

B. If the two rescuers are part of the crew of a BLS ambulance already at the scene AND an ALS unit is en route to the scene with an ESTIMATED TIME OF ARRIVAL LESS THAN 8 MINUTES:

- **WAIT FOR THE ARRIVAL OF THE ALS UNIT.**

C. If the two rescuers are part of a first responder unit:

- **WAIT FOR THE ARRIVAL OF THE BLS OR ALS UNIT, AS APPROPRIATE.**

D. If the two rescuers and the patient are already en route to the hospital:

- **RESUME TRANSPORT IMMEDIATELY.**

If one rescuer is present:

E. If the rescuer is part of a first responder unit:

- **WAIT FOR THE ARRIVAL OF THE BLS OR ALS UNIT, AS APPROPRIATE.**

Management of a Recurrent Cardiac Arrest—One or Two Rescuers

ALGORITHM 11
PROTOCOL 11

ALGORITHM 11: Management of a Recurrent Cardiac Arrest—One or Two Rescuers

If
RECURRENT
CARDIAC ARREST

If
TWO RESCUERS
Go to:
Algorithm 3:
"Initial Management
Witnessed Arrest—
Two Rescuers"

If
ONE RESCUER
Go to:
Algorithm 6:
"Initial Management
Pre-arrival/witnessed
Arrest —One Rescuer"

PROTOCOL 11: Management of a Recurrent Cardiac Arrest—One or Two Rescuers.

If two rescuers are present:

1. Proceed to **PROTOCOL 3:** Initial Management of EMT/FR-D-witnessed Cardiac Arrest while on the Scene or en Route—Two Rescuers.

If one rescuer is present:

2. Proceed to **PROTOCOL 6:** Initial Management of Pre-arrival Cardiac Arrest or EMT/FR-D-witnessed Cardiac Arrest while on the Scene—One Rescuer, without Bystander CPR.

Appendix

Protocols for Specific Automated External Defibrillators

The protocols included in the **Appendix** detail the use of specific semi- and fully automatic external defibrillators in the management of the following conditions:

A. Management of a persistent shockable rhythm:
   1. Ventricular fibrillation (V-Fib)
   2. Pulseless ventricular tachycardia (V-Tach)
B. Management of a nonshockable rhythm:
   1. Ventricular asystole
   2. Electromechanical dissociation (EMD)
C. Management of a perfusing rhythm

The automated external defibrillators (AEDs) for which protocols are provided include:
- Laerdal Heartstart 2000 (with ECG screen)
- Laerdal Heartstart 2000 (without ECG screen)
- Laerdal Heartstart 3000
- Laerdal Heartstart 1000s/Rapid Zap 1000s
- Laerdal Heartstart 1000s—SE Protocol
- Laerdal Heartstart 1000/Rapid Zap 1000
- First Medic 610
- First Medic 510
- Marquette Series 1200 Responder
- Physio-Control Lifepak 250 automatic advisory defibrillator with Lifepak Monitor
- Physio-Control Lifepak 200 Automatic Advisory Defibrillator
- Physio-Control Lifepak 300 Automatic Advisory Defibrillator

---

NOTE!

These protocols may be modified in accordance with the local prehospital defibrillation protocols.

This section on the protocols for using the AEDS is not intended to be studied in its entirety by the EMT/FR-D student. Only the protocols that pertain to the specific model of AED designated for use in the prehospital defibrillation program in which the student will participate should be studied.

Laerdal

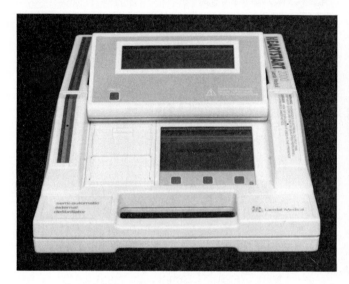

Laerdal Heartstart 2000 (with ECG screen)

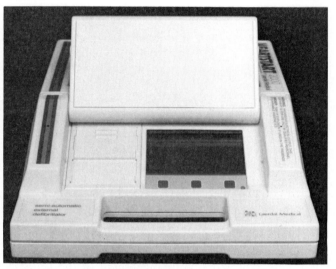

Laerdal Heartstart 2000 (without ECG screen)

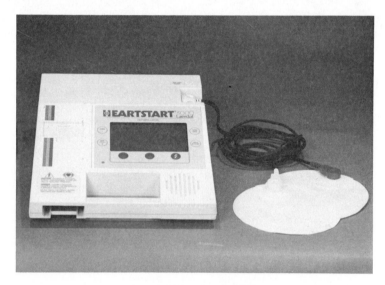

Laerdal Heartstart 3000

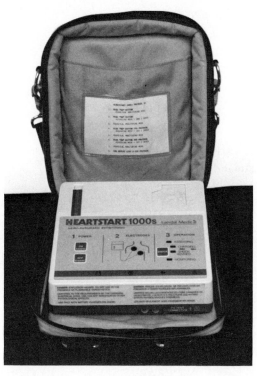

Laerdal Heartstart 1000s/Rapid Zap 1000s

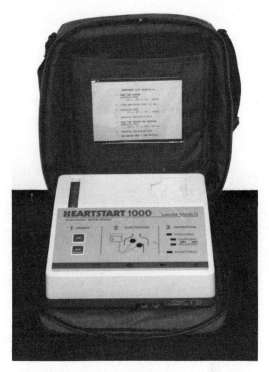

Laerdal Heartstart 1000/Rapid Zap 1000

Laerdal Heartstart 2000 (with ECG Screen)

A. Management of a persistent shockable rhythm: **1. Ventricular fibrillation (V-FIB)**
2. Pulseless ventricular tachycardia (V-TACH)

- Recognize the **situation.**
- Verify **cardiac arrest.**
- Start **one- or two-rescuer CPR.**

Rescuer one (CPR trained)	Rescuer two (EMT/FR-D)	Command screen messages	Verbal messages
1. Continue CPR.	1. Insert the **Medical Control Module** and, if appropriate, the **tape cassette.**		
	2. Verify that a **fully charged battery** is in place.		
	Note: Steps 1 and 2 should be done before arrival at the scene, preferably, during shift check.		
	3. Connect the **color-coded cables** to the defibrillator electrode pads. **White cable connector** to the **right electrode;** the **red cable connector** to the **left electrode.**		
	AND		
	Attach the **defibrillator electrode pads** to the **patient's chest.**		

Continued.

Laerdal Heartstart 2000 (with ECG Screen), cont'd

A. Management of a persistent shockable rhythm: 1. Ventricular fibrillation (V-FIB)

2. Pulseless ventricular tachycardia (V-TACH)

Rescuer one (CPR trained)	Rescuer two (EMT/FR-D)	Command screen messages	Verbal messages
	4. Turn on the **SAED** by flipping up the lid.	**ON**	
	5. Record the **NAMES** of the **RESCUERS,** the **TIME** displayed on the **Command Screen,** and the **AGE, SEX,** and **CONDITION** of the patient, including the **PATIENT'S PULSE.***	**SELF TEST OK**	
2. Stop **CPR** and **STAND CLEAR!**	**6.** State: **"STOP CPR! STAND CLEAR!"**	**PRESS TO ANALYZE**	
	7. Record the **TIME.*** (Palpate the **PATIENT'S PULSE— OPTIONAL.)**		
NO PULSE V-FIB OR V-TACH **SHOCKABLE RHYTHM**	**8.** Press the **"ANALYZE" BUTTON** for the **FIRST TIME** while analyzing the **ECG** on the ECG screen.	**ANALYZING** **STAND CLEAR**	**"STAND CLEAR!"**
	9. State: **"V-FIB (OR V-TACH) PRESENT!"**	**SHOCK INDICATED**	**"BEEP"**
	NOTE! If **"NO SHOCK"** is indicated now or at any time, PALPATE THE PATIENT'S PULSE. If the PULSE IS ABSENT, indicating a "NONPERFUSING RHYTHM," proceed to B: MANAGEMENT OF A NONSHOCKABLE RHYTHM.	**CHARGING** **200 J SELECTED**	**"CHARGING TONE"**
	10. Verify immediately that the energy setting is **"200 JOULES."**	**PRESS TO CHANGE ENERGY**	
	11. State: **"STAND CLEAR! DEFIBRILLATE AT 200 JOULES!"** while making sure that **no one is touching the patient.**	**READY PRESS TO SHOCK**	**"READY TONE"** **"PRESS TO SHOCK"**
	12. Press the **"SHOCK" BUTTON** for the **FIRST TIME** while observing the **ECG** on the ECG screen.	**1 SHOCK**	
	13. Record the **TIME** noted on the **Command Screen** after the delivery of the **first shock.*** (Palpate the **PATIENT'S PULSE— OPTIONAL.)**	**PRESS TO ANALYZE**	

*Omit voice recording of narrative if not required by local protocol.

Continued.

Laerdal Heartstart 2000 (with ECG Screen), cont'd

A. Management of a persistent shockable rhythm: 1. Ventricular fibrillation (V-FIB)
2. Pulseless ventricular tachycardia (V-TACH)

Rescuer one (CPR trained)	Rescuer two (EMT/FR-D)	Command screen messages	Verbal messages
NO PULSE V-FIB **OR** V-TACH **SHOCKABLE RHYTHM**	**14.** Press the "ANALYZE" BUTTON for the SECOND TIME while analyzing the ECG on the ECG screen. **15.** State: "V-FIB (OR V-TACH) STILL PRESENT!" **NOTE!** If "NO SHOCK" is indicated now or at any time, PALPATE THE PATIENT'S PULSE. If a SPONTANEOUS PULSE is present, indicating a "PERFUSING RHYTHM," proceed to C: MANAGEMENT OF A PERFUSING RHYTHM. **16.** Verify immediately that the energy setting is "200 JOULES." **17.** State: "STAND CLEAR! DEFIBRILLATE AT 200 JOULES!" while making sure that **no one is touching the patient.** **18.** Press the "SHOCK" BUTTON for the SECOND TIME while observing the ECG on the ECG screen. **19.** Record the TIME noted on the Command screen after the delivery of the second shock.* (Palpate the PATIENT'S PULSE—OPTIONAL.)	ANALYZING STAND CLEAR SHOCK INDICATED CHARGING 200 J SELECTED PRESS TO CHANGE ENERGY READY PRESS TO SHOCK 2 SHOCKS PRESS TO ANALYZE	 "STAND CLEAR!" "BEEP" "CHARGING TONE" "READY TONE" "PRESS TO SHOCK"
NO PULSE V-FIB **OR** V-TACH **SHOCKABLE RHYTHM**	**20.** Press the "ANALYZE" BUTTON for the THIRD TIME while analyzing the ECG on the ECG screen. **21.** State: "V-FIB (OR V-TACH) STILL PRESENT!" **22.** Verify immediately that the energy setting is "360 JOULES." **23.** State: "STAND CLEAR! DEFIBRILLATE AT 360 JOULES!" while making sure that **no one is touching the patient.**	ANALYZING STAND CLEAR SHOCK INDICATED CHARGING 360 J SELECTED PRESS TO CHANGE ENERGY READY PRESS TO SHOCK	 "STAND CLEAR!" "BEEP" "CHARGING TONE" "READY TONE" "PRESS TO SHOCK"

*Omit voice recording of narrative if not required by local protocol.

Continued.

Laerdal Heartstart 2000 (with ECG Screen), cont'd

A. Management of a persistent shockable rhythm: 1. Ventricular fibrillation (V-FIB)
2. Pulseless ventricular tachycardia (V-TACH)

Rescuer one (CPR trained)	Rescuer two (EMT/FR-D)	Command screen messages	Verbal messages
	24. Press the **"SHOCK" BUTTON** for the **THIRD TIME** while observing the **ECG on the ECG screen.**	<u>**3 SHOCKS**</u>	
	25. Record the **TIME** noted on the **Command Screen** after the delivery of the **third shock.***	**PRESS TO ANALYZE**	
NO PULSE V-FIB	**26.** Palpate the **patient's carotid artery** while analyzing the **ECG on the ECG screen.**		
OR V-TACH	**27.** State: **"V-FIB (OR V-TACH) STILL PRESENT! NO PULSE!"**		
SHOCKABLE RHYTHM **3.** Resume **CPR.** **4. TRANSPORT THE PATIENT IMMEDIATELY OR WAIT FOR THE BLS OR ALS UNIT, AS APPROPRIATE.**	**28.** State: **"CONTINUE CPR,"** and, if appropriate, **"TRANSPORT!"** **OR** Repeat **Steps 6 through 28,** as appropriate. The **subsequent shocks** are delivered in a sequence of **360, 360,** and **360 joules.**		

> **NOTE!**
>
> The **ENERGY LEVELS** and the **TOTAL NUMBER OF SHOCKS DELIVERED** may depend on the local protocol.

29. Continue **performing CPR, reanalyzing the ECG rhythm, delivering shocks,** and **checking the patient's pulse,** according to local protocol.

30. Record the **TIME** noted on the **Command Screen** upon relinquishing the patient to an **AEMT** or upon arrival at the **emergency department.***

---

*Omit voice recording of narrative if not required by local protocol.

Laerdal Heartstart 2000 (with ECG Screen)

B. Management of a nonshockable rhythm: 1. Ventricular asystole
2. Electromechanical dissociation (EMD)

IF "NO SHOCK" IS INDICATED AND A PULSE IS ABSENT, INDICATING A NONPERFUSING RHYTHM:

Rescuer one (CPR trained)	Rescuer two (EMT/FR-D)	Command screen messages	Verbal messages
NO PULSE Asystole OR EMD	**1.** Palpate the patient's carotid artery. **2.** State: "**ASYSTOLE (OR EMD) PRESENT! NO PULSE!**"	NO SHOCK INDICATED PRESS TO ANALYZE	
NONSHOCKABLE RHYTHM **1.** Resume **CPR,** and continue for 1 minute. **2.** Stop **CPR** and **STAND CLEAR!**	**3.** State: "**CONTINUE CPR!**" **4.** State: "**STOP CPR! STAND CLEAR!**" **5.** Record the **TIME** noted on the **Command Screen.*** (Palpate the **PATIENT'S PULSE—OPTIONAL.**)		
NO PULSE Asystole OR EMD	**6.** Press the "**ANALYZE**" **BUTTON** for the **SECOND TIME** while analyzing the **ECG on the ECG screen.** **7.** Palpate the **patient's carotid artery.**	<u>ANALYZING</u> STAND CLEAR NO SHOCK INDICATED PRESS TO ANALYZE	"**STAND CLEAR!**"
NONSHOCKABLE RHYTHM **3.** Resume **CPR.** **4. TRANSPORT THE PATIENT IMMEDIATELY OR WAIT FOR THE BLS OR ALS UNIT, AS APPROPRIATE.**	**8.** State: "**ASYSTOLE (OR EMD) STILL PRESENT! NO PULSE!**" **9.** State: "**CONTINUE CPR!**" and, if appropriate, "**TRANSPORT!**" **10.** Continue **performing CPR, reanalyzing the ECG rhythm,** and **checking the patient's pulse,** according to locol protocol. **11.** Record the **TIME** noted on the **Command Screen** upon relinquishing the patient to an **AEMT** or upon arrival at the **emergency department.***		

*Omit voice recording of narrative if not required by local protocol.

Laerdal Heartstart 2000 (with ECG Screen)

C. Management of a perfusing rhythm

IF "NO SHOCK" IS INDICATED AND A SPONTANEOUS PULSE IS PRESENT, INDICATING A PERFUSING RHYTHM:

Rescuer one (CPR trained)	Rescuer two (EMT/FR-D)	Command screen messages	Verbal messages
PULSE PRESENT Organized ECG rhythm **PERFUSING RHYTHM** 1. Open and maintain an **open airway** while administering **high concentration oxygen.** 2. Assist **ventilation** while administering **supplemental high concentration oxygen** if necessary. 3. **TRANSPORT THE PATIENT IMMEDIATELY OR WAIT FOR THE BLS OR ALS UNIT, AS APPROPRIATE.**	1. Palpate the patient's carotid artery. 2. State: **"PULSE AND ECG PRESENT!"** 3. State: **"ADMINISTER OXYGEN"** and **"TRANSPORT!"** 4. Obtain the initial **vital signs** and repeat them as often as the situation indicates, and, if appropriate, record them.* 5. **Monitor** the **patient's ECG** using the SAED. If cardiac arrest recurs **at the scene or en route:** • State: **"STAND CLEAR!"** AND • Repeat **Steps 8 through 25, A: MANAGEMENT OF A PERSISTENT SHOCKABLE RHYTHM,** as appropriate, until the shockable rhythm is converted into a perfusing rhythm or up to a total of **6 shocks** are delivered. The first shock of this series is delivered at the same energy level that was successful in terminating the dysrhythmia the last time. Subsequent shocks are delivered at 360 joules. --- **NOTE!** **The ENERGY LEVELS and the TOTAL NUMBER OF SHOCKS DELIVERED may depend on the local protocol.** --- 6. Record the **TIME** noted on the **Command Screen** upon relinquishing the patient to an **AEMT** or upon arrival at the **emergency department.***	**NO SHOCK INDICATED** **PRESS TO ANALYZE**	

*Omit voice recording of narrative if not required by local protocol.

Laerdal Heartstart 2000 (without ECG screen)

A. **Management of a persistent shockable rhythm: 1. Ventricular fibrillation (V-FIB)**
                                                 2. Pulseless ventricular tachycardia (V-TACH)

- Recognize the **situation.**
- Verify **cardiac arrest.**
- Start **one- or two-rescuer CPR.**

Rescuer one (CPR trained)	Rescuer two (EMT/FR-D)	Command screen messages	Verbal messages
1. Continue **CPR.**	1. Insert the **Medical Control Module** and, if appropriate, the **tape cassette.**		
	2. Verify that a **fully charged battery** is in place.		
	Note: Steps 1 and 2 should be done before arrival at the scene, preferably, during shift check.		
	3. Connect the **color-coded cables** to the defibrillator electrode pads. **White cable connector** to the **right electrode;** the **red cable connector** to the **left electrode.** **AND** Attach the **defibrillator electrode pads** to the **patient's chest.**		
	4. Turn on the **SAED** by flipping up the lid.	**ON**	
	5. Record the **NAMES** of the **RESCUERS,** the **TIME** displayed on the **Command Screen,** and the **AGE, SEX,** and **CONDITION** of the patient, including the **PATIENT'S PULSE.***	**SELF TEST OK**	
2. Stop **CPR** and **STAND CLEAR!**	6. State: **"STOP CPR! STAND CLEAR!"**	**PRESS TO ANALYZE**	
	7. Record the **TIME.*** (Palpate the **PATIENT'S PULSE—OPTIONAL.**)		
	8. Press the **"ANALYZE" BUTTON** for the **FIRST TIME.**	<u>**ANALYZING**</u>	
		STAND CLEAR	**"STAND CLEAR!"**
	NOTE! If **"NO SHOCK"** is indicated now or at any time, PALPATE THE PATIENT'S PULSE. If the PULSE IS ABSENT, indicating a **"NONPERFUSING RHYTHM,"** proceed to B: MANAGEMENT OF A NON-SHOCKABLE RHYTHM.	<u>**SHOCK INDICATED CHARGING**</u> **200 J SELECTED**	**"BEEP"** **"CHARGING TONE"**
	9. Verify immediately that the energy setting is **"200 JOULES."**	**PRESS TO CHANGE ENERGY**	

*Omit voice recording of narrative if not required by local protocol.   *Continued.*

Laerdal Heartstart 2000 (without ECG screen), cont'd

A. Management of a persistent shockable rhythm: 1. Ventricular fibrillation (V-FIB)
2. Pulseless ventricular tachycardia (V-TACH)

Rescuer one (CPR trained)	Rescuer two (EMT/FR-D)	Command screen messages	Verbal messages
	10. State: "STAND CLEAR! DEFIBRILLATE AT 200 JOULES!" while making sure that **no one is touching the patient.**	READY PRESS TO SHOCK	"READY TONE" "PRESS TO SHOCK"
	11. Press the "SHOCK" BUTTON for the FIRST TIME.	1 SHOCK	
	12. Record the TIME noted on the Command Screen after the delivery of the first shock.* (Palpate the PATIENT'S PULSE— OPTIONAL.)	PRESS TO ANALYZE	
	13. Press the "ANALYZE" BUTTON for the SECOND TIME.	ANALYZING	
		STAND CLEAR	"STAND CLEAR!"
	NOTE! If "NO SHOCK" is indicated now or at any time, PALPATE THE PATIENT'S PULSE. If a SPONTANEOUS PULSE is present, indicating a "PERFUSING RHYTHM," proceed to C: MANAGEMENT OF A PERFUSING RHYTHM.	SHOCK INDICATED	"BEEP"
		CHARGING	"CHARGING TONE"
		200 J SELECTED	
		PRESS TO CHANGE ENERGY	
	14. Verify immediately that the energy setting is "200 JOULES."		
	15. State: "STAND CLEAR! DEFIBRILLATE AT 200 JOULES!" while making sure that **no one is touching the patient.**	READY PRESS TO SHOCK	"READY TONE" "PRESS TO SHOCK"
	16. Press the "SHOCK" BUTTON for the SECOND TIME.	2 SHOCKS	
	17. Record the TIME noted on the Command screen after the delivery of the second shock.* (Palpate the PATIENT'S PULSE— OPTIONAL.)	PRESS TO ANALYZE	
	18. Press the "ANALYZE" BUTTON for the THIRD TIME.	ANALYZING	
		STAND CLEAR	"STAND CLEAR!"
		SHOCK INDICATED	"BEEP"
		CHARGING	"CHARGING TONE"
	19. Verify immediately that the energy setting is "360 JOULES."	360 J SELECTED	

---

*Omit voice recording of narrative if not required by local protocol.

Continued.

Laerdal Heartstart 2000 (without ECG screen), cont'd

A. Management of a persistent shockable rhythm: 1. Ventricular fibrillation (V-FIB)
2. Pulseless ventricular tachycardia (V-TACH)

Rescuer one (CPR trained)	Rescuer two (EMT/FR-D)	Command screen messages	Verbal messages
		PRESS TO CHANGE ENERGY	
	20. State: **"STAND CLEAR! DEFIBRILLATE AT 360 JOULES!"** while making sure that **no one is touching the patient.**	**READY PRESS TO SHOCK**	**"READY TONE" "PRESS TO SHOCK"**
	21. Press the **"SHOCK" BUTTON** for the **THIRD TIME.**	**3 SHOCKS**	
	22. Record the **TIME** noted on the **Command Screen** after the delivery of the **third shock.***	**PRESS TO ANALYZE**	
	23. Palpate the **patient's carotid artery.**		
	24. State: **"NO PULSE!"**		
3. Resume **CPR.**	25. State: **"CONTINUE CPR,"** and, if appropriate, **"TRANSPORT!"**		
4. **TRANSPORT THE PATIENT IMMEDIATELY OR WAIT FOR THE BLS OR ALS UNIT, AS APPROPRIATE.**	**OR** Repeat **Steps 6 through 25,** as appropriate. The **subsequent shocks** are delivered in a sequence of **360, 360, and 360 joules.**		

NOTE!

The ENERGY LEVELS and the TOTAL NUMBER OF SHOCKS DELIVERED may depend on the local protocol.

---

26. Continue **performing CPR, reanalyzing the ECG rhythm, delivering shocks,** and **checking the patient's pulse,** according to local protocol.

27. Record the **TIME** noted on the **Command Screen** upon relinquishing the patient to an **AEMT** or upon arrival at the **emergency department.***

*Omit voice recording of narrative if not required by local protocol.

Laerdal Heartstart 2000 (without ECG Screen)

B. Management of a nonshockable rhythm: 1. Ventricular asystole
2. Electromechanical dissociation (EMD)

IF "NO SHOCK" IS INDICATED AND A PULSE IS ABSENT, INDICATING A NONPERFUSING RHYTHM:

Rescuer one (CPR trained)	Rescuer two (EMT/FR-D)	Command screen messages	Verbal messages
	1. Palpate the patient's carotid artery.		
	2. State: "NO PULSE!"	NO SHOCK INDICATED	
1. Resume **CPR,** and continue for 1 minute.	3. State: "CONTINUE CPR!"	PRESS TO ANALYZE	
2. Stop **CPR** and **STAND CLEAR!**	4. State: "STOP CPR! STAND CLEAR!"		
	5. Record the **TIME** noted on the **Command Screen.***		
	(Palpate the **PATIENT'S PULSE— OPTIONAL.**)		
	6. Press the "ANALYZE" BUTTON for the SECOND TIME.	ANALYZING STAND CLEAR	"STAND CLEAR!"
	7. Palpate the **patient's carotid artery.**	NO SHOCK INDICATED	
	8. State: "NO PULSE!""		
3. Resume **CPR.**	9. State: "CONTINUE CPR!" and, if appropriate, "TRANSPORT!"	PRESS TO ANALYZE	
4. **TRANSPORT THE PATIENT IMMEDIATELY OR WAIT FOR THE BLS OR ALS UNIT, AS APPROPRIATE.**	10. Continue **performing CPR, reanalyzing the ECG rhythm,** and **checking the patient's pulse,** according to locol protocol.		
	11. Record the **TIME** noted on the **Command Screen** upon relinquishing the patient to an **AEMT** or upon arrival at the **emergency department.***		

*Omit voice recording of narrative if not required by local protocol.

Laerdal Heartstart 2000 (without ECG screen)

C. Management of a perfusing rhythm

IF "NO SHOCK" IS INDICATED AND A SPONTANEOUS PULSE IS PRESENT, INDICATING A PERFUSING RHYTHM:

Rescuer one (CPR trained)	Rescuer two (EMT/FR-D)	Command screen messages	Verbal messages
1. Open and maintain an **open airway** while administering **high concentration oxygen.**	1. Palpate the patient's carotid artery.	**NO SHOCK INDICATED**	
2. Assist **ventilation** while administering **supplemental high concentration oxygen** if necessary.	2. State: **"PULSE PRESENT!"**	**PRESS TO ANALYZE**	
3. **TRANSPORT THE PATIENT IMMEDIATELY OR WAIT FOR THE BLS OR ALS UNIT, AS APPROPRIATE.**	3. State: **"ADMINISTER OXYGEN"** and **"TRANSPORT!"**		
	4. Obtain the initial **vital signs** and repeat them as often as the situation indicates, and, if appropriate, record them.*		

If cardiac arrest recurs at the scene or en route:

- State: **"STAND CLEAR!"**

AND

- Repeat **Steps 8 through 25, A: MANAGEMENT OF A PERSISTENT SHOCKABLE RHYTHM,** as appropriate, until the shockable rhythm is converted into a perfusing rhythm or up to a total of **6 shocks** are delivered. The first shock of this series is delivered at the same energy level that was successful in terminating the dysrhythmia the last time. Subsequent shocks are delivered at 360 joules.

NOTE!

The ENERGY LEVELS and the TOTAL NUMBER OF SHOCKS DELIVERED may depend on the local protocol.

---

5. Record the **TIME** noted on the **Command Screen** upon relinquishing the patient to an **AEMT** or upon arrival at the **emergency department.***

*Omit voice recording of narrative if not required by local protocol.

Laerdal Heartstart 3000

A. Management of a persistent shockable rhythm: 1. Ventricular fibrillation (V-FIB)
2. Pulseless ventricular tachycardia (V-TACH)

- Recognize the **situation.**
- Verify **cardiac arrest.**
- Start **one- or two-rescuer CPR.**

Rescuer one (CPR trained)	Rescuer two (EMT/FR-D)	Command screen messages	Verbal messages
1. Continue **CPR.**	1. Insert the **Medical Control Module** and, if appropriate, the **tape cassette.**		
	2. Verify that a **fully charged battery** is in place.		
	Note: Steps 1 and 2 should be done before arrival at the scene, preferably, during shift check.		
	3. Connect the **color-coded cables** to the defibrillator electrode pads. **White cable connector** to the **right electrode;** the **red cable connector** to the **left electrode.**		
	AND		
	Attach the **defibrillator electrode pads** to the **patient's chest.**		
	4. Turn on the **SAED** by pressing the **"ON" BUTTON.**	SELFTEST IN PROGRESS	"BEEP"
	5. Record the **NAMES** of the **RESCUERS,** the **TIME** displayed on the **Command Screen,** and the **AGE, SEX,** and **CONDITION** of the patient, including the **PATIENT'S PULSE.***	SELFTEST OK	
2. Stop **CPR** and **STAND CLEAR!**	6. State: **"STOP CPR! STAND CLEAR!"**	SELECTED 200 J	
	7. Record the **TIME.***	ANALYZE CHECK PATIENT	
	(Palpate the **PATIENT'S PULSE— OPTIONAL.**)	(CHECK PATIENT)†	("CHECK PATIENT")†
NO PULSE	8. Press the **"ANALYZE" BUTTON** for the **FIRST TIME** while analyzing the ECG on the ECG screen.	STAND CLEAR ANALYZING	"STAND CLEAR!"
V-FIB	9. State: **"V-FIB (OR V-TACH) PRESENT!"**	ENERGY SELECT	
OR			
V-TACH	**NOTE!** If **"NO SHOCK"** is indicated now or at any time, PALPATE THE PATIENT'S PULSE. If the PULSE IS ABSENT, indicating a "NONPERFUSING RHYTHM," proceed to B: MANAGEMENT OF A NONSHOCKABLE RHYTHM.	CHARGING	"CHARGING TONE"
SHOCKABLE RHYTHM			

*Omit voice recording of narrative if not required by local protocol.

†"CHECK PATIENT" messages appear within 10 seconds if "ANALYZE" button is not pressed.

Laerdal Heartstart 3000, cont'd

A. Management of a persistent shockable rhythm: 1. Ventricular fibrillation (V-FIB)
2. Pulseless ventricular tachycardia (V-TACH)

Rescuer one (CPR trained)	Rescuer two (EMT/FR-D)	Command screen messages	Verbal messages
	10. Verify immediately that the energy setting is **"200 JOULES."**		
	11. State: **"STAND CLEAR! DEFIBRILLATE AT 200 JOULES!"** while making sure that **no one is touching the patient.**	READY SHOCK	"READY TONE" "PRESS TO SHOCK"
	12. Press the **"SHOCK" BUTTON** for the **FIRST TIME** while observing the **ECG** on the **ECG screen.**	1 SHOCK	
	13. Record the **TIME** noted on the **Command Screen** after the delivery of the **first shock.***	SELECTED 200 J ANALYZE	
	(Palpate the **PATIENT'S PULSE— OPTIONAL.**)	(CHECK PATIENT)	("CHECK PATIENT")
NO PULSE	**14.** Press the **"ANALYZE" BUTTON** for the **SECOND TIME** while analyzing the **ECG** on the **ECG screen.**	STAND CLEAR ANALYZING	"STAND CLEAR!"
V-FIB	**15.** State: **"V-FIB (OR V-TACH) STILL PRESENT!"**	ENERGY SELECT	
OR			
V-TACH		CHARGING	"CHARGING TONE"
SHOCKABLE RHYTHM			

> **NOTE!**
>
> If **"NO SHOCK"** is indicated now or at any time, PALPATE THE PATIENT'S PULSE. If a SPONTANEOUS PULSE is present, indicating a **"PERFUSING RHYTHM,"** proceed to C: MANAGEMENT OF A PERFUSING RHYTHM.

Rescuer one (CPR trained)	Rescuer two (EMT/FR-D)	Command screen messages	Verbal messages
	16. Verify immediately that the energy setting is **"200 JOULES."**		
	17. State: **"STAND CLEAR! DEFIBRILLATE AT 200 JOULES!"** while making sure that **no one is touching the patient.**	READY SHOCK	"READY TONE" "PRESS TO SHOCK"
	18. Press the **"SHOCK" BUTTON** for the **SECOND TIME** while observing the **ECG** on the **ECG screen.**	2 SHOCKS	
	19. Record the **TIME** noted on the **Command Screen** after the delivery of the second **shock.***	SELECTED 360 J ANALYZE	
	(Palpate the **PATIENT'S PULSE— OPTIONAL.**)	(CHECK PATIENT)	("CHECK PATIENT")

*Omit voice recording of narrative if not required by local protocol.

Continued.

Laerdal Heartstart 3000, cont'd

A. Management of a persistent shockable rhythm: 1. Ventricular fibrillation (V-FIB)
2. Pulseless ventricular tachycardia (V-TACH)

Rescuer one (CPR trained)	Rescuer two (EMT/FR-D)	Command screen messages	Verbal messages
NO PULSE V-FIB OR V-TACH SHOCKABLE RHYTHM	**20.** Press the "**ANALYZE**" **BUTTON** for the **THIRD TIME** while observing the **ECG on the ECG screen.**	STAND CLEAR ANALYZING	"STAND CLEAR!"
	21. State: "**V-FIB (OR V-TACH) STILL PRESENT!**"	ENERGY SELECT	
	22. Verify immediately that the energy setting is "**360 JOULES.**"	CHARGING	"CHARGING TONE
	23. State: "**STAND CLEAR! DEFIBRIL-LATE AT 360 JOULES!**" while making sure that **no one is touching the patient.**	READY SHOCK	"READY TONE" "PRESS TO SHOCK"
NO PULSE V-FIB OR V-TACH SHOCKABLE RHYTHM	**24.** Press the "**SHOCK**" **BUTTON** for the **THIRD TIME** while observing the **ECG on the ECG screen.**	3 SHOCKS	
	25. Record the **TIME** noted on the **Command Screen** after the delivery of the **third shock.***	SELECTED 360 J ANALYZE	
	26. Palpate the **patient's carotid artery** while analyzing the **ECG on the ECG screen.**	CHECK PATIENT	"CHECK PATIENT"
	27. State: "**V-FIB (OR V-TACH) STILL PRESENT! NO PULSE!**"		

*Omit voice recording of narrative if not required by local protocol.

Laerdal Heartstart 3000, cont'd

A. Management of a persistent shockable rhythm: 1. Ventricular fibrillation (V-FIB)
2. Pulseless ventricular tachycardia (V-TACH)

Rescuer one (CPR trained)	Rescuer two (EMT/FR-D)	Command screen messages	Verbal messages
3. Resume **CPR**. 4. **TRANSPORT THE PATIENT IMMEDIATELY OR WAIT FOR THE BLS OR ALS UNIT, AS APPROPRIATE.**	28. State: **"Continue CPR,"** and, if appropriate, **TRANSPORT!"** **OR** **Repeat Steps 6 through 28,** as appropriate. The **subsequent shocks** are delivered in a sequence of **360, 360,** and **360 joules.**		

> **NOTE!**
>
> The **ENERGY LEVELS and the TOTAL NUMBER OF SHOCKS DELIVERED may depend on the local protocol.**

	29. Continue **performing CPR, reanalyzing the ECG rhythm, delivering shocks,** and **checking the patient's pulse,** according to local protocol. 30. Record the **TIME** noted on the **Command Screen** upon relinquishing the patient to an **AEMT** or upon arrival at the **emergency department.***		

*Omit voice recording of narrative if not required by local protocol.

Laerdal Heartstart 3000

B. Management of a nonshockable rhythm: 1. Ventricular asystole
2. Electromechanical dissociation (EMD)

IF "NO SHOCK" IS INDICATED AND A PULSE IS ABSENT, INDICATING A NONPERFUSING RHYTHM:			
Rescuer one (CPR trained)	Rescuer two (EMT/FR-D)	Command screen messages	Verbal messages
	1. Palpate the patient's carotid artery.	NO SHOCK INDICATED	
NO PULSE Asystole **OR** EMD **NONSHOCKABLE RHYTHM**	2. State: "ASYSTOLE (OR EMD) PRESENT! NO PULSE!"	CHECK PULSE	"CHECK PULSE!"
		SELECTED 200 J (or 360 J)	
		ANALYZE	
1. Resume **CPR,** and continue for 1 minute.	3. State: "CONTINUE CPR!"		
2. Stop **CPR** and **STAND CLEAR!**	4. State: "STOP CPR! STAND CLEAR!"		
	5. Record the **TIME** noted on the **Command Screen.*** (Palpate the **PATIENT'S PULSE— OPTIONAL.**)		
	6. Press the **"ANALYZE" BUTTON** for the **SECOND TIME** while analyzing the **ECG** on the ECG screen.	STAND CLEAR	"STAND CLEAR!"
		ANALYZING	
		ENERGY SELECT	
		NO SHOCK INDICATED	

*Omit voice recording of narrative if not required by local protocol.

Laerdal Heartstart 3000, cont'd

B. Management of a nonshockable rhythm: 1. Ventricular asystole
2. Electromechanical dissociation (EMD)

Rescuer one (CPR trained)	Rescuer two (EMT/FR-D)	Command screen messages	Verbal messages
NO PULSE Asystole **OR** EMD **NONSHOCKABLE RHYTHM** 3. Resume **CPR**. 4. **TRANSPORT THE PATIENT IMMEDIATELY OR WAIT FOR THE BLS OR ALS UNIT, AS APPROPRIATE.**	7. Palpate the **patient's carotid artery.** 8. State: **"ASYSTOLE (OR EMD) STILL PRESENT! NO PULSE!"** 9. State: **"CONTINUE CPR!"** and, if appropriate, **"TRANSPORT!"** 10. Continue **performing CPR, reanalyzing the ECG rhythm,** and **checking the patient's pulse,** according to local protocol. 11. Record the **TIME** noted on the **Command Screen** upon relinquishing the patient to an **AEMT** or upon arrival at the **emergency department.***	**CHECK PULSE**	**"CHECK PULSE!"**

*Omit voice recording of narrative if not required by local protocol.

Laerdal Heartstart 3000

C. Management of a perfusing rhythm

IF "NO SHOCK" IS INDICATED AND A SPONTANEOUS PULSE IS PRESENT, INDICATING A PERFUSING RHYTHM:

Rescuer one (CPR trained)	Rescuer two (EMT/FR-D)	Command screen messages	Verbal messages
	1. Palpate the carotid artery.	**NO SHOCK INDICATED**	
PULSE PRESENT Organized ECG rhythm **PERFUSING RHYTHM**	**2.** State: **"PULSE AND ECG PRESENT!"**	**CHECK PULSE** **SELECTED 200 J (or 360 J)** **ANALYZE**	**"CHECK PULSE!"**

1. Open and maintain an **open airway** while administering **high concentration oxygen.**

3. State: **"ADMINISTER OXYGEN"** and **"TRANSPORT!"**

2. Assist **ventilation** while administering **supplemental high concentration oxygen** if necessary.

4. Obtain the initial **vital signs** and repeat them as often as the situation indicates, and, if appropriate, record them.*

3. TRANSPORT THE PATIENT IMMEDIATELY OR WAIT FOR THE BLS OR ALS UNIT, AS APPROPRIATE.

5. Monitor the **patient's ECG** using the SAED.

If cardiac arrest recurs at the scene or en route:

- State: **"STAND CLEAR!"**

AND

- Repeat **Steps 8 through 28, A: MANAGEMENT OF A PERSISTENT SHOCKABLE RHYTHM,** as appropriate, until the shockable rhythm is converted into a perfusing rhythm or up to a total of **6 shocks** is delivered. The first shock of this series is delivered at the same energy level that was successful in terminating the dysrhythmia the last time. Subsequent shocks are delivered at 360 joules.

NOTE!

The ENERGY LEVELS and the TOTAL NUMBER OF SHOCKS DELIVERED may depend on the local protocol.

---

6. Record the **TIME** noted on the **Command Screen** upon relinquishing the patient to an **AEMT** or upon arrival at the **emergency department.***

*Omit voice recording of narrative if not required by local protocol.

Laerdal Heartstart 1000s/Rapid Zap 1000s

A. Management of a persistent shockable rhythm: 1. Ventricular fibrillation (V-FIB)
2. Pulseless ventricular tachycardia (V-TACH)

- Recognize the **situation.**
- Verify **cardiac arrest.**
- Start **one-** or **two-rescuer CPR.**

Rescuer one (CPR trained)	Rescuer two (EMT/FR-D)	Command screen messages	Verbal messages
1. Continue **CPR.**	**1.** Insert the **tape cassette,** if appropriate.		
	2. Verify that a **fully charged battery** is in place.		
	Note: Steps 1 and 2 should be done before arrival at the scene, preferably, during shift check.		
	3. Connect the **color-coded cables** to the defibrillator electrode pads. **White cable connector** to the **right electrode;** the **red cable connector** to the **left electrode.** AND Attach the **defibrillator electrode pads** to the **patient's chest.**		
	4. Turn on the **SAED** by pressing the **POWER ON/ASSESS** switch.	<u>MONITORING</u>	"CHECK BREATHING AND PULSE"
	5. Record the **NAMES** of the **RESCUERS,** and the **AGE, SEX,** and **CONDITION** of the patient, including the **PATIENT'S PULSE.***		
2. Stop **CPR** and **STAND CLEAR!**	**6.** State: **"STOP CPR! STAND CLEAR!"**		
	7. Record the **TIME.*** (Palpate the **PATIENT'S PULSE—OPTIONAL**)		
	8. Press the **POWER ON/ASSESS** switch for the **FIRST TIME.**	<u>ASSESSING</u>	"ASSESSING, HANDS OFF!"
	┌─────────────────────────┐ │ **NOTE!** │ │ **If "MONITORING" and "CHECK BREATHING AND PULSE" are indicated following "ASSESSING" now or at any time, PALPATE THE PATIENT'S PULSE. If the PULSE IS ABSENT, indicating a "NONPERFUSING RHYTHM," proceed to B: MANAGEMENT OF A NONSHOCKABLE RHYTHM.** └─────────────────────────┘	<u>CHARGING</u> 200 J	"STAND BACK!" "CHARGING TONE"
	9. State: **"STAND CLEAR! DEFIBRILLATE AT 200 JOULES!"** while making sure that **no one is touching the patient.**	**SHOCK ADVISED**	"READY TONE" "STAND BACK"

*Omit voice recording of narrative if not required by local protocol.

Continued.

Laerdal Heartstart 1000s/Rapid Zap 1000s, cont'd

A. Management of a persistent shockable rhythm: 1. Ventricular fibrillation (V-FIB)
2. Pulseless ventricular tachycardia (V-TACH)

Rescuer one (CPR trained)	Rescuer two (EMT/FR-D)	Command screen messages	Verbal messages
	10. Press the **"SHOCK" SWITCH** for the **FIRST TIME.**		**"SHOCK DELIVERED"**
	11. Record the **TIME** after the delivery of the **first shock.*** (Palpate the **PATIENT'S PULSE—OPTIONAL**)	**MONITORING**	**"CHECK BREATHING AND PULSE"**
	12. Press the **POWER ON/ASSESS** switch for the **SECOND TIME.**	**ASSESSING**	**"ASSESSING, HANDS OFF!"**
	NOTE! If **"MONITORING"** and **"CHECK BREATHING AND PULSE"** are indicated following **"ASSESSING"** now or at any time, PALPATE THE PATIENT'S PULSE. If the PULSE IS PRESENT, indicating a **"PERFUSING RHYTHM,"** proceed to **B: MANAGEMENT OF A PERFUSING RHYTHM.**	**CHARGING** 200 J	**"STAND BACK!"** **"CHARGING TONE"**
	13. State: **"STAND CLEAR! DEFIBRILLATE AT 200 JOULES!"** while making sure that **no one is touching the patient.**	**SHOCK ADVISED**	**"READY TONE"** **"STAND BACK"**
	14. Press the **"SHOCK" SWITCH** for the **SECOND TIME.**		**"SHOCK DELIVERED"**
	15. Record the **TIME** after the delivery of the **second shock.*** (Palpate the **PATIENT'S PULSE—OPTIONAL**)	**MONITORING**	**"CHECK BREATHING AND PULSE"**
	16. Press the **POWER ON/ASSESS** switch for the **THIRD TIME.**	**ASSESSING**	**"ASSESSING, HANDS OFF!"**
		CHARGING 360 J	**"STAND BACK!"** **"CHARGING TONE"**
	17. State: **"STAND CLEAR! DEFIBRILLATE AT 360 JOULES!"** while making sure that **no one is touching the patient.**	**SHOCK ADVISED**	**"READY TONE"** **"STAND BACK"**
	18. Press the **"SHOCK" SWITCH** for the **THIRD TIME.**		**"SHOCK DELIVERED"**
	19. Record the **TIME** after the delivery of the **third shock.***	**MONITORING**	**"CHECK BREATHING AND PULSE"**

*Omit voice recording of narrative if not required by local protocol.

Laerdal Heartstart 1000s/Rapid Zap 1000s, cont'd

A. Management of a persistent shockable rhythm: 1. Ventricular fibrillation (V-FIB)
2. Pulseless ventricular tachycardia (V-TACH)

Rescuer one (CPR trained)	Rescuer two (EMT/FR-D)	Command screen messages	Verbal messages
	20. Palpate the **patient's carotid artery.**		
	21. State: **"NO PULSE!"**		
3. Resume **CPR.**	**22.** State: **"CONTINUE CPR!"**		**"CHECK BREATHING AND PULSE"**
4. Stop **CPR** and **STAND CLEAR!**	**23.** State: **"STOP CPR! STAND CLEAR!"**		
	24. Record the **TIME.*** (Palpate the **PATIENT'S PULSE—OPTIONAL**)		
	25. Press the **POWER ON/ASSESS** switch for the **FOURTH TIME.**	**ASSESSING**	**"ASSESSING, HANDS OFF!"**
		CHARGING 360 J	**"STAND BACK!"** **"CHARGING TONE"**
	26. State: **"STAND CLEAR! DEFIBRILLATE AT 360 JOULES!"** while making sure that **no one is touching the patient.**	**SHOCK ADVISED**	**"READY TONE"** **"STAND BACK"**
	27. Press the **"SHOCK" SWITCH** for the **FOURTH TIME.**		**"SHOCK DELIVERED"**
	28. Record the **TIME** after the delivery of the **fourth shock.*** (Palpate the **PATIENT'S PULSE—OPTIONAL**)	**MONITORING**	**"CHECK BREATHING AND PULSE"**
	29. Press the **POWER ON/ASSESS** switch for the **FIFTH TIME.**	**ASSESSING**	**"ASSESSING, HANDS OFF!"**
		CHARGING 360 J	**"STAND BACK!"** **"CHARGING TONE"**
	30. State: **"STAND CLEAR! DEFIBRILLATE AT 360 JOULES!"** while making sure that **no one is touching the patient.**	**SHOCK ADVISED**	**"READY TONE"** **"STAND BACK!"**
	31. Press the **"SHOCK" SWITCH** for the **FIFTH TIME.**		**"SHOCK DELIVERED"**
	32. Record the **TIME** after the delivery of the **fifth shock.*** (Palpate the **PATIENT's PULSE—OPTIONAL**)	**MONITORING**	**"CHECK BREATHING AND PULSE"**

*Omit voice recording of narrative if not required by local protocol.

Continued.

Laerdal Heartstart 1000s/Rapid Zap 1000s, cont'd

A. Management of a persistent shockable rhythm: 1. Ventricular fibrillation (V-FIB)
2. Pulseless ventricular tachycardia (V-TACH)

Rescuer one (CPR trained)	Rescuer two (EMT/FR-D)	Command screen messages	Verbal messages
	33. Press the **POWER ON/ASSESS** switch for the **SIXTH TIME.**	<u>ASSESSING</u>	"ASSESSING, HANDS OFF!"
		<u>CHARGING</u> 360 J	"STAND BACK!" "CHARGING TONE"
	34. State: "STAND CLEAR! DEFIBRILLATE AT 360 JOULES!" while making sure that **no one is touching the patient.**	SHOCK ADVISED	"READY TONE" "STAND BACK"
	35. Press the "SHOCK" SWITCH for the **SIXTH TIME.**		"SHOCK DELIVERED"
	36. Record the **TIME** after the delivery of the **sixth shock.***	<u>MONITORING</u>	"CHECK BREATHING AND PULSE"
	37. Palpate the **patient's carotid artery.**		
	38. State: "NO PULSE!"		
	39. Continue "MONITORING" or turn off the SAED, according to local protocol.		

AND

5. Resume **CPR.**	State: "CONTINUE CPR," and, if appropriate, "TRANSPORT!"		
6. TRANSPORT THE PATIENT IMMEDIATELY OR WAIT FOR THE BLS OR ALS UNIT, AS APPROPRIATE.			

> **NOTE!**
>
> **The ENERGY LEVELS and the TOTAL NUMBER OF SHOCKS DELIVERED may depend on the local protocol.**

40. Continue **performing CPR, reanalyzing the ECG rhythm, delivering shocks, and checking the patient's pulse,** according to local protocol.

41. Record the **TIME** upon relinquishing the patient to an **AEMT** or upon arrival at the **emergency department.***

*Omit voice recording of narrative if not required by local protocol.

Laerdal Heartstart 1000s/Rapid Zap 1000s

B. Management of a nonshockable rhythm: 1. Ventricular asystole
2. Electromechanical dissociation (EMD)

IF "MONITORING" AND "CHECK BREATHING AND PULSE" ARE INDICATED FOLLOWING "ASSESSING" AND A PULSE IS ABSENT, INDICATING A NONPERFUSING RHYTHM:

Rescuer one (CPR trained)	Rescuer two (EMT/FR-D)	Command screen messages	Verbal messages
	1. Palpate the patient's carotid artery.	**MONITORING**	**"CHECK BREATHING AND PULSE"**
1. Resume **CPR,** and continue it for 1 minute.	2. State: **"NO PULSE!" "CONTINUE CPR!"**		
2. Stop **CPR** and **STAND CLEAR!**	3. State: **"STOP CPR! STAND CLEAR!"**		
	4. Record the **TIME***		
	5. Press the **POWER ON/ASSESS** switch.	**ASSESSING**	**"ASSESSING, HANDS OFF"**
	6. Palpate the **patient's carotid artery.**	**MONITORING**	**"CHECK BREATHING AND PULSE"**
	7. State: **"NO PULSE!"**		
	8. Continue **"MONITORING"** or turn off the **SAED** according to local protocol.		
	AND		
3. Resume **CPR.**	State: **"CONTINUE CPR,"** and, if appropriate, **"TRANSPORT!"**		
4. **TRANSPORT THE PATIENT IMMEDIATELY OR WAIT FOR THE BLS OR ALS UNIT, AS APPROPRIATE.**	9. Continue **performing CPR, reanalyzing the ECG rhythm,** and **checking the patient's pulse,** according to local protocol.		
	10. Record the **TIME** upon relinquishing the patient to an **AEMT** or upon arrival at the **emergency department.***		

*Omit voice recording of narrative if not required by local protocol.

Laerdal Heartstart 1000s/Rapid Zap 1000s

C. Management of a perfusing rhythm

IF "MONITORING" AND "CHECK BREATHING AND PULSE" ARE INDICATED FOLLOWING "ASSESSING" AND A SPONTANEOUS PULSE IS PRESENT, INDICATING A PERFUSING RHYTHM:

Rescuer one (CPR trained)	Rescuer two (EMT/FR-D)	Command screen messages	Verbal messages
	1. Palpate the patient's carotid artery.	<u>MONITORING</u>	**"CHECK BREATHING AND PULSE"**
	2. State: **"PULSE PRESENT!"**		
	3. Continue **"MONITORING"** or turn off the **SAED,** according to local protocol.		
1. Open and maintain an **open airway** while administering **high concentration oxygen.**	4. State: **"ADMINISTER OXYGEN"** and **"TRANSPORT!"**		
2. Assist **ventilation** while administering **supplemental high concentration oxygen** if necessary.	5. Obtain the initial **vital signs** and repeat them as often as the situation indicates, and, if appropriate, record them.*		
3. **TRANSPORT THE PATIENT IMMEDIATELY OR WAIT FOR THE BLS OR ALS UNIT, AS APPROPRIATE.**	**If cardiac arrest recurs at the scene or en route:**		
	• State: **"STAND CLEAR!"**		
	<div align="center">**AND**</div>		
	• Turn on the **SAED,** if the **SAED** had been turned off, and repeat **Steps 7 through 21, A: MANAGEMENT OF A PERSISTENT SHOCKABLE RHYTHM,** as appropriate, until the shockable rhythm is converted into a perfusing rhythm or up to a total of **6 shocks** are delivered.		

> **NOTE!**
>
> The **ENERGY LEVELS** and the **TOTAL NUMBER OF SHOCKS DELIVERED** may depend on the local protocol.

6. Record the **TIME** upon relinquishing the patient to an **AEMT** or upon arrival at the **emergency department.***

---

*Omit voice recording of narrative if not required by local protocol.

Laerdal Heartstart 1000s—SE Protocol

A. Management of a persistent shockable rhythm: 1. Ventricular fibrillation (V-FIB)
2. Pulseless ventricular tachycardia (V-TACH)

- Recognize the **situation.**
- Verify **cardiac arrest.**
- Start **one- or two-rescuer CPR.**

Rescuer one (CPR trained)	Rescuer two (EMT/FR-D)	Command screen messages	Audible messages/tones
1. Continue **CPR.**	1. Insert the **tape cassette,** if appropriate.		
	2. Verify that a **fully charged battery** is in place.		
	Note: Steps 1 and 2 should be done before arrival at the scene, preferably, during shift check.		
	3. Connect the **color-coded cables** to the defibrillator electrode pads. **White cable connector** to the **right electrode;** the **red cable connector** to the **left electrode.**		
	AND		
	Attach the **defibrillator electrode pads** to the **patient's chest.**		
	4. Turn on the **SAED** by pressing the **POWER ON/ASSESS** switch.	ASSESSING	"ASSESSING, HANDS OFF!"
2. Stop **CPR** and **STAND CLEAR!**	5. State: "STOP CPR! STAND CLEAR!"	CHARGING	"STAND BACK!"
	6. Record the **NAMES** of the **RESCUERS** and the **AGE, SEX,** and **CONDITION** of the patient, including the **PATIENT'S PULSE.***	200 J	"CHARGING TONE"
	7. Record the **TIME.***	SHOCK ADVISED	"READY TONE" "STAND BACK"
	8. Press the **"SHOCK" SWITCH** for the **FIRST TIME.**		"SHOCK DELIVERED"
	9. Record the **TIME** after the delivery of the **first shock.***	ASSESSING	

> **NOTE!**
>
> If "MONITORING" and "CHECK BREATHING AND PULSE" are indicated following "ASSESSING" now or at any time, PALPATE THE PATIENT'S PULSE. If the PULSE IS ABSENT, indicating a "NONPERFUSING RHYTHM," proceed to B: MANAGEMENT OF A NONSHOCKABLE RHYTHM.

		Command screen messages	Audible messages/tones
		CHARGING	"STAND BACK!"
		200 J	"CHARGING TONE"
		SHOCK ADVISED	"READY TONE" "STAND BACK!"

*Omit voice recording of narrative if not required by local protocol.

Continued.

A. Management of a persistent shockable rhythm: 1. Ventricular fibrillation (V-FIB)
2. Pulseless ventricular tachycardia (V-TACH)

Rescuer one (CPR trained)	Rescuer two (EMT/FR-D)	Command screen messages	Audible messages/tones
	10. Press the **"SHOCK" SWITCH** for the **SECOND TIME**.		**"SHOCK DELIVERED"**
	11. Record the **TIME** after the delivery of the **second shock.***	**ASSESSING**	
	NOTE! If **"MONITORING"** and **"CHECK BREATHING AND PULSE"** are indicated following **"ASSESSING"** now or at any time, **PALPATE THE PATIENT'S PULSE. If the PULSE IS PRESENT,** indicating a **"PERFUSING RHYTHM,"** proceed to **B: MANAGEMENT OF A PERFUSING RHYTHM.**	**CHARGING** **360 J**	**"STAND BACK!"** **"CHARGING TONE"**
	12. Press the **"SHOCK" SWITCH** for the **THIRD TIME**.	**SHOCK ADVISED**	**"READY TONE"** **"STAND BACK!"**
	13. Record the **TIME** after the delivery of the **third shock.***		**"SHOCK DELIVERED"**
	14. Palpate the **patient's carotid artery**.	**MONITORING**	**"CHECK BREATHING AND PULSE"**
	15. State: **"NO PULSE!"**		
3. Resume **CPR**.	16. State: **"CONTINUE CPR!"**		
4. Stop **CPR** and **STAND CLEAR!**	17. State: **"STOP CPR! STAND CLEAR!"**		**"CHECK BREATHING AND PULSE"**
	18. Record the **TIME.***		
	19. Press the **POWER/ON ASSESS** switch.	**ASSESSING**	**"ASSESSING, HANDS OFF!"**
		CHARGING **360 J**	**"STAND BACK!"** **"CHARGING TONE"**
		SHOCK ADVISED	**"READY TONE"** **"STAND BACK!"**
	20. Press the **"SHOCK" SWITCH** for the **FOURTH TIME**.		**"SHOCK DELIVERED"**
	21. Record the **TIME** after the delivery of the **fourth shock.***	**ASSESSING**	
		CHARGING **360 J**	**"STAND BACK!"** **"CHARGING TONE"**
		SHOCK ADVISED	**"READY TONE"** **"STAND BACK!"**

*Omit voice recording of narrative if not required by local protocol.

Continued.

Laerdal Heartstart 1000s—SE Protocol, cont'd

A. Management of a persistent shockable rhythm: 1. Ventricular fibrillation (V-FIB)
2. Pulseless ventricular tachycardia (V-TACH)

Rescuer one (CPR trained)	Rescuer two (EMT/FR-D)	Command screen messages	Audible messages/tones
	22. Press the **"SHOCK" SWITCH** for the **FIFTH TIME.**	**"SHOCK DELIVERED"**	
	23. Record the **TIME** after the delivery of the **fifth shock.***	ASSESSING	
		CHARGING **360 J**	**"STAND BACK!"** **"CHARGING TONE"**
		SHOCK ADVISED	**"READY TONE"** **"STAND BACK!"**
	24. Press the **"SHOCK" SWITCH** for the **SIXTH TIME.**		**"SHOCK DELIVERED"**
	25. Record the **TIME** after the delivery of the **sixth shock.***	MONITORING	**"CHECK BREATHING AND PULSE"**
	26. Palpate the **patient's carotid artery.**		
	27. State: **"NO PULSE!"**		
	28. Continue **"MONITORING"** or turn off the **SAED,** according to local protocol.		
	AND		
5. Resume **CPR.**	State: **"CONTINUE CPR,"** and, if appropriate, **"TRANSPORT!"**		
6. **TRANSPORT THE PATIENT IMMEDIATELY OR WAIT FOR THE BLS OR ALS UNIT, AS APPROPRIATE.**			

> **NOTE!**
>
> **The ENERGY LEVELS and the TOTAL NUMBER OF SHOCKS DELIVERED may depend on the local protocol.**

29. Continue **performing CPR, reanalyzing the ECG rhythm, delivering shocks,** and **checking the patient's pulse,** according to local protocol.

30. Record the **TIME** upon relinquishing the patient to an **AEMT** or upon arrival at the **emergency department.***

---

*Omit voice recording of narrative if not required by local protocol.

Laerdal Heartstart 1000s—SE Protocol

B. Management of a nonshockable rhythm: 1. Ventricular asystole
2. Electromechanical dissociation (EMD)

IF "MONITORING" AND "CHECK BREATHING AND PULSE" ARE INDICATED FOLLOWING "ASSESSING" AND A PULSE IS ABSENT, INDICATING A NONPERFUSING RHYTHM:

Rescuer one (CPR trained)	Rescuer two (EMT/FR-D)	Command screen messages	Verbal messages
	1. Palpate the **patient's carotid artery.**	<u>**MONITORING**</u>	**"CHECK BREATHING AND PULSE"**
1. Resume **CPR,** and continue for 1 minute.	2. State: **"NO PULSE! CONTINUE CPR!"**		
2. Stop **CPR** and **STAND CLEAR!**	3. State: **"STOP CPR! STAND CLEAR!"**		
	4. Record the **TIME.***		
	5. Press the **POWER ON/ASSESS** switch.	<u>**ASSESSING**</u>	**"ASSESSING, HANDS OFF!"**
	6. Palpate the **patient's carotid artery.**	<u>**MONITORING**</u>	**"CHECK BREATHING AND PULSE"**
	7. State: **"NO PULSE!"**		
	8. Continue **"MONITORING"** or turn off the **SAED,** according to local protocol.		
	AND		
3. Resume **CPR.**	State: **"CONTINUE CPR,"** and, if appropriate, **"TRANSPORT!"**		
4. **TRANSPORT THE PATIENT IMMEDIATELY OR WAIT FOR THE BLS OR ALS UNIT, AS APPROPRIATE.**	9. Continue **performing CPR, reanalyzing the ECG rhythm,** and **checking the patient's pulse,** according to local protocol.		
	10. Record the **TIME** upon relinquishing the patient to an **AEMT** or upon arrival at the **emergency department.***		

*Omit voice recording of narrative if not required by local protocol.

Laerdal Heartstart 1000s—SE Protocol

C. Management of a perfusing rhythm

IF "MONITORING" AND "CHECK BREATHING AND PULSE" ARE INDICATED FOLLOWING "ASSESSING" AND A PULSE IS PRESENT, INDICATING A PERFUSING RHYTHM:

Rescuer one (CPR Trained)	Rescuer two (EMT/FR-D)	Command screen messages	Verbal messages
	1. Palpate the **patient's carotid artery.**	MONITORING	"CHECK BREATHING AND PULSE"
	2. State: **"PULSE PRESENT!"**		
	3. Continue **"MONITORING"** or turn off the **SAED,** according to local protocol.		
1. Open and maintain an **open airway** while administering **high concentration oxygen.**	4. State: **"ADMINISTER OXYGEN"** and **"TRANSPORT!"**		
2. Assist **ventilation** while administering **supplemental high concentration oxygen** if necessary.	5. Obtain the initial **vital signs** and repeat them as often as the situation indicates, and, if appropriate, record them.*		
	If cardiac arrest recurs at the scene or en route:		
	• State: **"STAND CLEAR!"**		
3. **TRANSPORT THE PATIENT IMMEDIATELY OR WAIT FOR THE BLS OR ALS UNIT, AS APPROPRIATE.**	**AND**		
	• Press the **POWER/ON ASSESS** switch and repeat **Steps 7 through 28, A: MANAGEMENT OF A PERSISTENT SHOCKABLE RHYTHM,** as appropriate, until the shockable rhythm is converted into a perfusing rhythm or until up to a total of **6 shocks** are delivered.		

> **NOTE!**
>
> The ENERGY LEVELS and the TOTAL NUMBER OF SHOCKS DELIVERED may depend on the local protocol.

6. Record the **TIME** upon relinquishing the patient to an **AEMT** or upon arrival at the **emergency department.***

---

*Omit voice recording of narrative if not required by local protocol.

Laerdal Heartstart 1000/Rapid Zap 1000

A. Management of a persistent shockable rhythm: 1. Ventricular fibrillation (V-FIB)
2. Pulseless ventricular tachycardia (V-TACH)

- Recognize the **situation.**
- Verify **cardiac arrest.**
- Start **one- or two-rescuer CPR.**

Rescuer one (CPR trained)	Rescuer two (EMT/FR-D)	Command screen messages	Verbal messages
1. Continue **CPR.**	**1.** Insert the **tape cassette,** if appropriate.		
	2. Verify that a **fully charged battery** is in place.		
	Note: Steps 1 and 2 should be done before arrival at the scene, preferably, during shift check.		
	3. Connect the **color-coded cabbles** to the defibrillator electrode pads. **White cable connector** to the **right electrode;** the **red cable connector** to the **left electrode.**		
	AND		
	Attach the **defibrillator electrode pads** to the **patient's chest.**		
	4. Turn on the **AED** by pressing the **POWER ON** switch.	ASSESSING	"ASSESSING, HANDS OFF!"
			"STAND BACK!"
2. Stop **CPR** and **STAND CLEAR!**	**5.** State: "**STOP CPR! STAND CLEAR!**"	CHARGING	"CHARGING TONE"
	6. Record the **NAMES** of the **RESCUERS,** the **TIME** displayed on the **Command Screen,** and the **AGE, SEX,** and **CONDITION** of the patient, including the **PATIENT'S PULSE.***	200 J	
	7. Record the **TIME.***		

> **NOTE!**
>
> If "MONITORING" and CHECK BREATHING AND PULSE" are indicated following "ASSESSING" now or at any time, PALPATE THE PATIENT'S PULSE, If the PULSE IS ABSENT, indicating a "NONPERFUSING RHYTHM," proceed to B: MANAGEMENT OF A NONSHOCKABLE RHYTHM.

			"READY TONE"
	(First shock delivered)	DELIVERED 200 J	"SHOCK DELIVERED"

*Omit voice recording of narrative if not required by local protocol.

Laerdal Heartstart 1000/Rapid Zap 1000, cont'd

A. Management of a persistent shockable rhythm: 1. Ventricular fibrillation (V-FIB)
2. Pulseless ventricular tachycardia (V-TACH)

Rescuer one (CPR trained)	Rescuer two (EMT/FR-D)	Command screen messages	Verbal messages
	8. Record the **TIME.***	ASSESSING	"ASSESSING, HANDS OFF!"
	NOTE! If "MONITORING" and "CHECK BREATHING AND PULSE" are indicated following "ASSESSING" now or at any time, PALPATE THE PATIENT'S PULSE. If the PULSE IS PRESENT, indicating a "PERFUSING RHYTHM," proceed to C: MANAGEMENT OF A PERFUSING RHYTHM.	CHARGING 200 J	"STAND BACK!" "CHARGING TONE"
			"READY TONE"
	(Second shock delivered)	DELIVERED 200 J	"SHOCK DELIVERED"
	9. Record the **TIME.***	ASSESSING	"ASSESSING, HANDS OFF!"
		CHARGING 360 J	"STAND BACK!" "CHARGING TONE"
			"READY TONE"
	(Third shock delivered.)	DELIVERED 360 J	"SHOCK DELIVERED"
	10. Record the **TIME.***		
	11. Palpate the **patient's carotid artery.**	MONITORING	"CHECK BREATHING AND PULSE"
	12. State: "NO PULSE!"		
	13. State: "CONTINUE CPR!"		"STOP CPR"
3. Resume **CPR.**	14. State: "STOP CPR! STAND CLEAR!"	ASSESSING	"ASSESSING, HANDS OFF!"
4. Stop **CPR** and **STAND CLEAR!**	15. Record the **TIME.***		
		CHARGING 360 J	"STAND BACK!" "CHARGING TONE" "READY TONE"
	(Fourth shock delivered.)	DELIVERED 360 J	"SHOCK DELIVERED"
	16. Record the **TIME.***	ASSESSING	"STAND BACK!" "CHARGING TONE"
		CHARGING 360 J	
			"READY TONE"

*Omit step if voice recording of narrative is not required by local protocol.

Continued.

Laerdal Heartstart 1000/Rapid Zap 1000, cont'd

A. Management of a persistent shockable rhythm: 1. Ventricular fibrillation (V-FIB)
2. Pulseless ventricular tachycardia (V-TACH)

Rescuer one (CPR trained)	Rescuer two (EMT/FR-D)	Command screen messages	Verbal messages
	(Fifth shock delivered)	**DELIVERED** 360 J	"SHOCK DELIVERED"
	17. Record the **TIME**.*	**ASSESSING**	"STAND BACK!"
		CHARGING 360 J	"CHARGING TONE"
			"READY TONE"
	(Sixth shock delivered.)	**DELIVERED** 360 J	"SHOCK DELIVERED"
	18. Record the **TIME**.*	**MONITORING**	"CHECK BREATHING AND PULSE"
	19. Palpate the **patient's carotid artery.**		
	20. State: **"NO PULSE!"**		
	21. Continue **MONITORING** or turn off the **AED,** according to local protocol.		

AND

5. Resume **CPR.**	State: **"CONTINUE CPR,"** and, if appropriate, **"TRANSPORT!"**		
6. **TRANSPORT THE PATIENT IMMEDIATELY OR WAIT FOR THE BLS OR ALS UNIT, AS APPROPRIATE.**			

> **NOTE!**
>
> The **ENERGY LEVELS** and **TOTAL NUMBER OF SHOCKS DELIVERED** may depend on the local protocol.

22. Continue **performing CPR, reanalyzing ECG rhythm, delivering shocks,** and **checking the patient's pulse,** according to local protocol.

23. Record the **TIME** upon relinquishing the patient to an **AEMT** or upon arrival at the **emergency department.***

*Omit voice recording of narrative if not required by local protocol.

Laerdal Heartstart 1000/Rapid Zap 1000

B. Management of a nonshockable rhythm: 1. Ventricular asystole
2. Electromechanical dissociation (EMD)

IF "MONITORING" AND "CHECK BREATHING AND PULSE" ARE INDICATED FOLLOWING "ASSESSING" AND A PULSE IS ABSENT, INDICATING A NONPERFUSING RHYTHM:

Rescuer one (CPR trained)	Rescuer two (EMT/FR-D)	Command screen messages	Verbal messages
1. Resume **CPR,** and continue it for 1 minute.	1. Palpate the patient's carotid artery.	**MONITORING**	**"CHECK BREATHING AND PULSE"**
	2. State: **"NO PULSE!" "CONTINUE CPR!"**		
2. Stop **CPR** and **STAND CLEAR!**	3. State: **"STOP CPR! STAND CLEAR!"**		**"STOP CPR!"**
	4. Record the **TIME.***		
	5. If **"ASSESSING"** does not appear after 1 minute of **"MONITORING,"** press the **POWER ON** switch to initiate **"ASSESSING."**	**ASSESSING**	**"ASSESSING, HANDS OFF!"**
	6. Palpate the **patient's carotid artery.**	**MONITORING**	**"CHECK BREATHING AND PULSE"**
	7. State: **"NO PULSE!"**		
	8. Continue **"MONITORING"** or turn off the **AED,** according to local protocol.		
	AND		
3. Resume **CPR.**	State: **"CONTINUE CPR,"** and, if appropriate, **"TRANSPORT!"**		
4. **TRANSPORT THE PATIENT IMMEDIATELY OR WAIT FOR THE BLS OR ALS UNIT, AS APPROPRIATE.**	9. Continue **performing CPR, reanalyzing the ECG rhythm** and **checking the patient's pulse,** according to local protocol.		
	10. Record the **TIME** upon relinquishing the patient to an **AEMT** or upon arrival at the **emergency department.***		

*Omit voice recording of narrative if not required by local protocol.

Laerdal Heartstart 1000/Rapid Zap 1000

C. Management of a perfusing rhythm

Rescuer one (CPR trained)	Rescuer two (EMT/FR-D)	Command screen messages	Verbal messages
	IF "MONITORING" AND "CHECK BREATHING AND PULSE" ARE INDICATED FOLLOWING "ASSESSING" AND A SPONTANEOUS PULSE IS PRESENT, INDICATING A PERFUSING RHYTHM:		

Rescuer one (CPR trained)	Rescuer two (EMT/FR-D)	Command screen messages	Verbal messages
	1. Palpate the patient's carotid artery.	<u>**MONITORING**</u>	**"CHECK BREATHING AND PULSE"**
	2. State: **"PULSE PRESENT!"**		
	3. Continue **"MONITORING"** or turn off the **AED,** according to local protocol.		
1. Open and maintain an **open airway** while administering **high concentration oxygen.**	State: **"ADMINISTER OXYGEN"** and **"TRANSPORT!"**		
2. Assist **ventilation** while administering **supplemental high concentration oxygen** if necessary.	4. Obtain the initial **vital signs** and repeat them as often as the situation indicates, and, if appropriate, record them.*		
	If cardiac arrest recurs at the scene or en route:		
3. **TRANSPORT THE PATIENT IMMEDIATELY OR WAIT FOR THE BLS OR ALS UNIT, AS APPROPRIATE.**	• State: **"STAND CLEAR!"**		
	AND		
	• Turn on the **SAED,** if the **SAED** had been turned off, and repeat **Steps 7 through 21, A: MANAGEMENT OF A PERSISTENT SHOCKABLE RHYTHM,** as appropriate, until the shockable rhythm is converted into a perfusing rhythm or up to a total of **6 shocks** are delivered.		

> **NOTE!**
>
> **The ENERGY LEVELS and the TOTAL NUMBER OF SHOCKS DELIVERED may depend on the local protocol.**

5. Record the **TIME** upon relinquishing the patient to an **AEMT** or upon arrival at the **emergency department.***

---

*Omit voice recording of narrative if not required by local protocol.

First Medic*

- First Medic 610, pp. 225-230
- First Medic 510, pp. 231-235

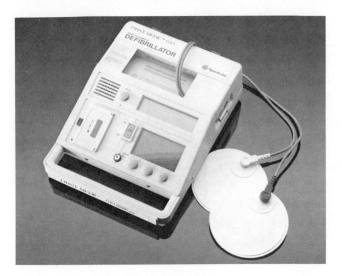

First Medic 610

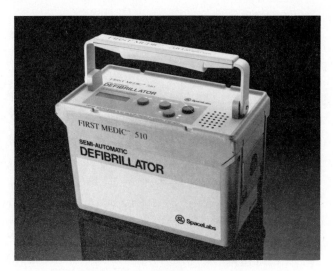

First Medic 510

*The set of protocols detailed here for First Medic 610 and First Medic 510 represents one of several protocols available from the manufacturer.

First Medic 610

A. Management of a persistent shockable rhythm: 1. Ventricular fibrillation (V-FIB)
2. Pulseless ventricular tachycardia (V-TACH)

- Recognize the situation.
- Verify **cardiac arrest.**
- Start **one- or two-rescuer CPR.**

Rescuer one (CPR trained)	Rescuer two (EMT/FR-D)	Command screen messages	Verbal messages
1. Continue **CPR.**	1. Insert the **Memory Module** and, if appropriate, the **tape cassette.**		
	2. Verify that a **fully charged battery** is in place.		
	Note: Steps 1 and 2 should be done before arrival at the scene, prefereably, during shift check.		
	3. Connect the **color-coded cables** to the defibrillator electrode pads. **White cable connector** to the **right electrode;** the **red cable connector** to the **left electrode.**		
	AND		
	Attach the **defibrillator electrode pads** to the **patient's chest.**		
	4. Turn on the **SAED** by pressing the **POWER ON** switch.	**ON**	

Continued.

First Medic 610, cont'd

A. Management of a persistent shockable rhythm: 1. Ventricular fibrillation (V-FIB)
2. Pulseless ventricular tachycardia (V-TACH)

Rescuer one (CPR trained)	Rescuer two (EMT/FR-D)	Command screen messages	Verbal messages
	5. Record the **NAMES** of the **RESCUERS**, the **TIME** displayed on the **Command Screen**, and the **AGE, SEX**, and **CONDITION** of the patient, including the **PATIENT's PULSE.***	**SELF TEST OK**	
2. Stop **CPR** and **STAND CLEAR!**	**6.** State: **"STOP CPR! STAND CLEAR!"**		
	7. Record the **TIME.*** (Palpate the **PATIENT'S PULSE—OPTIONAL.**)	**PRESS TO ANALYZE**	
NO PULSE	**8.** Press the **"ANALYZE" BUTTON** for the **FIRST TIME** while analyzing the **ECG** on the ECG screen.	<u>**ANALYZING**</u> **STAND CLEAR**	**"STAND CLEAR!"**
V-FIB OR V-TACH	**9.** State: **"V-FIB (OR V-TACH) PRESENT!"**		
SHOCKABLE RHYTHM	**NOTE!** If "NO SHOCK" is indicated now or at any time, PALPATE THE PATIENT'S PULSE. If the PULSE IS ABSENT, indicating a "NONPERFUSING RHYTHM," proceed to B: MANAGEMENT OF A NONSHOCKABLE RHYTHM.	**SHOCK INDICATED**	
	10. Verify immediately that the energy setting is **"200 JOULES."**	<u>**CHARGING**</u> **200 J SELECTED** **PRESS TO CHANGE ENERGY**	**"CHARGING TONE"**
	11. State: **"STAND CLEAR! DEFIBRILLATE AT 200 JOULES!"** while making sure that **no one** is **touching the patient.**	**READY PRESS TO SHOCK**	**"READY TONE" "PRESS TO SHOCK"**
	12. Press the **"SHOCK" BUTTON** for the **FIRST TIME** while observing the **ECG** on the ECG screen.	<u>**1 SHOCK**</u>	
	13. Record the **TIME** noted on the **Command Screen** after the delivery of the **first shock.*** (Palpate the **PATIENT'S PULSE—OPTIONAL.**)	**PRESS TO ANALYZE**	

---

*Omit voice recording of narrative if not required by local protocol.

Continued.

First Medic 610, cont'd

A. Management of a persistent shockable rhythm: 1. Ventricular fibrillation (V-FIB)
2. Pulseless ventricular tachycardia (V-TACH)

Rescuer one (CPR trained)	Rescuer two (EMT/FR-D)	Command screen messages	Verbal messages
NO PULSE V-FIB **OR** V-TACH **SHOCKABLE RHYTHM**	**14.** Press the **"ANALYZE" BUTTON** for the **SECOND TIME** while analyzing the ECG on the ECG screen. **15.** State: **"V-FIB (OR V-TACH) STILL PRESENT!"**	ANALYZING STAND CLEAR	"STAND CLEAR!"
	NOTE! If **"NO SHOCK"** is indicated now or at any time, **PALPATE THE PATIENT'S PULSE.** If a **SPONTANEOUS PULSE** is present, indicating a **"PERFUSING RHYTHM,"** proceed to C: MANAGEMENT OF A PERFUSING RHYTHM.	SHOCK INDICATED	
	16. Verify immediately that the energy setting is **"200 JOULES."**	CHARGING 200 J SELECTED PRESS TO CHANGE ENERGY	"CHARGING TONE"
	17. State: **"STAND CLEAR! DEFIBRILLATE AT 200 JOULES!"** while making sure that **no one is touching the patient.**	READY PRESS TO SHOCK	"READY TONE" "PRESS TO SHOCK"
	18. Press the **"SHOCK" BUTTON** for the **SECOND TIME** while observing the ECG on the ECG screen.	2 SHOCKS	
	19. Record the **TIME** noted on the **Command Screen** after the delivery of the second shock.* (Palpate the **PATIENT'S PULSE— OPTIONAL.**)	PRESS TO ANALYZE	
NO PULSE V-FIB **OR** V-TACH **SHOCKABLE RHYTHM**	**20.** Press the **"ANALYZE" BUTTON** for the **THIRD TIME** while analyzing the ECG on the ECG screen. **21.** State: **"V-FIB (OR V-TACH) STILL PRESENT!"**	ANALYZING STAND CLEAR SHOCK INDICATED	"STAND CLEAR!"
	22. Verify immediately that the energy setting is **"360 JOULES."**	CHARGING 360 J SELECTED PRESS TO CHANGE ENERGY	"CHARGING TONE"

*Omit voice recording of narrative if not required by local protocol.

Continued.

First Medic 610, cont'd

A. Management of a persistent shockable rhythm: 1. Ventricular fibrillation (V-FIB)
2. Pulseless ventricular tachycardia (V-TACH)

Rescuer one (CPR trained)	Rescuer two (EMT/FR-D)	Command screen messages	Verbal messages
	23. State: "STAND CLEAR! DEFIBRIL-LATE AT 360 JOULES!" while making sure that **no one is touching the patient.**	READY PRESS TO SHOCK	"READY TONE" "PRESS TO SHOCK"
	24. Press the "SHOCK" BUTTON for the THIRD TIME while observing the ECG on the ECG screen.	3 SHOCKS	
	25. Record the TIME noted on the Command Screen after the delivery of the third shock.*	PRESS TO ANALYZE	
NO PULSE	26. Palpate the **patient's carotid artery** while analyzing the ECG on the ECG screen.		
V-FIB	27. State: "V-FIB (OR V-TACH) STILL PRESENT! NO PULSE!"		
OR			
V-TACH			
SHOCKABLE RHYTHM			
3. Resume CPR.	28. State: "CONTINUE CPR," and, if appropriate, "TRANSPORT!"		
4. TRANSPORT THE PATIENT IMMEDIATELY OR WAIT FOR THE BLS OR ALS UNIT, AS APPROPRIATE.	OR Repeat Steps 6 through 28, as appropriate.		

> **NOTE!**
>
> The ENERGY LEVELS and the TOTAL NUMBER OF SHOCKS DELIVERED may depend on the local protocol.

29. Continue **performing CPR, reanalyzing the ECG rhythm, delivering shocks, and checking the patient's pulse,** according to local protocol.

30. Record the TIME noted on the Command Screen upon relinquishing the patient to an AEMT or upon arrival at the emergency department.*

*Omit voice recording of narrative if not required by local protocol.

B. Management of a nonshockable rhythm: 1. Ventricular asystole
2. Electromechanical dissociation (EMD)

IF "NO SHOCK" IS INDICATED AND A PULSE IS ABSENT, INDICATING A NONPERFUSING RHYTHM:

Rescuer one (CPR trained)	Rescuer two (EMT/FR-D)	Command Screen messages	Verbal messages
NO PULSE *Asystole* **OR** *EMD*	1. Palpate the patient's carotid artery. 2. State: **"ASYSTOLE (OR EMD) PRESENT! NO PULSE!"**	**NO SHOCK INDICATED** **PRESS TO ANALYZE**	"BEEP"
NONSHOCKABLE RHYTHM 1. Resume **CPR**, and continue for 1 minute. 2. Stop **CPR** and **STAND CLEAR!**	3. State: **"CONTINUE CPR!"** 4. State: **"STOP CPR! STAND CLEAR!"** 5. Record the **TIME** noted on the **Command Screen.*** (Palpate the **PATIENT'S PULSE—OPTIONAL.**)		
NO PULSE *Asystole* **OR** *EMD*	6. Press the **"ANALYZE" BUTTON** for the **SECOND TIME** while analyzing the **ECG on the ECG screen.** 7. Palpate the **patient's carotid artery.** 8. State: **"ASYSTOLE (OR EMD) STILL PRESENT! NO PULSE!"**	**ANALYZING** **STAND CLEAR** **NO SHOCK INDICATED** **PRESS TO ANALYZE**	"STAND CLEAR!" "BEEP"
NONSHOCKABLE RHYTHM 3. Resume **CPR.** 4. **TRANSPORT THE PATIENT IMMEDIATELY OR WAIT FOR THE BLS OR ALS UNIT, AS APPROPRIATE.**	9. State: **"CONTINUE CPR!"** and, if appropriate, **"TRANSPORT!"** 10. Continue **performing CPR, reanalyzing the ECG rhythm,** and **checking the patient's pulse,** according to local protocol. 11. Record the **TIME** noted on the **Command Screen** upon relinquishing the patient to an **AEMT** or upon arrival at the **emergency department.***		

*Omit voice recording of narrative if not required by local protocol.

First Medic 610

C. Management of a perfusing rhythm.

**IF "NO SHOCK" IS INDICATED
AND A SPONTANEOUS PULSE IS PRESENT,
INDICATING A PERFUSING RHYTHM:**

Rescuer one (CPR trained)	Rescuer two (EMT/FR-D)	Command screen messages	Verbal messages
	1. Palpate the patient's carotid artery.	**NO SHOCK INDICATED**	**"BEEP"**
PULSE PRESENT	2. State: **"PULSE AND ECG PRESENT!"**	**PRESS TO ANALYZE**	

Organized ECG rhythm

PERFUSING RHYTHM

1. Open and maintain an **open airway** while administering **high concentration oxygen.**

2. Assist **ventilation** while administering **supplemental high concentration oxygen** if necessary.

3. **TRANSPORT THE PATIENT IMMEDIATELY OR WAIT FOR THE BLS OR ALS UNIT, AS APPROPRIATE.**

3. State: **"ADMINISTER OXYGEN"** and **"TRANSPORT!"**

4. Obtain the initial **vital signs** and repeat them as often as the situation indicates, and, if appropriate, record them.*

5. **Monitor the patient's ECG** using the **SAED.**

If cardiac arrest recurs at the scene or en route:

- State: **"STAND CLEAR!"**

AND

- Repeat **Steps 6 through 28, A: MANAGEMENT OF A PERSISTENT SHOCKABLE RHYTHM,** as appropriate, until the shockable rhythm is converted into a perfusing rhythm or up to a total of **6 shocks** is delivered. The first shock of this series is delivered at the same energy level that was successful in terminating the dysrhythmia the last time. Subsequent shocks are delivered at 360 joules.

NOTE!

The ENERGY LEVELS and the TOTAL NUMBER OF SHOCKS DELIVERED may depend on the local protocol.

---

6. Record the **TIME** noted on the **Command Screen** upon relinquishing the patient to an **AEMT** or upon arrival at the **emergency department.**

---

*Omit voice recording of narrative if not required by local protocol.

First Medic 510

A. Management of a persistent shockable rhythm: 1. Ventricular fibrillation (V-FIB)
2. Pulseless ventricular tachycardia (V-TACH)

- Recognize the situation.
- Verify cardiac arrest.
- Start one- or two-rescuer CPR.

Rescuer one (CPR trained)	Rescuer two (EMT/FR-D)	Command screen messages	Verbal messages
1. Continue **CPR**	1. Insert the **Memory Module** and, if appropriate, the **tape cassette.**		
	2. Verify that a **fully charged battery** is in place.		
	Note: Steps 1 and 2 should be done before arrival at the scene, prefereably, during shift check.		
	3. Connect the **color-coded cables** to the defibrillator electrode pads. **White cable connector** to the **right electrode;** the **red cable connector** to the **left electrode.**		
	AND		
	Attach the **defibrillator electrode pads** to the **patient's chest.**		
	4. Turn on the **SAED** by pressing the **POWER ON** switch.	ON	
	5. Record the **NAMES** of the **RESCUERS,** the **TIME** displayed on the **Command Screen,** and the **AGE, SEX,** and **CONDITION** of the patient, including the **PATIENT's PULSE.***	SELF TEST OK	
2. Stop **CPR** and **STAND CLEAR!**	6. State: **"STOP CPR! STAND CLEAR!"**		
	7. Record the **TIME.*** (Palpate the **PATIENT'S PULSE—OPTIONAL.**)	PRESS TO ANALYZE	
	8. Press the **"ANALYZE" BUTTON** for the **FIRST TIME.**	<u>ANALYZING</u> STAND CLEAR SHOCK INDICATED	"STAND CLEAR!"

> **NOTE!**
>
> If "NO SHOCK" is indicated now or at any time, PALPATE THE PATIENT'S PULSE. If the PULSE IS ABSENT, indicating a "NONPERFUSING RHYTHM," proceed to B: MANAGEMENT OF A NONSHOCKABLE RHYTHM.

*Omit voice recording of narrative if not required by local protocol.

Continued.

First Medic 510, cont'd

A. Management of a persistent shockable rhythm: 1. Ventricular fibrillation (V-FIB)
2. Pulseless ventricular tachycardia (V-TACH)

Rescuer one (CPR trained)	Rescuer two (EMT/FR-D)	Command screen messages	Verbal messages
	9. Verify immediately that the energy setting is "200 JOULES."	**CHARGING** **200 J SELECTED** **PRESS TO CHANGE ENERGY**	"CHARGING TONE"
	10. State: "STAND CLEAR! DEFIBRILLATE AT 200 JOULES!" while making sure that **no one is touching the patient.**	**READY PRESS TO SHOCK**	"READY TONE" "PRESS TO SHOCK"
	11. Press the "SHOCK" BUTTON for the **FIRST TIME.**	**SHK #1**	
	12. Record the **TIME** noted on the **Command Screen** after the delivery of the **first shock.*** (Palpate the **PATIENT'S PULSE—OPTIONAL.**)	**PRESS TO ANALYZE**	
	13. Press the "ANALYZE" BUTTON for the **SECOND TIME.**	**ANALYZING** **STAND CLEAR** **SHOCK INDICATED**	"STAND CLEAR!"
	NOTE! If "NO SHOCK" is indicated now or at any time, PALPATE THE PATIENT'S PULSE. If a SPONTANEOUS PULSE is present, indicating a "PERFUSING RHYTHM," proceed to C: MANAGEMENT OF A PERFUSING RHYTHM.		
	14. Verify immediately that the energy setting is "200 JOULES."	**CHARGING** **200 J SELECTED** **PRESS TO CHANGE ENERGY**	"CHARGING TONE"
	15. State: "STAND CLEAR! DEFIBRILLATE AT 200 JOULES!" while making sure that **no one is touching the patient.**	**READY PRESS TO SHOCK**	"READY TONE" "PRESS TO SHOCK"
	16. Press the "SHOCK" BUTTON for the **SECOND TIME.**	**SHK #2**	
	17. Record the **TIME** noted on the **Command Screen** after the delivery of the **second shock.*** (Palpate the **PATIENT'S PULSE—OPTIONAL.**)	**PRESS TO ANALYZE**	

*Omit voice recording of narrative if not required by local protocol.

Continued.

First Medic 510, cont'd

A. Management of a persistent shockable rhythm: 1. Ventricular fibrillation (V-FIB)
2. Pulseless ventricular tachycardia (V-TACH)

Rescuer one (CPR trained)	Rescuer two (EMT/FR-D)	Command screen messages	Verbal messages
	18. Press the **"ANALYZE" BUTTON** for the **THIRD TIME.**	ANALYZING	
		STAND CLEAR	"STAND CLEAR!"
		SHOCK INDICATED	
	19. Verify immediately that the energy setting is **"360 JOULES."**	CHARGING	"CHARGING TONE"
		360 J SELECTED	
		PRESS TO CHANGE ENERGY	
	20. State: **"STAND CLEAR! DEFIBRILLATE AT 360 JOULES!"** while making sure that **no one is touching the patient.**	READY PRESS TO SHOCK	"READY TONE" "PRESS TO SHOCK"
	21. Press the **"SHOCK" BUTTON** for the **THIRD TIME.**	SHK #3	
	22. Record the **TIME** noted on the **Command Screen** after the delivery of the **third shock.***	PRESS TO ANALYZE	
	23. Palpate the **patient's carotid artery.**		
	24. State: **"NO PULSE!"**		
3. Resume **CPR.**	**25.** State: **"CONTINUE CPR,"** and, if approprite, **"TRANSPORT!"**		
4. TRANSPORT THE PATIENT IMMEDIATELY OR WAIT FOR THE BLS OR ALS UNIT, AS APPROPRIATE.	**OR** Repeat **Steps 6 through 25,** as appropriate.		

> **NOTE!**
>
> **The ENERGY LEVELS and the TOTAL NUMBER OF SHOCKS DELIVERED may depend on the local protocol.**

26. Continue **performing CPR, reanalyzing the ECG rhythm, delivering shocks, and checking the patient's pulse,** according to local protocol.

27. Record the **TIME** noted on the **Command Screen** upon relinquishing the patient to an **AEMT** or upon arrival at the **emergency department.***

---

*Omit voice recording of narrative if not required by local protocol.

First Medic 510

B. Management of a nonshockable rhythm: 1. Ventricular asystole
2. Electromechanical dissociation (EMD)

IF "NO SHOCK" IS INDICATED AND A PULSE IS ABSENT, INDICATING A NONPERFUSING RHYTHM:

Rescuer one (CPR trained)	Rescuer two (EMT/FR-D)	Command screen messages	Verbal messages
	1. Palpate patient's carotid artery.	**NO SHOCK INDICATED**	"BEEP"
	2. State: **"ASYSTOLE (OR EMD) PRESENT! NO PULSE!"**	**PRESS TO ANALYZE**	
1. Resume **CPR,** and continue for 1 minute.	3. State: **"CONTINUE CPR!"**		
2. Stop **CPR** and **STAND CLEAR!**	4. State: **"STOP CPR! STAND CLEAR!"**		
	5. Record the **TIME** noted on the **Command Screen.***		
	(Palpate the **PATIENT'S PULSE— OPTIONAL.**)		
	6. Press the **ANALYZE" BUTTON** for the **SECOND TIME.**	ANALYZING STAND CLEAR	"STAND CLEAR!"
	7. Palpate the **patient's carotid artery.**	**NO SHOCK INDICATED**	"BEEP"
	8. State: **"NO PULSE!"**	**PRESS TO ANALYZE**	
3. Resume **CPR.**	9. State: **"CONTINUE CPR!"** and, if appropriate, **"TRANSPORT!"**		
4. **TRANSPORT THE PATIENT IMMEDIATELY OR WAIT FOR THE BLS OR ALS UNIT, AS APPROPRIATE.**	10. Continue **performing CPR, reanalyzing the ECG rhythm,** and **checking the patient's pulse,** according to locol protocol.		
	11. Record the **TIME** noted on the **Command Screen** upon relinquishing the patient to an **AEMT** or upon arrival at the **emergency department.***		

*Omit voice recording of narrative if not required by local protocol.

First Medic 510

C. Management of a perfusing rhythm

IF "NO SHOCK" IS INDICATED AND A SPONTANEOUS PULSE
IS PRESENT, INDICATING A PERFUSING RHYTHM":

Rescuer one (CPR trained)	Rescuer two (EMT/FR-D)	Command screen messages	Verbal messages
	1. Palpate the patient's carotid artery.	**NO SHOCK INDICATED**	"BEEP"
1. Open and maintain an **open airway** while administering **high concentration oxygen.**	2. State: **"PULSE AND ECG PRESENT!"**	**PRESS TO ANALYZE**	
2. **Assist ventilation** while administering **supplemental high concentration oxygen** if necessary.	3. State: **"ADMINISTER OXYGEN"** and **"TRANSPORT!"**		
3. **TRANSPORT THE PATIENT IMMEDIATELY OR WAIT FOR THE BLS OR ALS UNIT, AS APPROPRIATE.**	4. Obtain the initial **vital signs** and repeat them as often as the situation indicates, and, if appropriate, record them.*		

If cardiac arrest recurs at the scene or en route:

- State **"STAND CLEAR!"**

AND

- Repeat **Steps 6 through 25, A: MANAGEMENT OF A PERSISTENT SHOCKABLE RHYTHM,** as appropriate, until the shockable rhythm is converted into a perfusing rhythm or up to a total of **6 shocks** are delivered. The first shock of this series is delivered at the same energy level that was successful in terminating the dysrhythmia the last time. Subsequent shocks are delivered at 360 joules.

> **NOTE!**
>
> **The ENERGY LEVELS and the TOTAL NUMBER OF SHOCKS DELIVERED may depend on the local protocol.**

5. Record the **TIME** noted on the **Command Screen** upon relinquishing the patient to an **AEMT** or upon arrival at the **emergency department.***

*Omit voice recording of narrative if not required by local protocol.

Marquette

- Marquette Series 1200 Responder, pp. 236-241

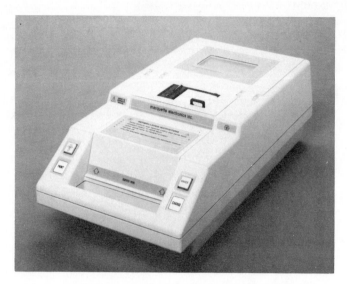

Marquette Series 1200 Responder

Marquette Series 1200 Responder

A. Management of a persistent shockable rhythm: 1. Ventricular fibrillation (V-FIB)
2. Pulseless ventricular tachycardia (V-TACH)

- Recognize the **situation.**
- Verify **cardiac arrest.**
- Start **one- or two-rescuer CPR.**

Rescuer one (CPR trained)	Rescuer two (EMT/FR-D)	Display panel messages	Audible signals
1. Continue **CPR.**	1. Insert the **Patient Event Card** and, if appropriate, the **tape.**		
	2. Verify that a **fully charged battery** is in place.		
	Note: Steps 1 and 2 should be done before arrival at the scene, preferably, during shift check.		
	3. Connect the **patient cables** to the **defibrillator electrode pads.** The **sternum cable connector** is connected to the **sternum defibrillator pad;** the **apex cable connector** to the **apex defibrillator pad.**		
	AND		
	Attach the **defibrillator pads** to the patient's chest.		

Continued.

Marquette Series 1200 Responder, cont'd

A. Management of a persistent shockable rhythm: 1. Ventricular fibrillation (V-FIB)
2. Pulseless ventricular tachycardia (V-TACH)

Rescuer one (CPR trained)	Rescuer two (EMT/FR-D)	Display panel messages	Audible signals
2. Stop **CPR** and **STAND CLEAR!**	**4.** State: **"STOP CPR! STAND CLEAR!"**		
	5. Turn on the **SAED**.	**TESTS 1-6 OK**	
	6. Turn on the **tape recorder,** if appropriate.	**PADS** **ANALYZING**	
	7. Record the **NAMES** of the **RESCUERS,** the **TIME,** and the **AGE, SEX,** and **CONDITION** of the patient, including the **PATIENT'S PULSE.*** (Palpate the **PATIENT'S PULSE—OPTIONAL.**)	**ALERT: CHARGE IF PATIENT UNCONSCIOUS**	"SLOW BEEP"
NO PULSE V-FIB **OR** V-TACH **SHOCKABLE RHYTHM**	**8.** Press the **"CHARGE" KEY** for the **FIRST TIME** while analyzing the **ECG** on the ECG screen, **AND** State: **"CHARGING!"**	**CHARGING TO 200 J** **DO NOT TOUCH PATIENT**	"MODERATELY FAST BEEP"
	NOTE! If **"NO SHOCK"** is advised now or at any time, **PALPATE THE PATIENT'S PULSE. If the PULSE IS ABSENT,** indicating a **"NONPERFUSING RHYTHM,"** proceed to B: MANAGEMENT OF A NONSHOCKABLE RHYTHM.		
	9. State: **"V-FIB (OR V-TACH) PRESENT!"**		
	10. Verify that the energy setting is **"200 JOULES."**		
	11. State: **"STAND CLEAR! DEFIBRILLATE AT 200 JOULES!"** while making sure that **no one is touching the patient.**	**STAND CLEAR**	"FAST BEEP"
	12. Press the **"SHOCK" SWITCH** for the **FIRST TIME** while observing the **ECG** on the ECG screen.	**SHOCK NOW!**	
	13. Record the **TIME** after the delivery of the **first shock.*** (Palpate the **PATIENT'S PULSE—OPTIONAL.**)	**ANALYZING** **ALERT: CHARGE IF PATIENT UNCONSCIOUS**	"SLOW BEEP"

*Omit voice recording of narrative if not required by local protocol.

Continued.

A. Management of a persistent shockable rhythm: 1. Ventricular fibrillation (V-FIB)

2. Pulseless ventricular tachycardia (V-TACH)

Rescuer one (CPR trained)	Rescuer two (EMT/FR-D)	Display panel messages	Audible signals
NO PULSE V-FIB **OR** V-TACH **SHOCKABLE RHYTHM**	**14.** Press the **"CHARGE" KEY** for the **SECOND TIME** while analyzing the ECG on the ECG screen, **AND** State: **"CHARGING!"**	**CHARGING TO 200 J**	**"MODERATELY FAST BEEP"**
	15. State: **"V-FIB (OR V-TACH) PRESENT!"**	**DO NOT TOUCH PATIENT**	
	NOTE! If **"NO SHOCK"** is advised now or at any time, PALPATE THE PATIENT'S PULSE. If a SPONTANEOUS PULSE is present, indicating a **"PERFUSING RHYTHM,"** proceed to C: MANAGEMENT OF A PERFUSING RHYTHM.		
	16. Verify that the energy setting is **"200 JOULES."**		
	17. State: **"STAND CLEAR! DEFIBRILLATE AT 200 JOULES!"** while making sure that **no one is touching the patient.**	**STAND CLEAR**	**"FAST BEEP"**
	18. Press the **"SHOCK" SWITCH** for the **SECOND TIME** while observing the ECG on the ECG screen.	**SHOCK NOW!**	
	19. Record the **TIME** after the delivery of the **second shock.***	<u>**ANALYZING**</u>	
	(Palpate the **PATIENT'S PULSE— OPTIONAL.**)	**ALERT: CHARGE IF PATIENT UNCONSCIOUS**	**"SLOW BEEP"**
NO PULSE V-FIB **OR** V-TACH **SHOCKABLE RHYTHM**	**20.** Press the **"CHARGE" KEY** for the **THIRD TIME** while analyzing the ECG on the ECG screen, **AND** State: **"CHARGING!"**	**CHARGING TO 360 J**	**"MODERATELY FAST BEEP"**
	21. State: **"V-FIB (OR V-TACH) PRESENT!"**		
	22. Verify that the energy setting is **"360 JOULES."**	**DO NOT TOUCH PATIENT**	

*Omit voice recording of narrative if not required by local protocol.

Marquette Series 1200 Responder, cont'd

A. Management of a persistent shockable rhythm: 1. Ventricular fibrillation (V-FIB)
2. Pulseless ventricular tachycardia (V-TACH)

Rescuer one (CPR trained)	Rescuer two (EMT/FR-D)	Display panel messages	Audible signals
	23. State: **"STAND CLEAR! DEFIBRILLATE AT 360 JOULES!"** while making sure that **no one is touching the patient.**	**STAND CLEAR** **SHOCK NOW!**	**"FAST BEEP"**
	24. Press the **"SHOCK" SWITCH** for the **THIRD TIME** while observing the **ECG on the ECG screen.**		
	25. Record the **TIME** after the delivery of the **third shock.***	<u>ANALYZING</u>	
NO PULSE	**26.** Palpate the **patient's carotid artery** while analyzing the **ECG on the ECG screen.**	**ALERT: CHARGE IF PATIENT UNCONSCIOUS**	**"SLOW BEEP"**
V-FIB	**27.** State: **"V-FIB (OR V-TACH) STILL PRESENT! NO PULSE!"**		
OR			
V-TACH			
SHOCKABLE RHYTHM			
3. Resume **CPR.**	**28.** State: **"CONTINUE CPR,"** and, if appropriate, **"TRANSPORT!"**		
4. TRANSPORT THE PATIENT IMMEDIATELY OR WAIT FOR THE BLS OR ALS UNIT, AS APPROPRIATE.	**OR** Repeat **Steps 8 through 28,** as appropriate. The **subsequent shocks** are delivered in a sequence of **360, 360,** and **360 joules.**		

NOTE!

The ENERGY LEVELS and the TOTAL NUMBER OF SHOCKS DELIVERED may depend on the local protocol.

---

29. Continue **performing CPR, reanalyzing the ECG rhythm, delivering shocks,** and **checking the patient's pulse,** according to local protocol.

30. Record the **TIME** upon relinquishing the patient to an **AEMT** or upon arrival at the **emergency department.***

---

*Omit step if voice recording of narrative is not required by local protocol.

Marquette Series 1200 Responder

B. Management of a nonshockable rhythm: 1. Ventricular asystole
2. Electromechanical dissociation (EMD)

	IF "NO SHOCK" IS ADVISED AND A PULSE IS ABSENT, INDICATING A NONPERFUSING RHYTHM:		
Rescuer one (CPR trained)	Rescuer two (EMT/FR-D)	Display panel messages	Audible signals
NO PULSE 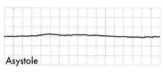 OR 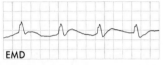	1. Palpate the patient's carotid artery. 2. State: "ASYSTOLE (OR EMD) PRESENT! NO PULSE!"	**NO SHOCK ADVISED**	
NONSHOCKABLE RHYTHM 1. Resume **CPR**, and continue for 1 minute. 2. Stop **CPR** and **STAND CLEAR!**	3. State: "CONTINUE CPR!" 4. State: "STOP CPR! STAND CLEAR!"		
NO PULSE 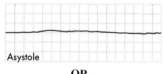 OR 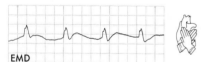	5. Palpate the **patient's carotid artery** while analyzing the **ECG on the ECG screen.** 6. State: "ASYSTOLE (OR EMD) STILL PRESENT! NO PULSE!"	**NO SHOCK ADVISED**	
NONSHOCKABLE RHYTHM 3. Resume **CPR.** 4. **TRANSPORT THE PATIENT IMMEDIATELY OR WAIT FOR THE BLS OR ALS UNIT, AS APPROPRIATE.**	7. State: "CONTINUE CPR!" and, if appropriate, "TRANSPORT" 8. Continue **performing CPR, reanalyzing the ECG rhythm,** and **checking the patient's pulse,** according to locol protocol. 9. Record the **TIME** upon relinquishing the patient to an **AEMT** on upon arrival at the **emergency department***		

*Omit voice recording of narrative if not required by local protocol.

Marquette Series 1200 Responder

C. Management of a perfusing rhythm

IF "NO SHOCK" IS ADVISED AND A SPONTANEOUS PULSE IS PRESENT, INDICATING A PERFUSING RHYTHM:

Rescuer one (CPR trained)	Rescuer two (EMT/FR-D)	Display panel messages	Audible signals
	1. Palpate the patient's carotid artery.	**NO SHOCK ADVISED**	

PULSE PRESENT

2. State: **"PULSE AND ECG PRESENT!"**

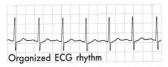

Organized ECG rhythm

PERFUSING RHYTHM

1. Open and maintain an **open airway** while administering **high concentration oxygen.**

2. Assist **ventilation while** administering **supplemental high concentration oxygen** if necessary.

3. **TRANSPORT THE PATIENT IMMEDIATELY OR WAIT FOR THE BLS OR ALS UNIT, AS APPROPRIATE.**

3. State: **"ADMINISTER OXYGEN"** and **"TRANSPORT!"**

4. **Obtain the initial vital signs** and repeat them as often as the situation indicates, and, if appropriate, record them.*

5. Monitor the patient's ECG using the **SAED.**

If cardiac arrest recurs at the scene or en route:

- State: **"STAND CLEAR!"**

  AND

- Repeat **Steps 8 through 28, A: MANAGEMENT OF A PERSISTENT SHOCKABLE RHYTHM,** as appropriate, until the shockable rhythm is converted into a perfusing rhythm or until up to a total of **6 shocks** are delivered.

> **NOTE!**
>
> The **ENERGY LEVELS** and the **TOTAL NUMBER OF SHOCKS DELIVERED** may depend on the local protocol.

6. Record the **TIME** upon relinquishing the patient to an **AEMT** or upon arrival at the emergency department.*

*Omit voice recording of narrative if not required by local protocol.

Physio-Control

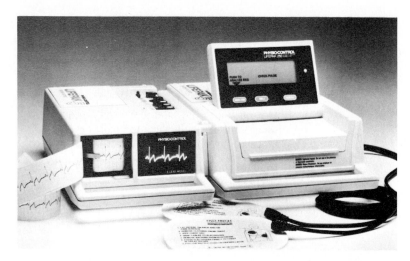

Physio-Control Lifepak 250 automatic advisory defibrillator with Lifepak monitor.

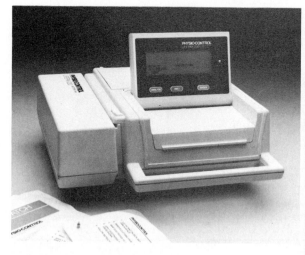

Physio-Control Lifepak 200 automatic advisory defibrillator.

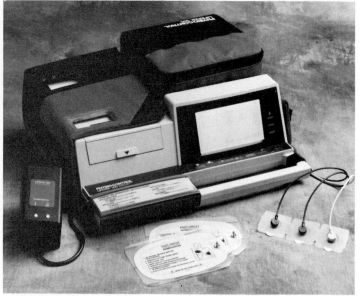

Physio-Control Lifepak 200 automatic advisory defibrillator.

Physio-Control Lifepak 250 Automatic Advisory Defibrillator with Lifepak Monitor

A. Management of persistent shockable rhythm: 1. Ventricular fibrillation (V-FIB)
2. Pulseless ventricular tachycardia (V-TACH)

- Recognize the **situation.**
- Verify **cardiac arrest.**
- Start **one- or two-rescuer CPR.**

Rescuer one (CPR trained)	Rescuer two (EMT/FR-D)	Message screen	Audible tones
1. Continue **CPR.**	1. Connect the **patient cables** to the **defibrillator electrodes.** **AND** Attach the **defibrillator electrodes** to the **patient's chest.**		
	2. Lift open the **display module** to turn on the **SAED.**	**PUSH TO ANALYZE ECG**	1 "BEEP"
	3. Insert the **tape,** if appropriate. **Note:** This should be done before arrival at the scene, preferable, during shift check.	**CHECK PULSE**	
	4. Record the **NAMES** of the **RESCUERS,** the **TIME,** and the **AGE, SEX,** and **CONDITION** of the patient, including the **PATIENT'S PULSE.***		
2. Stop **CPR** and **STAND CLEAR!**	5. State: **"STOP CPR! STAND CLEAR!"** (Palpate the **PATIENT'S PULSE—OPTIONAL.**)		
NO PULSE	6. Press the **"ANALYZE" SWITCH** for the **FIRST TIME** while analyzing the **ECG** on the **ECG** screen.	**DETECTOR ON**	2 "BEEPS"
V-FIB **OR** V-TACH **SHOCKABLE RHYTHM**	**NOTE!** If **"NO SHOCK"** is advised now or at any time, **PALPATE THE PATIENT'S PULSE. If the PULSE IS ABSENT,** indicating a **"NONPERFUSING RHYTHM,"** proceed to B: MANAGEMENT OF A NONSHOCKABLE RHYTHM.	**DO NOT TOUCH PATIENT** **SHOCK ADVISED** **CHARGING 200 J** **PUSH FOR 360 J**	4 "BEEPS"
	7. State: **"V-FIB (OR V-TACH) PRESENT!"**		
	8. Verify immediately that the energy setting is **"200 JOULES."**		
	9. State: **"STAND CLEAR! DEFIBRILLATE AT 200 JOULES!"** while making sure that **no one is touching the patient.**	**DO NOT TOUCH PATIENT** **200 J**	5 "BEEPS"

*Omit voice recording of narrative if not required by local protocol.

Continued.

Physio-Control Lifepak 250 Automatic Advisory Defibrillator with Lifepak Monitor, cont'd

A. Management of persistent shockable rhythm: 1. Ventricular fibrillation (V-FIB)

2. Pulseless ventricular tachycardia (V-TACH)

Rescuer one (CPR trained)	Rescuer two (EMT/FR-D)	Message screen	Audible tones
	10. Press the **"SHOCK" SWITCH** for the **FIRST TIME** while observing the **ECG** on the ECG screen.	**SHOCK NOW!**	**"STEADY TONE"**
	11. Record the **TIME** after the delivery of the **first shock.** *	**PUSH TO ANALYZE ECG**	1 "BEEP"
	(Palpate the **PATIENT'S PULSE— OPTIONAL.**)	**CHECK PULSE**	
NO PULSE	12. Press the **"ANALYZE" SWITCH** for the **SECOND TIME** while analyzing the **ECG** on the ECG screen.	**DETECTOR ON**	2 "BEEPS"
V-FIB	13. State: **"V-FIB (OR V-TACH) STILL PRESENT!"**	**DO NOT TOUCH PATIENT**	
OR	**NOTE!** If **"NO SHOCK"** is advised now or at any time, PALPATE THE PATIENT'S PULSE. If a SPONTANEOUS PULSE is present, indicating a **"PERFUSING RHYTHM,"** proceed to C: MANAGEMENT OF A PERFUSING RHYTHM.	**SHOCK ADVISED** **CHARGING 200 J** **PUSH FOR 360 J** **DO NOT TOUCH PATIENT**	4 "BEEPS"
V-TACH **SHOCKABLE RHYTHM**			
	14. Verify immediately that the energy setting is **"200 JOULES."**	**200 J**	5 "BEEPS"
	15. State: **"STAND CLEAR! DEFIBRILLATE AT 200 JOULES!"** while making sure that **no one is touching the patient.**	**SHOCK NOW!**	**"STEADY TONE"**
	16. Press the **"SHOCK" SWITCH** for the **SECOND TIME** while observing the **ECG** on the ECG screen.	**PUSH TO ANALYZE ECG**	1 "BEEP"
	17. Record the **TIME** after the delivery of the **second shock.** *		
	(Palpate the **PATIENT'S PULSE— OPTIONAL.**)	**CHECK PULSE**	

*Omit voice recording of narrative if not required by local protocol.

Continued.

Physio-Control Lifepak 250 Automatic Advisory Defibrillator with Lifepak Monitor, cont'd

A. Management of persistent shockable rhythm: 1. Ventricular fibrillation (V-FIB)
2. Pulseless ventricular tachycardia (V-TACH)

Rescuer one (CPR trained)	Rescuer two (EMT/FR-D)	Message screen	Audible tones
NO PULSE V-FIB **OR** V-TACH **SHOCKABLE RHYTHM**	**18.** Press the **"ANALYZE" SWITCH** for the **THIRD TIME** while analyzing the ECG on the ECG screen. **19.** State: **"V-FIB (OR V-TACH) STILL PRESENT!"**	DETECTOR ON DO NOT TOUCH PATIENT SHOCK ADVISED CHARGING 200 J	2 "BEEPS" 4 "BEEPS"
	20. Press the **"360 J" SWITCH** while the defibrillator is charging. **21.** Verify immediately that the energy setting is **"360 JOULES."** **22.** State: **"STAND CLEAR! DEFIBRILLATE AT 360 JOULES!"** while making sure that **no one is touching the patient.**	PUSH FOR 360 J CHARGING 360 J DO NOT TOUCH PATIENT 360 J	 5 "BEEPS"
	23. Press the **"SHOCK" SWITCH** for the **THIRD TIME** while observing the **ECG** on the ECG screen. **24.** Record the **TIME** after the delivery of the **third shock.***	SHOCK NOW! PUSH TO ANALYZE ECG	"STEADY TONE" 1 "BEEP"
NO PULSE V-FIB **OR** V-TACH **SHOCKABLE RHYTHM**	**25.** Palpate the **patient's carotid artery** while analyzing the **ECG** on the ECG screen. **26.** State: **"V-FIB (OR V-TACH) STILL PRESENT! NO PULSE!"**	CHECK PULSE	

*Omit voice recording of narrative if not required by local protocol.

Continued.

Physio-Control Lifepak 250 Automatic Advisory Defibrillator with Lifepak Monitor, cont'd

A. Management of persistent shockable rhythm: 1. Ventricular fibrillation (V-FIB)
2. Pulseless ventricular tachycardia (V-TACH)

Rescuer one (CPR trained)	Rescuer two (EMT/FR-D)	Message screen	Audible tones
3. Resume **CPR**. 4. **TRANSPORT THE PATIENT IMMEDIATELY OR WAIT FOR THE BLS OR ALS UNIT, AS APPROPRIATE.**	27. State: **"CONTINUE CPR,"** and, if appropriate, **"TRANSPORT!"** **OR** Repeat **Steps 5 through 27,** as appropriate. The **subsequent shocks** are delivered in a sequence of **360, 360,** and **360 joules.** ┌─────────────────────────┐ **NOTE!** The **ENERGY LEVELS** and the **TOTAL NUMBER OF SHOCKS DELIVERED** may depend on the local protocol. └─────────────────────────┘ 28. Continue **performing CPR, reanalyzing the ECG rhythm, delivering shocks,** and **checking the patient's pulse,** according to local protocol. 29. Record the **TIME** upon relinquishing the patient to an **AEMT** or upon arrival at the **emergency department.***		

*Omit voice recording of narrative if not required by local protocol.

Physio-Control Lifepak 250 Automatic Advisory Defibrillator with Lifepak Monitor

B. Management of a nonshockable rhythm: 1. Ventricular asystole
2. Electromechanical dissociation (EMD)

If "NO SHOCK" IS ADVISED AND A PULSE IS ABSENT, INDICATING A NONPERFUSING RHYTHM:

Rescuer one (CPR trained)	Rescuer two (EMT/FR-D)	Message screen	Audible tones
	1. Palpate the patient's carotid artery.	NO SHOCK ADVISED	3 "BEEPS"
NO PULSE	2. State: "ASYSTOLE (OR EMD) PRESENT! NO PULSE!"	PUSH TO ANALYZE ECG	1 "BEEP"
Asystole		CHECK PULSE	
OR			
EMD			
NONSHOCKABLE RHYTHM			
1. Resume **CPR,** and continue for 1 minute.	3. State: "CONTINUE CPR!"		
2. Stop **CPR** and **STAND CLEAR!**	4. State: "STOP CPR! STAND CLEAR!" (Palpate the **PATIENT'S PULSE—OPTIONAL.**)		
NO PULSE	5. Press the **"ANALYZE" SWITCH** for the **SECOND TIME** while analyzing the **ECG on the ECG screen.**	DETECTOR ON DO NOT TOUCH PATIENT	2 "BEEPS"
Asystole	6. Palpate the patient's carotid artery.	NO SHOCK ADVISED	3 "BEEPS"
OR	7. State: "ASYSTOLE (OR EMD) STILL PRESENT! NO PULSE!"	PUSH TO ANALYZE ECG	1 "BEEP"
EMD			
NONSHOCKABLE RHYTHM			
3. **Resume CPR.**	8. State: "CONTINUE CPR!" and, if appropriate, "TRANSPORT!"	CHECK PULSE	
4. **TRANSPORT THE PATIENT IMMEDIATELY OR WAIT FOR THE BLS OR ALS UNIT, AS APPROPRIATE.**	9. Continue **performing CPR, reanalyzing the ECG rhythm,** and **checking the patient's pulse,** according to locol protocol.		
	10. Record the **TIME** upon relinquishing the patient to an **AEMT** or upon arrival at the **emergency department.***		

*Omit voice recording of narrative if not required by local protocol.

Physio-Control Lifepak 250 Automatic Advisory Defibrillator with Lifepak Monitor

C. Management of a perfusing rhythm

**IF "NO SHOCK" IS ADVISED AND A SPONTANEOUS PULSE
IS PRESENT, INDICATING A PERFUSING RHYTHM:**

Rescuer one (CPR trained)	Rescuer two (EMT/FR-D)	Message screen	Audible tones
	1. Palpate the patient's carotid artery.	PUSH TO ANALYZE ECG	3 "BEEPS"
PULSE PRESENT	**2.** State **"PULSE AND ECG PRESENT!"**	NO SHOCK ADVISED	1 "BEEP"

Organized ECG rhythm

PERFUSING RHYTHM

CHECK PULSE

Rescuer one (CPR trained)	Rescuer two (EMT/FR-D)
1. Open and maintain an **open airway** while administering **high concentration oxygen.**	**3.** State: **"ADMINISTER OXYGEN"** and **"TRANSPORT!"**
2. Assist **ventilation** while administering **supplemental high concentration oxygen** if necessary.	**4.** Obtain the initial **vital signs and repeat them as often as the situation indicates, and, if appropriate, record them.***
3. TRANSPORT THE PATIENT IMMEDIATELY OR WAIT FOR THE BLS OR ALS UNIT, AS APPROPRIATE.	**5. Monitor the patient's ECG** using the **SAED.**

If cardiac arrest recurs at the scene or en route:

- State **"STAND CLEAR!"**

AND

- Repeat **Steps 5 through 27, A: MANAGEMENT OF A PERSISTENT SHOCKABLE RHYTHM,** as appropriate, until the shockable rhythm is converted into a perfusing rhythm or up to a total of **6 shocks** are delivered. The first shock of this series is delivered at the same energy level that was successful in terminating the dysrhythmia the last time. Subsequent shocks are delivered at 360 joules.

> **NOTE!**
>
> The **ENERGY LEVELS** and the **TOTAL NUMBER OF SHOCKS DELIVERED may depend on the local protocol.**

6. Record the **TIME** upon relinquishing the patient to an **AEMT** or upon arrival at the **emergency department.***

---

*Omit voice recording of narrative if not required by local protocol.

Physio-Control Lifepak 200 Automatic Advisory Defibrillator or Physio-Control Lifepak 250 Automatic Advisory Defibrillator without Lifepak Monitor

A. Management of a persistent shockable rhythm: 1. Ventricular fibrillation (V-FIB)
2. Pulseless ventricular tachycardia (V-TACH)

- Recognize the **situation.**
- Verify **cardiac arrest.**
- Start **one- or two-rescuer CPR.**

Rescuer one (CPR trained)	Rescuer two (EMT/FR-D)	Message screen	Audible tones
1. Continue **CPR.**	1. Connect the **patient cables** to the **defibrillator electrodes.** **AND** Attach the **defibrillator electrodes** to the **patient's chest.**		
	2. Lift open the **display module** to turn on the **SAED.** 3. Insert the **tape,** if appropriate.	PUSH TO ANALYZE ECG	1 "BEEP"
	Note: This should be done before arrival at the scene, preferably, during shift check.	CHECK PULSE	
	4. Record the **NAMES** of the **RESCUERS,** the **TIME,** and the **AGE, SEX,** and **CONDITION** of the patient, including the **PATIENT'S PULSE.***		
2. Stop **CPR** and **STAND CLEAR!**	5. State: **"STOP CPR! STAND CLEAR!"** (Palpate the **PATIENT'S PULSE—OPTIONAL.**)		
	6. Press the **"ANALYZE" SWITCH** for the **FIRST TIME.**	DETECTOR ON	2 "BEEPS"
		DO NOT TOUCH PATIENT	
	┌─────────────────────────────┐ **NOTE!** If **"NO SHOCK"** is advised now or at any time, PALPATE THE PATIENT'S PULSE. If the PULSE IS ABSENT, indicating a **"NONPERFUSING RHYTHM,"** proceed to B: MANAGEMENT OF A NONSHOCKABLE RHYTHM. └─────────────────────────────┘	SHOCK ADVISED	4 "BEEPS"
		CHARGING 200 J	
		PUSH FOR 360 J	
		DO NOT TOUCH PATIENT	
	7. Verify immediately that the energy setting is **"200 JOULES."**	200 J	5 "BEEPS"
	8. State: **"STAND CLEAR! DEFIBRILLATE AT 200 JOULES!"** while making sure that **no one is touching the patient.**	SHOCK NOW!	"STEADY TONE"

*Omit voice recording of narrative if not required by local protocol.

Continued.

Physio-Control Lifepak 200 Automatic Advisory Defibrillator or Physio-Control Lifepak 250 Automatic Advisory Defibrillator without Lifepak Monitor, cont'd

A. Management of a persistent shockable rhythm: 1. Ventricular fibrillation (V-FIB)
2. Pulseless ventricular tachycardia (V-TACH)

Rescuer one (CPR trained)	Rescuer two (EMT/FR-D)	Message screen	Audible tones
	9. Press the "SHOCK" SWITCH for the FIRST TIME.		
	10. Record the TIME after the delivery of the first shock.*	PUSH TO ANALYZE ECG	1 "BEEP"
	(Palpate the PATIENT'S PULSE—OPTIONAL.)	CHECK PULSE	
	11. Press the "ANALYZE" SWITCH for the SECOND TIME.	DETECTOR ON	2 "BEEPS"
	NOTE! If "NO SHOCK" is advised now or at any time, PALPATE THE PATIENT'S PULSE. If a SPONTANEOUS PULSE is present, indicating a "PERFUSING RHYTHM," proceed to C: MANAGEMENT OF A PERFUSING RHYTHM.	DO NOT TOUCH PATIENT	
		SHOCK ADVISED	4 "BEEPS"
		CHARGING 200 J	
		PUSH FOR 360 J	
		DO NOT TOUCH PATIENT	
	12. Verify immediately that the energy setting is "200 JOULES."	200 J	5 "BEEPS"
	13. State: "STAND CLEAR! DEFIBRILLATE AT 200 JOULES!" while making sure that no one is touching the patient.	SHOCK NOW!	"STEADY TONE"
	14. Press the "SHOCK" SWITCH for the SECOND TIME.		
	15. Record the TIME after the delivery of the second shock.*	PUSH TO ANALYZE ECG	1 "BEEP"
	(Palpate the PATIENT'S PULSE—OPTIONAL.)	CHECK PULSE	
	16. Press the "ANALYZE" SWITCH for the THIRD TIME.	DETECTOR ON	2 "BEEPS"
		DO NOT TOUCH PATIENT	
		SHOCK ADVISED	4 "BEEPS"

*Omit voice recording of narrative if not required by local protocol.

Continued.

A. Management of a persistent shockable rhythm: 1. Ventricular fibrillation (V-FIB)
2. Pulseless ventricular tachycardia (V-TACH)

Rescuer one (CPR trained)	Rescuer two (EMT/FR-D)	Message screen	Audible tones
		CHARGING 200 J	
	17. Press the "360 J" SWITCH while the defibrillator is charging.	PUSH FOR 360 J	
		CHARGING 360 J	
		DO NOT TOUCH PATIENT	
	18. Verify immediately that the energy setting is "360 JOULES."	360 J	5 "BEEPS"
	19. State: "STAND CLEAR! DEFIBRILLATE AT 360 JOULES!" while making sure that **no one is touching the patient.**	SHOCK NOW!	"STEADY TONE"
	20. Press the "SHOCK" SWITCH for the THIRD TIME.		
	21. Record the TIME after the delivery of the **third shock.***	PUSH TO ANALYZE ECG	1 "BEEP"
	22. Palpate the **patient's carotid artery.**	CHECK PULSE	
	23. State: "NO PULSE!"		
3. Resume **CPR.**	24. State: "**CONTINUE CPR,**" and, if appropriate, "**TRANSPORT!**"		
4. TRANSPORT THE PATIENT IMMEDIATELY OR WAIT FOR THE BLS OR ALS UNIT, AS APPROPRIATE.	**OR** Repeat **Steps 5 through 24,** as appropriate. The **subsequent shocks** are delivered in a sequence of **360, 360,** and **360 joules.**		

> **NOTE!**
>
> The **ENERGY LEVELS** and the **TOTAL NUMBER OF SHOCKS DELIVERED** may depend on the local protocol.

25. Continue **performing CPR, reanalyzing the ECG rhythm, delivering shocks, and checking the patient's pulse,** according to local protocol.

26. Record the TIME upon relinquishing the patient to an **AEMT** or upon arrival at the **emergency department.***

*Omit voice recording of narrative if not required by local protocol.

Physio-Control Lifepak 200 Automatic Advisory Defibrillator or Physio-Control Lifepak 250 Automatic Advisory Defibrillator without Lifepak Monitor

B. Management of a nonshockable rhythm: 1. Ventricular asystole
2. Electromechanical dissociation (EMD)

IF "NO SHOCK" IS ADVISED AND A PULSE IS ABSENT, INDICATING A NONPERFUSING RHYTHM:

Rescuer one (CPR trained)	Rescuer two (EMT/FR-D)	Message screen	Audible tones
1. Resume **CPR,** and continue it for 1 minute.	1. Palpate the patient's carotid artery.	**NO SHOCK ADVISED**	3 "BEEPS"
	2. State: **"NO PULSE!"**		
	3. State: **"CONTINUE CPR!"**	**PUSH TO ANALYZE ECG**	1 "BEEP"
2. Stop **CPR** and **STAND CLEAR!**	4. State: **"STOP CPR! STAND CLEAR!"** (Palpate the **PATIENT'S PULSE—OPTIONAL.**)	**CHECK PULSE**	
	5. Press the **"ANALYZE" SWITCH** for the **SECOND TIME.**	**DETECTOR ON** **DO NOT TOUCH PATIENT**	2 "BEEPS"
	6. Palpate the patient's carotid artery.	**NO SHOCK ADVISED**	3 "BEEPS"
	7. State, **"NO PULSE!"**		
3. Resume **CPR.**	8. State: **"CONTINUE CPR!"** and, if appropriate, **"TRANSPORT!"**	**PUSH TO ANALYZE ECG**	1 "BEEP"
4. **TRANSPORT THE PATIENT IMMEDIATELY OR WAIT FOR THE BLS OR ALS UNIT, AS APPROPRIATE.**	9. Continue **performing CPR, reanalyzing the ECG rhythm,** and **checking the patient's pulse,** according to locol protocol.	**CHECK PULSE**	
	10. Record the **TIME** upon relinquishing the patient to an **AEMT** or upon arrival at the **emergency department.***		

*Omit voice recording of narrative if not required by local protocol.

Physio-Control Lifepak 200 Automatic Advisory Defibrillator or Physio-Control Lifepak 250 Automatic Advisory Defibrillator without Lifepak Monitor

C. Management of a perfusing rhythm

IF "NO SHOCK" IS ADVISED AND A SPONTANEOUS PULSE IS PRESENT, INDICATING A PERFUSING RHYTHM:

Rescuer one (CPR trained)	Rescuer two (EMT/FR-D)	Message screen	Audible tones
	1. Palpate the patient's carotid artery.	**NO SHOCK ADVISED**	3 "BEEPS"
	2. State: **"PULSE PRESENT!"**		
1. Open and maintain an **open airway** while administering **high concentration oxygen.**	3. State: **"ADMINISTER OXYGEN"** and **"TRANSPORT!"**	**PUSH TO ANALYZE ECG**	1 "BEEP"
2. Assist **ventilation** while administering **supplemental high concentration oxygen** if necessary.	4. Obtain the initial **vital signs** and repeat them as often as the situation indicates, and, if appropriate, record them.*	**CHECK PULSE**	
3. **TRANSPORT THE PATIENT IMMEDIATELY OR WAIT FOR THE BLS OR ALS UNIT, AS APPROPRIATE.**	**If cardiac arrest recurs at the scene or en route:**		
	• State **"STAND CLEAR!"**		
	AND		
	• Repeat **Steps 5 through 24, A: MANAGEMENT OF A PERSISTENT SHOCKABLE RHYTHM,** as appropriate, until the shockable rhythm is converted into a perfusing rhythm or up to a total of **6 shocks** are delivered. The first shock of this series is delivered at the same energy level that was successful in terminating the dysrhythmia the last time. Subsequent shocks are delivered at 360 joules.		

> **NOTE!**
>
> **The ENERGY LEVELS and the TOTAL NUMBER OF SHOCKS DELIVERED may depend on the local protocol.**

5. Record the **TIME** upon relinquishing the patient to an **AEMT** or upon arrival at the **emergency department.***

*Omit voice recording of narrative if not required by local protocol.

Physio-Control Lifepak 300 Automatic Advisory Defibrillator

A. Management of persistent shockable rhythm: 1. Ventricular fibrillation (V-FIB)
2. Pulseless ventricular tachycardia (V-TACH)

- Recognize the **situation.**
- Verify **cardiac arrest.**
- Start **one- or two-rescuer CPR.**

Rescuer one (CPR trained)	Rescuer two (EMT/FR-D)	Message screen	Audible messages/tones
1. Continue **CPR.**	**1.** Connect the **defibrillation cables** to the **defibrillation electrodes.** **AND** Attach the **black "Stern" and the red "Apex" defibrillation electrodes** to the **patient's chest.**		
	2. Push the **"ON"** switch to turn on the **SAED.**	**PERFORMING SELF TESTS...**	
	3. Insert the **tape,** if appropriate.		
	4. Verify that a **fully charged battery** is in place.	**PUSH TO ANALYZE**	"BEEP(S)"
	Note: This should be done before arrival at the scene, preferably, during shift check.		
	5. Record the **NAMES** of the **RESCUERS,** the **TIME,** and the **AGE, SEX,** and **CONDITION** of the patient, including the **PATIENT'S PULSE.***		
2. Stop **CPR** and **STAND CLEAR!**	**6.** State: **"STOP CPR! STAND CLEAR!"** (Palpate the **PATIENT'S PULSE—OPTIONAL.**)		
NO PULSE V-FIB **OR** V-TACH **SHOCKABLE RHYTHM**	**7.** Press the **"PUSH TO ANALYZE" BUTTON** for the **FIRST TIME** while analyzing the **ECG** on the ECG screen. **NOTE** If "NO SHOCK" is advised now or at any time, PALPATE THE PATIENT'S PULSE. If the PULSE IS ABSENT, indicating a "NONPERFUSING RHYTHM," proceed to B: MANAGEMENT OF A NONSHOCKABLE RHYTHM.	**STAND CLEAR** **ANALYZING NOW** **SHOCK ADVISED** **CHARGING TO 200 J**	**2 BEEPS** "STAND CLEAR" **2 BEEPS** "SHOCK ADVISED" "CHARGING TONE"
	8. State: **"V-FIB (OR V-TACH) PRESENT!"**	**STAND CLEAR**	
	9. Verify immediately that the energy setting is **"200 JOULES."**	**200 J AVAILABLE**	

*Omit voice recording of narrative if not required by local protocol.

Continued.

A. Management of persistent shockable rhythm: 1. Ventricular fibrillation (V-FIB)
2. Pulseless ventricular tachycardia (V-TACH)

Rescuer one (CPR trained)	Rescuer two (EMT/FR-D)	Message screen	Audible messages/tones
	10. State: "STAND CLEAR! DEFIBRIL-LATE AT 200 JOULES!" while making sure that **no one is touching the patient.**	PUSH TO SHOCK	2 BEEPS "PUSH TO SHOCK" "READY TONE"
	11. Press the "PUSH TO SHOCK" BUTTON for the **FIRST TIME** while observing the **ECG on the ECG screen.**	ENERGY DELIVERED 1	
	12. Record the **TIME** after the delivery of the **first shock.***	PUSH TO ANALYZE	
	(Palpate the **PATIENT'S PULSE—OPTIONAL.**)		
NO PULSE V-FIB	13. Press the "PUSH TO ANALYZE" **BUTTON** for the **SECOND TIME** while analyzing the **ECG on the ECG screen.**	STAND CLEAR	2 BEEPS "STAND CLEAR"
OR	14. State: "V-FIB (OR V-TACH) STILL PRESENT!"	ANALYZING NOW	
V-TACH **SHOCKABLE RHYTHM**	**NOTE!** If "NO SHOCK" is advised now or at any time, **PALPATE THE PATIENT'S PULSE. If a SPONTANEOUS PULSE is present, indicating a "PERFUSING RHYTHM,"** proceed to C: MANAGEMENT OF A PERFUSING RHYTHM.	SHOCK ADVISED —— CHARGING TO 200 J —— STAND CLEAR	2 BEEPS "SHOCK ADVISED" "CHARGING TONE"
	15. Verify immediately that the energy setting is "**200 JOULES.**"	200 J AVAILABLE	
	16. State: "STAND CLEAR! DEFIBRIL-LATE AT 200 JOULES!" while making sure that **no one is touching the patient.**	PUSH TO SHOCK	2 BEEPS "PUSH TO SHOCK" "READY TONE"
	17. Press the "PUSH TO SHOCK" BUTTON for the **SECOND TIME** while observing the **ECG on the ECG screen.**	ENERGY DELIVERED 2	
	18. Record the **TIME** after the delivery of the **second shock.***	PUSH TO ANALYZE	
	(Palpate the **PATIENT'S PULSE—OPTIONAL.**)		
NO PULSE V-FIB	19. Press the "PUSH TO ANALYZE" **BUTTON** for the **THIRD TIME** while analyzing the **ECG on the ECG screen.**	STAND CLEAR	2 BEEPS "STAND CLEAR"
OR	20. State: "V-FIB (OR V-TACH) STILL PRESENT!"	ANALYZING NOW	
V-TACH **SHOCKABLE RHYTHM**			

*Omit voice recording of narrative if not required by local protocol.

Continued.

A. Management of persistent shockable rhythm: 1. Ventricular fibrillation (V-FIB)
2. Pulseless ventricular tachycardia (V-TACH)

Rescuer one (CPR trained)	Rescuer two (EMT/FR-D)	Message screen	Audible messages/tones
			2 BEEPS
		SHOCK ADVISED	**"SHOCK ADVISED"**
		CHARGING TO 360 J	**"CHARGING TONE"**
		STAND CLEAR	
	21. Verify immediately that the energy setting is **"360 JOULES."**	**360 J AVAILABLE**	
			2 BEEPS
	22. State: **"STAND CLEAR! DEFIBRILLATE AT 360 JOULES!"** while making sure that no one is touching the patient.	**PUSH TO SHOCK**	**"PUSH TO SHOCK" "READY TONE"**
	23. Press the **"PUSH TO SHOCK"** BUTTON for the **THIRD TIME** while observing the **ECG on the ECG screen.**	**ENERGY DELIVERED 3**	
	24. Record the **TIME** after the delivery of the **third shock.***	**PUSH TO ANALYZE**	
NO PULSE	25. Palpate the **patient's carotid artery** while analyzing the **ECG on the ECG screen.**	**CHECK PATIENT**	**2 BEEPS "CHECK PATIENT"**

V-FIB

OR

V-TACH

SHOCKABLE RHYTHM

3. Resume **CPR.**

4. **TRANSPORT THE PATIENT IMMEDIATELY OR WAIT FOR THE BLS OR ALS UNIT, AS APPROPRIATE.**

26. State: **"V-FIB (OR V-TACH) STILL PRESENT! NO PULSE!"**

27. State: **"CONTINUE CPR,"** and, if appropriate, **"TRANSPORT!"**

OR

Repeat **Steps 6 through 27,** as appropriate. The **subsequent shocks** are delivered in a sequence of **360, 360,** and **360** joules.

NOTE!

The **ENERGY LEVELS** and the **TOTAL NUMBER OF SHOCKS DELIVERED** may depend on the local protocol.

---

28. Continue **performing CPR, reanalyzing the ECG rhythm, delivering shocks,** and **checking the patient's pulse,** according to local protocol.

29. Record the **TIME** upon relinquishing the patient to an **AEMT** or upon arrival at the **emergency department.***

---

*Omit voice recording of narrative if not required by local protocol.

Physio-Control Lifepak 300 Automatic Advisory Defibrillator

B. Management of a nonshockable rhythm: 1. Ventricular asystole
2. Electromechanical dissociation (EMD)

If "NO SHOCK" is advised and a pulse is absent, indicating a NONPERFUSING RHYTHM:

Rescuer one (CPR trained)	Rescuer two (EMT/FR-D)	Message screen	Audible messages/tones
		NO SHOCK ADVISED	2 BEEPS
	1. Palpate the **patient's carotid artery.**	CHECK PULSE	"CHECK PULSE"
NO PULSE	2. State: **"ASYSTOLE (OR EMD) PRESENT! NO PULSE!"**	PUSH TO ANALYZE	

Asystole

OR

EMD

NONSHOCKABLE RHYTHM	3. State: **"CONTINUE CPR!"**		
1. Resume **CPR,** and continue for 1 minute.	4. State: **"STOP CPR! STAND CLEAR!"** (Palpate the **PATIENT'S PULSE— OPTIONAL.**)		
2. Stop **CPR** and **STAND CLEAR!**	5. Press the **"PUSH TO ANALYZE" BUTTON** for the **SECOND TIME** while analyzing the **ECG on the ECG screen.**	STAND CLEAR	2 BEEPS "STAND CLEAR"
		ANALYZING NOW	
		NO SHOCK ADVISED	2 BEEPS
	6. Palpate the patient's carotid artery.	CHECK PULSE	"CHECK PULSE"
NO PULSE	7. State: **"ASYSTOLE (OR EMD) STILL PRESENT! NO PULSE!"**	PUSH TO ANALYZE	

Asystole

OR

EMD

NONSHOCKABLE RHYTHM	8. State: **"CONTINUE CPR!"** and, if appropriate, **"TRANSPORT!"**		
3. Resume **CPR.**	9. Continue **performing CPR, reanalyzing the ECG rhythm,** and **checking the patient's pulse,** according to local protocol.		
4. **TRANSPORT THE PATIENT IMMEDIATELY OR WAIT FOR THE BLS OR ALS UNIT, AS APPROPRIATE.**	10. Record the **TIME** upon relinquishing the patient to an **AEMT** or upon arrival at the **emergency department.***		

*Omit voice recording of narrative if not required by local protocol.

Physio-Control Lifepak 300 Automatic Advisory Defibrillator

C. Management of a Perfusing Rhythm

Rescuer one (CPR trained)	Rescuer two (EMT/FR-D)	Message screen	Audible messages/tones
	If "NO SHOCK" is advised and a spontaneous pulse is present, indicating a perfusing rhythm:		
		NO SHOCK ADVISED	2 BEEPS
	1. Palpate the **patient's carotid artery.**	CHECK PULSE	"CHECK PULSE"
PULSE PRESENT	**2.** State: **"PULSE AND ECG PRESENT!"**	PUSH TO ANALYZE	

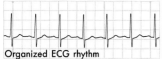

Organized ECG rhythm

PERFUSING RHYTHM

1. Open and maintain an **open airway** while administering **high concentration oxygen.**

2. Assist **ventilation** while administering **supplemental high concentration oxygen** if necessary.

3. TRANSPORT THE PATIENT IMMEDIATELY OR WAIT FOR THE BLS OR ALS UNIT, AS APPROPRIATE.

3. State: **"ADMINISTER OXYGEN"** and **"TRANSPORT!"**

4. Obtain the initial **vital signs** and repeat them as often as the situation indicates, and, if appropriate, record them.*

5. **Monitor** the **patient's ECG** using the **SAED.**

If cardiac arrest recurs at the scene or en route:

• State: **"STAND CLEAR!"**

AND

• Repeat **Steps 7 through 27, A: MANAGEMENT OF A PERSISTENT SHOCKABLE RHYTHM,** as appropriate, until the shockable rhythm is converted into a perfusing rhythm or up to a total of **6 shocks** are delivered. The first shock of this series is delivered at the same energy level that was successful in terminating the dysrhythmia the last time. Subsequent shocks are delivered at 360 joules.

NOTE!

The ENERGY LEVELS and the TOTAL NUMBER OF SHOCKS DELIVERED may depend on the local protocol.

---

6. Record the **TIME** upon relinquishing the patient to an **AEMT** or upon arrival at the **emergency department.***

---

*Omit voice recording of narrative if not required by local protocol.

Glossary

A

Acidosis A disturbance in the acid-base balance of the body caused by accumulation of excessive amounts of carbon dioxide (respiratory acidosis), lactic acid (metabolic acidosis), or both.

AC interference One of the causes of ECG artifacts.

Acute myocardial infarction (AMI) A heart condition that is present when part of the myocardium dies (necrosis) because of interruption of blood flow to the area.

Advanced emergency medical technician (AEMT) A prehospital emergency care provider capable of providing advanced life support (ALS) services.

Advanced life support (ALS) Emergency medical care beyond basic life support including one or more of the following: starting an IV, administering IV fluids, administering drugs, defibrillating, inserting an esophageal obturator airway or endotracheal tube, and monitoring and interpreting the ECG.

AED Abbreviation for automated external defibrillator.

AEMT Abbreviation for Advanced Emergency Medical Technician.

Agonal Occurring at the moment of or just before death.

AICD Abbreviation for automatic implantable cardiovascular defibrillator.

Alternating-current (AC) shock Obsolete method of terminating ventricular fibrillation.

Alveoli The tiny air sacs in the lungs. When these become filled with serum and foam because of left heart failure, pulmonary edema results.

Ambulatory Walking about.

AMI Abbreviation for acute myocardial infarction.

Aneurysm Localized dilatation or ballooning of the wall of a ventricle or an artery.

Angina pectoris Pain from myocardial ischemia caused by physical exertion or emotional stress. The pain is almost always present behind the sternum (substernal), often radiating to the arms (most commonly to the left one), neck, or abdomen. Usually, it lasts 3 to 5 minutes (rarely 30 minutes), disappearing with rest or nitroglycerin. **Stable angina** is characterized by recurrent pain with a predictable and similar pattern of onset and duration. **Unstable angina** is characterized by a changing pattern of onset and duration of pain, e.g., the pain occurs with less physical exertion or emotional stress or the pain is not relieved by the usual medication or rest.

Anorexia Loss of appetite.

Anoxia Absence or lack of oxygen.

Anterior In front of.

Anterior axillary line An imaginary line beginning in front of the axilla (armpit) and running parallel to the sternum just outside of the nipple.

Antidysrhythmic drugs Drugs that prevent or terminate cardiac dysrhythmias.

Anti-perspirant A common household product, such as Arrid Dry, used in its spray form to dry out sweaty skin before the attachment of defibrillator electrodes to ensure proper adhesion of the electrodes to the skin.

Aorta The main trunk of the arterial system of the body consisting of the ascending aorta, the aortic arch, and the descending aorta. The descending aorta is further divided into the thoracic and abdominal aorta.

Aortic valve The one-way valve between the left ventricle and the ascending aorta.

Apex of the heart The pointed lower end of the heart formed by the right and left ventricles.

Apical thrust of the heart The palpable thrust of the apex of the heart against the chest wall. It is normally palpated in the left fifth intercostal space in the midclavicular line.

Apnea Absence of breathing.

Arcing A band of sparks or flash of light that jumps between two electrodes when held too close or when a low-resistance path exists between the electrodes.

Artifacts (ECG) Abnormal waves and spikes in an ECG caused by muscle tremor, patient or ECG cable movement, AC interference, loose electrodes, and external chest compression.

Artificial pacemaker An electronic device used to stimulate the heart to beat when the heart's own pacemaker becomes very slow (bradycardia) or the electrical conduction system malfunctions causing a complete atrioventricular (AV) block with ventricular escape rhythm or ventricular asystole. An artificial pacemaker consists of an electronic pulse generator, a battery, and a wire lead that senses the electrical activity of the heart and delivers electrical impulses to the atria or ventricles or both when the pacemaker senses an absence of electrical activity. An artificial pacemaker may be permanent and implanted or external and temporary.

Asystole Absence of contractions of the ventricles or the entire heart.

Atherosclerosis The aging and destructive process within arteries causing them to become progressively narrow and hard and eventually to obstruct.

Atria The thin-walled chambers which receive the blood flowing to the heart on its way to the ventricles. The two atria form the upper part (or the base) of the heart and are separated from the ventricles by the mitral and tricuspid valves. The singular form of atria is atrium.

Atrioventricular (AV) junction The part of the electrical conduction system that normally conducts the electrical impulse from the atria to the ventricles. It consists of the AV node and bundle of His.

Atrioventricular (AV) node The part of the electrical conduction system, located in the posterior floor of the right atrium near the interatrial septum, through which the electrical impulses are normally conducted from the atria to the bundle of His.

Automated external defibrillator (AED) An electrical device capable of delivering direct-current (DC) shock to a patient in cardiac arrest after automatically analyzing the patient's electrocardiogram for a shockable rhythm. Used in terminating ventricular fibrillation and pulseless ventricular tachycardia with a rate of 120 to 200 per minute or greater.

Automatic implantable cardiovascular defibrillator (AICD) An implantable electronic device used to deliver one or more direct-current (DC) shocks to the patient's ventricles automatically when a shockable rhythm occurs.

Automaticity The property of cardiac cells to generate electrical pulses automatically.

AV Abbreviation for atrioventricular.

AV junction See Atrioventricular (AV) junction.

AV node See Atrioventricular (AV) node.

Axilla Armpit.

B

Backward failure of the left heart. A condition caused by the inability of a damaged left ventricle to pump blood forward effectively. The result is pulmonary congestion and edema.

"Bag of worms" Descriptive phrase used to describe the appearance of the ventricles in ventricular fibrillation. *See* "Quivering bowl of jelly."

Base *See* Base of the heart.

Base of the heart The upper part of the heart formed by the right and left atria.

Basic life support (BLS) Emergency care consisting of establishing and maintaining an open airway, providing ventilatory assistance, and performing cardiopulmonary resuscitation.

Benign complications of AMI Nonlife-threatening dysrhythmias and mild congestive heart failure.

Biological death Present when irreversible brain damage has occurred, usually within 5 to 10 minutes after cardiac arrest, if untreated.

Blood clot A soft mass of blood elements; a thrombus.

Blood electrolytes Mineral substances dissolved in the blood necessary for proper functioning of the body, including the electrical conduction system of the heart and the myocardium. Includes blood calcium and potassium.

Blood-tinged sputum One of the signs of pulmonary congestion and edema. Also called hemoptysis.

Bradycardia A heart rate of less than 60 beats per minute. Also a dysrhythmia with a heart rate below 35 to 60 beats per minute.

Bretylium tosylate Drug used to treat ventricular dysrhythmias such as pulseless ventricular tachycardia and ventricular fibril-

lation resistant to defibrillatory shock to improve the chances of defibrillation.

Bundle branches The part of the electrical conduction system in the ventricles consisting of the right and left bundle branch that conducts the electrical impulses from the bundle of His to the Purkinje network of the myocardium.

Bundle of His The part of the electrical conduction system located in the upper part of the interventricular septum that conducts the electrical impulses from the AV node to the right and left bundle branches. The bundle of His and the AV node form the AV junction.

Bystander A person at the scene of an emergency other than the rescuers.

Bystander CPR Performance of CPR by a family member, friend, police officer, fireman, nurse, EMT, or anyone at the scene of a witnessed or unwitnessed cardiac arrest before the arrival of the EMT/FR-D.

C

Calcium A mineral substance dissolved in the blood necessary for proper functioning of the heart, including the electrical conduction system of the heart and the myocardium.

Capacitor An electrical component present in all defibrillators used primarily for storage of electrical energy.

Capillary The smallest blood vessel in the body, connecting the arteries and arterioles with the venules and veins.

Capillary refill A simple diagnostic test to assess the ability of the circulatory system to recirculate blood through an area of the body temporarily deprived of blood, i.e., the adequacy of peripheral blood flow. It is performed by pressing firmly down with the thumb on an area of the patient's body such as the palm of the hand or the forehead, forcing the blood out of the skin and the subcutaneous tissue and causing them to blanch. The pressure is quickly released, and the time that it takes for the blanched area of the skin to return to its previous color intensity is noted, in seconds. Normally, the capillary refill is less than two seconds, indicating normal peripheral blood flow. A delayed capillary refill, greater than two seconds, indicates an abnormally sluggish blood flow as present in hypotension and shock.

Cardiac arrest The sudden and unexpected cessation of an adequate circulation to maintain life in a patient who was not expected to die. Its cause may be medical or traumatic.

Cardiac cells The cells of the heart: myocardial cells and the specialized cells of the electrical conduction system of the heart.

Cardiac output The amount of blood pumped out of the heart into the body's circulation per unit of time, usually calculated in liters of blood per minute.

Cardiac rupture A relatively rare but serious life-threatening complication of AMI in which the dead (necrotic) tissue is torn apart or disrupted. Rupture can occur in the papillary muscle, interventricular septum, or myocardium.

Cardiac standstill Absence of atrial and ventricular contractions. This term is used interchangeably with ventricular asystole.

Cardiac tamponade A condition which occurs when an excessive amount of fluid or blood accumulates in the pericardial cavity. When it occurs in acute myocardial infarction, its cause is usually myocardial rupture. Hypotension and shock with electromechanical dissociation (EMD) result from cardiac tamponade.

Cardiogenic Originating in the heart.

Cardiogenic shock Shock caused by severe damage to the heart, usually the left ventricle, from an AMI.

Cardiopulmonary resuscitation (CPR) Application of rescue breathing and external chest compression in patients with cardiac arrest to maintain some circulation to support life.

Cardiovascular disease Disease of the heart and blood vessels.

Chest burns One of the complications of defibrillation.

Cholesterol A fatty substance found in animal tissue, egg yolks, and various oils and fats felt to cause atherosclerosis of the coronary arteries when eaten in excessive amounts.

Chordae tendinea Fibrous strands attached to the papillary muscles at one end and the free edges of the valve leaflets of the mitral and tricuspid valves at the other end. These strands, which resemble the lines of a parachute, prevent the valve leaflets from ballooning backward into the atria.

Circulatory system The blood vessels in the body, including the systemic and pulmonary circulatory systems.

Clavicle The curved bone attached to the uppermost part of the sternum at a right angle, forming the anterior part of the shoulder girdle; the collarbone.

Clinical death Present the moment the patient's pulse and blood pressure are absent; occurs immediately with the onset of cardiac arrest.

Coarse ventricular fibrillation Ventricular fibrillation with large fibrillatory waves—greater than 3 mm in height.

Coarse ventricular fibrillatory waves Large fibrillatory waves, greater than 3 mm in height.

Collar bone *See* Clavicle.

Command circuit and screen An electronic component of a semi-automatic defibrillator providing information and guidance to the rescuer about whether or not to deliver a shock to the patient following the analysis of the patient's ECG.

Complexes See QRS complex.

Components of the electrocardiogram Includes the P wave, QRS complex, and T wave.

Conductive substance A substance, such as water, salt water or saline, wet sand, and nitroglycerine ointment, which conducts an electric current.

Conductivity The property of cardiac cells to conduct electrical impulses.

Congestive heart failure Excessive blood or tissue fluid in the lungs or body or both caused by the inefficient pumping of the heart.

Contractility The property of cardiac cells to contract when stimulated by an electrical impulse.

Control panel Usually a liquid crystal display (LCD) on a semi-automatic defibrillator that is used to display visual instructions to the rescuers.

Core temperature The temperature within the body as measured in the rectum.

Coronary arteries The arteries supplying blood to the heart.

Coronary circulation Passage of blood through the coronary arteries and their branches and the capillaries in the heart and then back to the right atrium via the coronary venules and veins and the coronary sinus.

Coronary heart disease (CHD) Progressive narrowing and eventual obstruction of the coronary arteries by atherosclerosis.

Coronary artery occlusion Blockage of a coronary artery by a blood clot, rupture or displacement of a plaque, or hemorrhage under an existing plaque.

Coronary sinus The outlet in the right atrium draining the venous system of the heart.

Costal cartilages The cartilages attached to the ends of the ribs connecting the ribs to the sternum.

Costochondral Pertaining to the cartilaginous ends of the ribs attached to the sternum.

Costochondral junction The point where the costal cartilages are united with the anterior tips of the ribs.

Cyanosis Presence of slightly bluish, grayish, slatelike, or purplish discoloration of the skin caused by the presence of unoxygenated blood.

Cyanotic Pertaining to cyanosis.

D

Decapitation Beheading or being beheaded: one of the criteria for not starting cardiopulmonary resuscitation and using the automated external defibrillator.

Dependent lividity *See* Livor mortis.

Defibrillation Application of a defibrillatory shock to the heart to terminate pulseless ventricular tachycardia and ventricular fibrillation.

Defibrillator An electronic device used by EMT/FR-Ds to deliver a direct-current (DC) shock across the chest to the heart to terminate pulseless ventricular tachycardia and ventricular fibrillation.

Defibrillator electrodes Disposable, self-adhesive pads with a metal electrode that are applied to the chest wall to detect the patient's ECG for analysis and to deliver shocks to the heart to terminate pulseless ventricular tachycardia and ventricular fibrillation. The negative electrode is applied to the upper right anterior chest in the angle formed by the right clavicle and the upper right border of the sternum. The positive electrode is attached to the left lower anterior chest wall, centered over the intersection of the left fourth intercostal space and the left anterior axillary line.

Diastole, ventricular The period of relaxation and distention of the ventricles between contractions, during which they fill with blood.

Direct-current (DC) shock The electrical current used in the treatment of pulseless ventricular tachycardia and ventricular fibrillation. Direct-current (DC) shock is commonly referred to as "defibrillatory shock" or simply as "shock."

Direct writer A mechanical device that records the patient's ECG and a log of events and the time of their occurrence on ECG paper. It is an option on some models of automated external defibrillators.

Display freeze feature Electronic circuitry which locks onto a segment of the ECG displayed on the ECG screen to permit more accurate visual analysis of the ECG. It is an option on some models of automated external defibrillators.

Dominant (primary) pacemaker of the heart The SA node.

Dual channel tape recorder An option supplied with some models of automated external defibrillators to enable the simultaneous recording of the operator's verbal narrative and the patient's ECG.

Dyspnea Difficulty in breathing caused by pulmonary congestion and edema, manifested by rapid shallow respiration. Dyspnea occcuring at rest or during physical exertion is called *exertional dyspnea;* dyspnea after a period of sleep while in a recumbent position, *paroxysmal nocturnal dyspnea.*

Dysrhythmia A rhythm other than a normal sinus rhythm. It is present when (1) the heart rate is less than 60 or greater than 100 beats per minute, (2) the rhythm is irregular, (3) premature contractions occur, or (4) the normal progression of the electrical impulse through the electrical conduction system is blocked. It includes escape and ectopic beats and rhythms. Also known as an arrhythmia, a less appropriate term, but one used as frequently.

E

ECG Abbreviation for electrocardiogram.

ECG analysis circuit A microprocessor circuit common to all automated external defibrillators which analyzes the patient's ECG for the presence of P waves, QRS complexes and their width and rate, and fibrillation waves to determine whether a shockable rhythm is present. Shockable rhythms are ventricular tachycardia with a rate of 120 to 200 beats per minute or greater and ventricular fibrillation. The rate at which ventricular tachycardia is considered to be "shockable" varies from manufacturer to manufacturer.

ECG electrodes (disposable) Disposable, self-adhesive pads with a metal or conductive plastic electrode that are applied to the chest wall to detect the patient's ECG for ECG monitoring and in addition in some models for analysis of the ECG to detect the sudden occurrence of a shockable rhythm.

ECG monitoring circuit An option that is available in some automated external defibrillators for continuous analysis of the patient's ECG to detect the sudden occurrence of a shockable rhythm.

ECG rhythm An ECG with waves and complexes.

ECG signal display screen An option, consisting of a liquid crystal display (LCD), available in some models of semi-automatic external defibrillators to provide a visual display of the patient's ECG.

Ectopic Refers to beats and rhythms originating in a pacemaker site other than the SA mode. Refers to something out-of-place.

Ectopic beat An abnormal beat (also referred to as a premature beat) originating in an ectopic pacemaker in the atria, AV junction, or ventricles, e.g., premature atrial contraction (PAC), premature junctional contraction (PJC), and premature ventricular contraction (PVC).

Ectopic pacemaker An abnormal pacemaker in the atria, AV junction, bundle branches, Purkinje network, or ventricular myocardium.

Ectopic rhythm A dysrhythmia originating in an ectopic pacemaker in the atria, AV junction, or ventricles, e.g., premature ventricular contractions (PVCs), ventricular tachycardia (VT, V-Tach), and ventricular fibrillation (VF, V-Fib).

Edema A condition in which the body tissues have accumulated excessive fluid (or exudate) as in congestive heart failure.

Effusion An abnormal accumulation of fluid in tissue or a body cavity such as the pericardial or abdominal cavity.

Electrical activity of the heart The electric current generated by the atria and ventricles, which can be graphically displayed on the ECG.

Electrical conduction system of the heart Includes the sinoatrial (SA) node, internodal atrial conduction tracts, atrioventricular (AV) node, bundle of His, right and left bundle branches, and Purkinje network.

Electrical impulse The tiny electric current that normally originates in the SA node automatically and is conducted through the electrical conduction system to the myocardial cells in the atria and ventricles, causing them to contract.

Electrical instability of the heart A condition of the atria and ventricles in which ectopic beats or rhythms are being generated by an ectopic pacemaker within the atria and ventricles, e.g., premature ventricular contractions, ventricular tachycardia, and ventricular fibrillation.

Electrocardiogram (ECG) The graphic display of the electrical activity of the heart. The ECG includes the P wave, QRS complex, and the T wave.

Electrocution Death by means of an electric current. One of the causes of ventricular fibrillation and cardiac arrest.

Electrode A sensing device that detects electrical activity such as that of the heart.

Electrolyte A substance that when in solution dissociates into cations and anions, thus becoming capable of conducting electricity. Examples are calcium and potassium.

Electrolyte imbalance Abnormal concentrations of serum electrolytes caused by excessive intake or loss of certain electrolytes such as calcium, potassium, carbonate, chloride, and sodium.

Electromechanical A term that refers to the electrical and mechanical activity of the haert. The electrical activity is represented by the electrocardiogram (ECG); the mechanical activity, by the contraction and relaxation of the ventricles, producing a cardiac output which results in the circulation of blood and a pulse and blood pressure.

Electromechanical dissociation (EMD) A condition of the heart in which the electrical activity of the heart is present and can be recorded on the ECG, but effective ventricular contractions (mechanical activity) are absent; consequently, a pulse and blood pressure are absent.

EMD Abbreviation for electromechanical dissociation.

EMT/FR-D Abbreviation for emergency medical technician/first responder-defibrillation. A generic term to identify both the emergency medical technician (EMT) and first responder (FR) trained in early defibrillation.

EMT/FR-D system An EMS system using EMT/FR-Ds as first responders or EMT-Ds as part of the staff of EMT-D ambulance units or both.

EMT/FR-D unit A basic life support emergency vehicle, either an ambulance or a first response vehicle, staffed by an EMT/FR-D.

EMT/FR-D-witnessed cardiac arrest A cardiac arrest occurring after the arrival of the EMT/FR-D on the scene.

Enzymes Organic catalysts. When cardiac tissue is anoxic or necrotic, enzymes normally present in myocardial cells are liberated into the bloodstream. Determining the blood levels of these enzymes is an important way of confirming the diagnosis of acute myocardial infarction.

Energy delivered Refers to the amount of energy in joules delivered to the patient. It is about 80% of the energy actually stored in the defibrillator's capacitor. The drop in energy is caused by electrical resistance in the electronic circuit, the electrodes and connecting cables and connectors, and the chest wall itself.

Epigastrium The upper, middle part of the abdomen that is located below the xiphoid process.

Epinephrine A drug that is used to treat ventricular dysrhythmias such as pulseless ventricular tachycardia and ventricular fibrillation resistant to defibrillatory shock to improve the chances of defibrillation.

Escape pacemaker A pacemaker that takes over pacing the heart when the pacemaker of the underlying rhythm slows to less than the escape pacemaker's inherent firing rate. Also called latent, secondary, or subsidiary pacemaker.

Escape rhythm Three or more consecutive QRS complexes that result when the underlying rhythm slows to less than the escape pacemakers's inherent firing rate and the escape pacemaker takes over. An example of an escape rhythm is ventricular escape rhythm.

External chest compression The method by which mechanical depression of the lower half of the sternum compresses the thoracic contents, squeezing the blood out into the systemic and pulmonary circulations.

F

Fibrillation Chaotic, disorganized beating of the myocardium in which each muscle fiber contracts and relaxes independently, producing rapid, tremulous, and ineffectual contractions. Fibrillation may occur in both the atria and ventricles. The difference between atrial and ventricular fibrillation is that QRS complexes are present in atrial fibrillation and absent in ventricular fibrillation.

Fibrillation waves (ventricular) Waves that are bizarre, irregularly shaped, rounded or pointed, and markedly dissimilar, originating in multiple ectopic pacemakers in the ventricles.

Fine ventricular fibrillation Ventricular fibrillation with small fibrillatory waves—less than 3 mm in height.

First responder unit A first response vehicle staffed by a first responder who may be an EMT/FR-D.

Flat line The flat line in an ECG during which electrical activity is absent.

Fully automatic external defibrillator An electronic device used by EMT/FR-Ds that analyzes the ECG of a patient in cardiac arrest to determine the presence of ventricular tachycardia with a rate of 120 to 200 per minute or greater or ventricular fibrillation and, if present, delivers a shock automatically.

H

Heart attack A lay person's term for acute myocardial infarction.

Heart rate The number of contractions of the ventricles per unit of time (usually a minute).

Heart sounds The audible vibrations produced by the opening and closing of the heart valves.

Hemoptysis Production of blood-tinged sputum.

Hypercarbia Excessive carbon dioxide in the blood.

Hypertension High blood pressure; generally considered to be a systolic blood pressure of 140 mm Hg or greater.

Hypotension Low blood pressure; generally considered to be a systolic blood pressure of 80 to 90 mm Hg or less.

Hypothermia A state of low body temperature.

Hypovolemia A reduced amount of blood in the body's cardiovascular system.

Hypovolemic cardiac arrest Cardiac arrest resulting from inadequate perfusion of the heart secondary to low cardiac output from low blood volume.

Hypoxia Reduced amount of oxygen. Hypoxia is used interchangeably with the term anoxia.

Hypoxic Refers to having a reduced amount of oxygen.

I

Impedance The resistance to the flow of an electric current measured in ohms.

Impedance measuring circuit Component of the automated external defibrillator which measures the impedance in ohms across the chest through the defibrillator electrodes. If no impedance is detected, the rescuer is warned that the electrodes are not properly applied.

Infarct Area of dead tissue.

Infarction Death (necrosis) of tissue caused by interruption of the blood supply to the affected tissue.

Inferior vena cava One of the two largest veins in the body that empty venous blood into the right atrium.

Inherent firing rate The rate at which a given dominant or escape pacemaker of the heart normally generates electrical impulses.

Interatrial septum The membranous wall dividing the right and left atria.

Intercostal space Area between two adjacent ribs, containing intercostal muscles, arteries, veins, and nerves.

Internal DC shock The direct-current (DC) shock, of up to 30 joules, delivered by the automatic implantable cardiovascular defibrillator (AICD) directly to the heart.

Internodal atrial conduction tracts Part of the electrical conduction system of the heart consisting of three bundles of specialized conducting tissue located in the walls of the right atrium between the SA node and AV node.

Interventricular septum The membranous, muscular wall dividing the heart into the right and left ventricles.

Irreversible brain damage Occurs usually within five to ten minutes after cardiac arrest if untreated. Occurs at the time of biological death.

Ischemia Reduced blood flow to tissue caused by narrowing or occlusion of the artery supplying blood to it. Ischemia results in tissue anoxia.

J

Joule Unit of electrical energy delivered for one second by an electrical source, such as a defibrillator. Used interchangeably with watt-seconds.

Joules of delivered energy The actual amount of electrical energy that is delivered to the patient's chest across the defibrillator paddles in comparison to the larger amount measured across the capacitor's terminals at the time of discharge. This drop in energy is due to the resistance in the paddles or electrodes, connecting cables, connectors, and the chest wall itself.

Jugular veins The large veins that are located in the neck which become distended and pulsate in congestive heart failure caused by right heart failure.

L

Landmarks of the chest Includes the anterior axillary line, the apical thrust of the heart, the midclavicular line, the midline of the sternum, and the precordium.

Latent (secondary, subsidiary) pacemaker cells *See* Escape pacemaker.

Lateral Away from the midline.

Lead II An ECG monitoring lead obtained by placing the negative electrode on the upper right anterior chest wall (or on the right shoulder or arm) and the positive electrode over the left lower anterior chest wall in the left anterior axillary line (or on the left leg).

Left atrium The thin-walled chamber on the left side of the heart which receives oxygenated blood from the lungs through the pulmonary veins and empties it into the left ventricle through the mitral valve.

Left anterior axillary line An imaginary line beginning in front of the left axilla (armpit) and running parallel to the left side of the sternum just outside of the left nipple.

Left bundle branch Part of the electrical conduction system located in the left ventricle connecting the bundle of His with the Purkinje network in the left ventricle.

Left heart The left side of the heart consisting of the left atrium and left ventricle which receives oxygenated blood from the lungs and pumps it into the systemic circulation.

Left heart failure Failure of the left ventricle to pump blood forward, effectively resulting in a backup of blood and tissue fluid in the lungs—pulmonary congestion and edema.

Left midclavicular line An imaginary line beginning in the middle of the left clavicle and running parallel to the sternum slightly inside the left nipple.

Left ventricle The thick-walled, muscular chamber on the left side of the heart which receives oxygenated blood from the left atrium and pumps it into the systemic circulation.

Lethal dysrhythmias Life-threatening dysrhythmias, including electromechanical dissociation (EMD), ventricular tachycardia, ventricular fibrillation, and ventricular asystole.

Lethal complication in AMI Include life-threatening dysrhythmias, mechanical pump failure, and rupture of the heart.

Lidocaine A drug that is used to treat ventricular dysrhythmias such as pulseless ventricular tachycardia and ventricular fibrillation resistant to defibrillatory shock to improve the chances of defibrillation.

Life-threatening dysrhythmias Include electromechanical dissociation (EMD), ventricular tachycardia, ventricular fibrillation, and ventricular asystole.

Lipid A fatty, organic substance that is found in the blood. Research has indicated that higher levels of lipids are involved in the formation of atherosclerosis of the coronary arteries.

Liquid crystal display (LCD) A low-energy output device used in automated external defibrillators to display the ECG and visual messages.

Livor mortis Dark, dull red discoloration of the skin appearing on dependent parts of the body 20 to 30 minutes after death, as a result of cessation of circulation and settling of the blood by gravity. Also called postmortem lividity. One of the criteria for not starting cardiopulmonary resuscitation and using the automated external defibrillator.

Loose electrodes A cause of ECG artifacts.

M

Manubrium The upper part of the sternum to which the clavicles are attached.

Mechanical activity of the heart The rhythmic contraction and relaxation of the atria and ventricles which produce the cardiac output responsible for the circulation of blood and the pulse and blood pressure.

Mechanical circulatory assistance Bypass of the heart and usually the lungs using a heart-lung bypass machine to support a failing heart.

Medial Pertaining to the middle; closer to the midline of the body or structure.

Medical control One of the most important components of an EMT/FR-D system provided by a physician who brings medical responsibility and direction to the EMT/FR-D program and under whose medical license the EMT/FR-Ds operate.

Memory module An electronic recording device used in some automated external defibrillators to store in memory such data as the patient's ECG rhythm before and after each ECG analysis, the time of each event, the messages and instructions generated by the automated external defibrillator, the date, and the serial number of the automated external defibrillator. Usually referred to as a plug-in memory module.

Microprocessor A computer chip with an ECG analysis circuit that is used in an automated external defibrillator to analyze the patient's ECG to detect the presence of a shockable rhythm.

Midclavicular line An imaginary line beginning in the middle of the clavicle and running parallel to the sternum slightly inside the nipple.

Midline An imaginary line that runs up and down the middle of the body.

Mitral valve The valve located between the left atrium and left ventricle.

Monitoring Lead II ECG *See* Lead II.

Muscle tremor Extraneous spikes and waves in the ECG caused by voluntary and involuntary muscle movement or shivering; often seen in elderly persons or in a cold environment.

Myocardial Pertaining to the muscular part of the heart.

Myocardial cells Cells of the heart having the ability to contract when electrically stimulated.

Myocardial infarction *See* Acute myocardial infarction.

Myocardial ischemia Reduced blood flow to myocardial tissue caused by narrowing or occlusion of the coronary artery supplying blood to it. Myocardial ischemia results in anoxia of the myocardial tissue which can result in angina pectoris and even acute myocardial infarction.

Myocardial rupture Breaking apart of the part of the myocardium damaged by an acute myocardial infarction, usually occurring several days after its onset. Myocardial rupture causes bleeding into the pericardial sac, resulting in cardiac tamponade and death if untreated.

Myocardium Cardiac muscle.

N

Necrosis Death of tissue.

Necrotic Refers to dead tissue.

Negative defibrillator electrode One of two electrodes used to deliver a shock across the chest to the heart to terminate a shockable rhythm. The negative electrode is attached to the upper right chest wall in the angle formed by the right clavicle and the right edge of the sternum.

Nitroglycerin A chemical compound with vasodilator properties that is useful in the treatment of angina pectoris. Available in sublingual, chewable, or oral, sustained-release forms and as an ointment and a transdermal patch for application to the skin. When found on the skin, the nitroglycerin ointment or patch must be removed as thoroughly as possible before the defibrillator electrodes are applied to prevent arcing during defibrillation.

Noise Extraneous spikes, waves, and complexes in the ECG signal caused by muscle tremor, 60-cycle AC interference, improperly attached electrodes, and motion.

Non-life-threatening dysrhythmias All ECG rhythms and dysrhythmias other than ventricular tachycardia, ventricular fibrillation, ventricular asystole, and electromechanical dissociation (EMD).

Nonperfusing rhythms All rhythms and dysrhythmias without a pulse. These include pulseless ventricular tachycardia, ventricular fibrillation, ventricular asystole, and electromechanical dissociation (EMD). The two *nonperfusing, shockable rhythms,* for which shock *is* indicated, are pulseless ventricular tachycardia with a rate of 120 to 200 per minute or greater and ventricular fibrillation. The three *nonperfusing, nonshockable rhythms,* for which shock *is not* indicated, are pulseless ventricular tachycardia with a rate of less than 120 to 200 per minute, ventricular asystole, and electromechanical dissociation (EMD).

Nonshockable rhythms All rhythms and dysrhythmias *except* ventricular fibrillation and pulseless ventricular tachycardia with a rate of 120 to 200 per minute or greater. Nonshockable rhythms may or may not have a pulse. The nonshockable rhythms without a pulse *(nonperfusing rhythms)* are ventricular asystole, electromechanical dissociation (EMD), and pulseless ventricular tachycardia with a rate of less than 120 to 200 per minute. All rhythms and dysrhythmias, including ventricular tachycardia, with a pulse regardless of their rate are nonshockable.

Nonshockable ventricular tachycardia Ventricular tachycardia with a rate of less than 120 to 200 per minute with or without a pulse.

Nonsustained ventricular tachycardia Short bursts of ventricular tachycardia (three or more consecutive abnormal QRS complexes) separated by the underlying rhythm. Paroxysmal ventricular tachycardia.

Normal sinus rhythm (NSR) Normal rhythm of the heart, originating in the SA node with a rate of 60 to 100 beats per minute.

O

Obviously dead One of the criteria for not starting cardiopulmonary resuscitation and using the automated external defibrillator.

Ohm Unit of electrical resistance.

Organized ECG rhythm The term used to indicate the presence of QRS complexes and, in most instances, T waves on the ECG, with or without P waves, indicating organized electrical activity of the heart. Includes all rhythms, including normal sinus rhythm (NSR), and dysrhythmias *except* ventricular tachycardia, ventricular fibrillation, and ventricular asystole.

Organized electrical activity of the heart Refers to the presence of an organized ECG rhythm.

Oscilloscope A display device with a screen for viewing an ECG and other physiologic data.

Oxygenated blood Blood high in oxygen, low in carbon dioxide. The prime example is arterial blood.

P

Pacemaker, artificial *See* Artificial pacemaker.

Pacemaker cells Normally, those of the SA node. Under certain conditions any cell of the electrical conduction system can function as a pacemaker cell and generate electrical impulses.

Pacemaker of the heart The SA node or an escape or ectopic pacemaker in the electrical conduction system of the heart or in the myocardium.

Pacemaker site The site of the origin of an electrical impulse. It can be the SA node or an escape or ectopic pacemaker in any part of the electrical conduction system of the heart or in the myocardium.

Pacemaker spikes Small, narrow, sharply pointed, upright or inverted blips on the ECG, generated by an artificial pacemaker usually at a rate between 60 and 75 per minute.

Palpable peripheral pulse A sign that a perfusing rhythm is present. A criteria used for not delivering a shock.

Palpitation Rapid or irregular beating of the heart or both as described by the patient.

Palpitations Sensation under the left breast or sternum commonly described by the patient as "skipping of the heart" resulting from premature contractions of the heart.

Papillary muscles Muscular protrusions of the myocardium into the ventricular cavities to which the chordae tendinea are anchored. The papillary muscles and attached chordae tendinea prevent the mitral and tricuspid valves from ballooning backward into the atria during ventricular contraction.

Parallel Running alongside in the same direction at a constant distance.

Paroxysmal ventricular tachycardia *See* Nonsustained ventricular tachycardia.

Patient or ECG cable movement A cause of ECG artifacts.

Perfusing rhythm An ECG rhythm or dysrhythmia accompanied by a palpable pulse. One that is nonshockable.

Perfusing, nonshockable rhythm All ECG rhythms and dysrhythmias with a spontaneous palpable pulse.

Pericardial effusion Accumulation of fluid in the pericardial sac or cavity.

Pericardium The tough fibrous outer membrane surrounding the heart.

Pericardial sac or cavity The space between the pericardium and the heart containing a small amount of lubricating fluid (pericardial fluid).

Peripheral edema The swelling of body tissue in congestive heart failure, usually found in the legs and sometimes in the lower back.

Permanent(ly) implanted artificial pacemaker An implantable electronic device used to deliver minute electrical impulses to the heart to stimulate it to beat when the heart's own pacemaker is not functioning.

Persistent shockable rhythm The continuation of pulseless ventricular tachycardia or ventricular fibrillation despite repeated delivery of shocks.

Placement of defibrillator electrodes The negative electrode is attached to the right upper chest wall in the angle formed by the right clavicle and the right edge of the sternum. The positive electrode is attached to the left lower anterior chest wall, centered over the intersection of the left fourth intercostal space and the left anterior axillary line.

Plaque With respect to coronary heart disease, a raised, usually hard patch on the inner surface of arteries caused by the atherosclerotic process.

Pleural effusion Accumulation of fluid in the pleural cavity.

Plug-in electronic memory module An electronic recording device available in some automated external defibrillators to store data. *See* memory module.

Pneumothorax Accumulation of air in the pleural cavity.

Portable defibrillator An electronic device used to deliver a shock across the chest to terminate pulseless ventricular tachycardia and ventricular fibrillation. The device may be manual or automatic.

Positive defibrillator electrode One of two electrodes used to deliver a shock across the chest to the heart to terminate a shockable rhythm. It is attached to the left lower anterior chest wall, centered over the intersection of the left fourth intercostal space and the left anterior axillary line.

Post-arrival arrest Cardiac arrest occurring after the arrival of the EMT/FR-D. Also called EMT/FR-D-witnessed cardiac arrest.

Posterior Pertaining to the back.

Post-mortem lividity. *See* Livor mortis.

Potassium A mineral substance dissolved in the blood necessary for proper functioning of the heart, including the electrical conduction system of the heart and the myocardium.

Pre-arrival cardiac arrest A cardiac arrest that has occurred before the arrival of the EMT/FR-D. It may be witnessed or unwitnessed. Bystander-CPR may or may not be in process.

Prearrest condition Refers to the physical, neurological, and mental conditon of the patient before cardiac arrest occurred.

Precordial Pertaining to the precordium.

Precordium The region of the thorax over the heart, the lower half of the sternum.

Prehospital cardiac arrest A cardiac arrest that has occurred before the patient has arrived at the emergency department. It may have occurred before the arrival of the EMT/FR-D (prearrival cardiac arrest) or after (post-arrival or EMT/FR-witnessed cardiac arrest).

Primary (dominant) pacemaker of the heart The SA node.

Premature ventricular contraction (PVC) An extra beat consisting of an abnormally wide and bizarre QRS complex originating in an ectopic pacemaker in the ventricles.

Property of automaticity The property of cardiac cells to generate electrical impulses automatically.

Property of conductivity The property of cardiac cells to conduct electrical impulses.

Property of contractility The property of cardiac cells to contract when they are stimulated by an electrical impulse.

Pulmonary artery The main blood vessel delivering unoxygenated blood from the right ventricle to the lungs.

Pulmonary arteries The arteries that deliver unoxygenated venous blood from the right ventricle to the lungs.

Pulmonary capillaries The tiniest blood vessels connecting the pulmonary arteries with the pulmonary veins. Delivery of oxygen to the blood and elimination of carbon dioxide occur at the capillary level.

Pulmonary circulation Passage of blood from the right ventricle through the pulmonary artery, all of its branches, and capillaries in the lungs and then back to the left atrium through the pulmonary venules and veins.

Pulmonary congestion Condition of the lungs when the pulmonary vessels become engorged and rigid with blood because of left heart failure.

Pulmonary edema Condition of the lungs when the alveoli become filled with fluid and foam following the appearance of pulmonary congestion because of severe left heart failure.

Pulmonary veins The veins that deliver oxygenated blood from the lungs to the left atrium.

Pulmonic valve The one-way valve between the right ventricle and the pulmonary artery.

Pulsating neck veins A sign of congestive heart failure caused by right heart failure.

Pulselessness An absent pulse. One of the criteria for making a determination of cardiac arrest. Also one of the criteria for making a determination of electromechanical dissociation (EMD) in the presence of an organized ECG rhythm, i.e., a pulseless ECG rhythm or dysrhythmia.

Pulseless ventricular tachycardia *See* Ventricular tachycardia.

Pump failure Partial or total failure of the heart to pump blood forward effectively, resulting in congestive heart failure or cardiogenic shock.

Purkinje network The part of the electrical conduction system between the bundle branches and the ventricular myocardium consisting of the Purkinje fibers and their terminal branches.

P wave Normally, the first wave of the P-QRS-T complex representing the electrical activity of the atria.

Q

QRS complex Normally, the wave following the P wave, consisting of the Q, R, and S waves and representing the electrical activity of the ventricles.

"Quivering bowl of jelly" Descriptive phrase used to describe the appearance of the ventricles in ventricular fibrillation. *See* "Bag of worms."

Q wave The first negative deflection of the QRS complex not preceded by an R wave.

R

Rales The fine "popping" sounds in the lungs caused by fluid and foam in the small air passages in the lungs.

Respiratory arrest A life-threatening condition caused by the cessation of breathing.

Respiratory insufficiency A life-threatening condition caused by the inability of the respiratory system to supply sufficient oxygen to the body to support life.

Resuscitation The restoration of life by artificial respiration and external chest compression.

Rhythm The regularity or irregularity of an ECG rhythm. An ECG rhythm.

Right anterior axillary line An imaginary line beginning in front of the right axilla (armpit) and running parallel to the right side of the sternum just outside of the right nipple.

Right atrium The thin-walled chamber on the right side of the heart which receives venous blood from the body through the inferior and superior vena cavae and from the heart through the coronary sinus and empties the blood into the ventricle through the tricuspid valve.

Right and left bundle branches Part of the electrical conduction system located in the ventricles between the bundle of His and the Purkinje network.

Right bundle branch Part of the electrical conduction system located in the right ventricle connecting the bundle of His with the Purkinje network in the right ventricle.

Right heart The part of the heart consisting of the right atrium and right ventricle which receives venous blood from the body and pumps it forward into the pulmonary vascular system.

Right heart failure The failure of the right ventricle to pump blood forward effectively, causing an accumulation of blood and fluid in the body tissue (peripheral edema).

Right ventricle The moderately thick, muscular-walled chamber that pumps blood it receives from the right atrium into the pulmonary circulation.

Rigor mortis Stiffening of the muscles 30 minutes to 6 hours or more (average 2 to 4 hours) after death. One of the criteria for not starting cardiopulmonary resuscitation and using the automated external defibrillator.

Rupture of the heart. *See* Cardiac rupture.

R wave The positive wave or deflection in the QRS complex.

S

SA Abbreviation for sinoatrial.

SAED Abbreviation for semi-automatic external defibrillator.

SA node The dominant pacemaker of the heart located in the wall of the right atrium near the inlet of the superior vena cava.

Secondary pacemaker of the heart *See* Escape pacemaker.

Semi-automatic external defibrillator (SAED) An electronic device used by EMT/FR-Ds that analyzes the ECG of a patient in cardiac arrest to determine the presence of ventricular tachycardia with a rate of 120 to 200 per minute or greater or ventricular fibrillation and, if present, instructs the EMT/FR-D to deliver a shock by pushing a discharge button or switch.

Septum A wall separating two cavities.

Serum The fluid part of the blood containing all the dissolved constituents except those used in clotting. The part of blood remaining after the formation of a clot and its removal.

Serum enzymes Refers to enzymes present in the blood. *See* Enzymes.

Shock A state of cardiovascular collapse caused by numerous factors such as severe AMI, hemorrhage, anaphylactic reaction, severe trauma, pain, strong emotions, drug toxicity, or other causes. A patient in decompensated shock typically has dulled senses and staring eyes, a pale and cyanotic color, cold and clammy skin, systolic blood pressure of 80 to 90 mm Hg or less, a feeble rapid pulse (over 110 beats per minute), and a delayed capillary refill of greater than 2 seconds.

Shockable rhythms Ventricular fibrillation and shockable ventricular tachycardia (i.e., ventricular tachycardia with a rate of 120 to 200 per minute or greater) without a pulse.

Shockable rhythm monitoring circuit See ECG rhythm monitoring circuit.

Shockable ventricular tachycardia Ventricular tachycardia with a rate of 120 to 200 per minute or greater. A pulse may or may not be present.

Signs Bodily evidence of disease found by physical examination.

"Silent" myocardial infarction An acute myocardial infarction without chest pain, occurring in 10 to 20 percent of the AMIs. Other signs and symptoms are usually present, such as extreme fatigue, weakness, lightheadedness, shortness of breath, nausea, vomiting, and dysrhythmias.

Sinoatrial (SA) node *See* SA node.

Specialized cells of the electrical conduction system of the heart Cells of the heart that generate electrical impulses automatically and conduct them to the myocardial cells throughout the heart.

Spikes Artifacts in the ECG. If numerous and occurring randomly, they are most likely caused by muscle tremor, AC interference, loose electrodes, or biotelemetry-related interference. If they are regular, occurring at a rate of about 60 to 75 per minute, they are most likely caused by an artificial pacemaker.

Spontaneous pulse A palpable pulse present without the benefit of CPR.

Sternum The long, flat, bladelike bone located in the midline in the anterior part of the chest.

Stored energy The amount of electrical charge or energy stored in the capacitor of the defibrillator before it is discharged.

Stroke volume The amount of blood pumped forward by the heart each time the ventricles contract.

Substernal(ly) Behind the sternum.

Sudden (cardiac) death Sudden and unexpected death usually from coronary heart disease in patients with relatively minor or vague premonitory symptoms, who appear well and are not expected to die.

Superior vena cava One of the largest veins in the body that empties venous blood into the right atrium.

Sustained ventricular tachycardia Ventricular tachycardia present continuously for a period of time.

S wave The first negative or downward wave or deflection of the QRS complex that is preceded by an R wave.

Symptoms Abnormal feeling of distress or other bodily disturbances. Includes fatigue, pain, shortness of breath (dyspnea), numbness, light-headedness, and so forth.

Systemic circulation Passage of blood from the left ventricle through the aorta, all its branches, and capillaries in the tissues of the body and then back to the right atrium through the venules, veins, and vena cavae.

Systole, ventricular The period during ventricular contraction and emptying of blood.

Systolic blood pressure The highest peak pressure exerted on the arterial walls during ventricular contraction, alternating with diastolic pressure.

T

T wave The part of the ECG following the QRS complex. It represents the electrical activity of the ventricles while they are finishing contracting and beginning to relax.

Tachycardia A heart rate greater than 100 beats per minute. Also a dysrhythmia with 3 or more beats occurring at a rate exceeding 100 beats per minute.

Tachypnea A respiratory rate over 25 breaths per minute.

Tension pneumothorax Accumulation of air in the pleural space under pressure as a result of a wound in the chest wall or lung, acting like a one-way valve.

Thorax The chest.

Thoracic cavity The cavity within the thorax.

Thoracic spine Part of the spine forming part of the posterior chest wall.

Thrombus A blood clot.

Tissue decomposition One of the criteria for not starting cardiopulmonary resuscitation and using the automated external defibrillator.

Tricuspid valve The valve between the right atrium and right ventricle.

U

Unconsciousness State of being unresponsive to sensory stimuli.

Underlying rhythm The basic rhythm interrupted by ectopic beats or overridden by an ectopic rhythm such as ventricular tachycardia.

Units of electrical energy Joules (watt-seconds).

Unoxygenated blood Blood low in oxygen, high in carbon dioxide. The prime example is venous blood.

Unresponsiveness State of being unresponsive to sensory stimuli.

Unwitnessed (cardiac) arrest A cardiac arrest not witnessed by a bystander or EMT/FR-D.

V

Vasodilation Dilation of blood vessels leading to increased blood flow to part of the body. One of the effects of nitroglycerin.

Ventricle The thick-walled muscular chamber which receives blood from the atrium and pumps it into the pulmonary or systemic circulation. The two ventricles form the larger lower part of the heart and the apex and are separated from the atria by the mitral and tricuspid valves.

Ventricular Pertaining to the ventricles.

Ventricular aneurysm A localized dilation or ballooning of the wall of the ventricle, usually the left one. An uncommon complication of AMI.

Ventricular dysrhythmia A dysrhythmia originating in an ectopic pacemaker in the ventricles.

Ventricular asystole (cardiac standstill) Cessation of ventricular contractions.

Ventricular diastole The interval or period during which the ventricles are relaxed and filling with blood. The period between ventricular contractions.

Ventricular escape rhythm A dysrhythmia originating in an escape pacemaker in the ventricles with a rate between 30 to 40 beats per minute or less.

Ventricular fibrillation A dysrhythmia originating in multiple ectopic pacemakers in the ventricles characterized by numerous ventricular fibrillatory waves and no QRS complexes.

Ventricular fibrillation (VF) waves Bizarre, irregularly shaped, rounded, or pointed, and markedly dissimilar waves originating in multiple ectopic pacemakers in the ventricles.

Ventricular systole The interval or period during which the ventricles are contracting and emptying of blood.

Ventricular tachycardia (VT, V-Tach) A dysrhythmia originating in an ectopic pacemaker in the ventricles with a rate between 110 and 250 beats per minute. It may occur in short bursts of three or more consecutive abnormal QRS complexes separated by the underlying rhythm (*nonsustained [or paroxysmal] ventricular tachycardia*) or continue for a period of time (*sustained ventricular tachycardia*). A pulse may or may not be present. Ventricular tachycardia with a pulse, regardless of the rate, is a *perfusing, nonshockable rhythm*. Ventricular tachycardia without a pulse, *pulseless ventricular tachycardia,* is a *nonperfusing rhythm,* regardless of the rate. Pulseless ventricular tachycardia with a rate of 120 to 200 per minute or greater is a *shockable rhythm*. Cardiopulmonary resuscitation is indicated for a pulseless ventricular tachycardia with a rate of less than 120 to 200 per minute.

VF, V-Fib Abbreviations for ventricular fibrillation.

Vital organs The brain, heart, and lungs.

Vital signs Physiologic measurements which include pulse, respiration, and blood pressure.

VT, V-Tach Abbreviations for ventricular tachycardia.

W

Watt-second Joule. A unit of electrical energy delivered by a source of energy, such as a defibrillator.

Witnessed (cardiac) arrest Cardiac arrest that was witnessed by a bystander or an EMT/FR-D.

Work capacity of the heart The ability of the heart to meet the demand of increased blood flow up to a certain point, above which the heart is unable to do so and fails.

Workload of the heart The amount of energy expended by the heart during myocardial contraction. Increases with increased heart rate and increased stroke volume (i.e., increased cardiac output) and with increased blood pressure.

X

Xiphoid process The small, arrowhead-shaped, cartilaginous, and bony portion of the sternum attached to the lower end of the body of the sternum.

Index